The Secrets to Great Health

from Your Nine Liver Dwarves

By Dr. Jonn Matsen, ND

Delicious New Recipes by Irene Hayton

Fully Illustrated by Nelson Dewey

PUBLISHED BY
Goodwin Books Ltd.
North Vancouver, B.C.

Distributed by
Gordon Soules Book Publishers Ltd.
1359 Ambleside Lane,
West Vancouver, BC, Canada V7T 2Y9
E-mail: books@gordonsoules.com
Web site: http://www.gordonsoules.com
(604) 922 6588 Fax: (604) 688 5442

© 1998 by Jonn Matsen. All rights reserved

Published by:
Goodwin Books, Ltd.
156 West 3rd Street
North Vancouver, B.C.
Canada V7M 1E8

Canadian Cataloguing in Publication Data

Matsen, Jonn, 1949–
    The secrets to great health

    Includes bibliographical references and index.
    ISBN 0-9682853-0-9

    1. Liver–Diseases–Diet therapy.   2. Liver–Diseases–Diet therapy–Recipes.   3. Digestive organs–Diseases–Diet therapy.
4. Diet in disease.   5. Naturopathy–Popular works.
I. Hayton, Irene.   II. Dewey, Nelson.   III. Title.
RC846.M38 1998   616.3'620654   C98-911144-X

I wish to thank my wife Maria, my daughter Jessie, and my son Michael for their love, support, and understanding during the many months of research and writing that I devoted to this book.

CONTENTS

- Tryptophan plays a crucial role in your brain function and emotions through the production of serotonin and melatonin.

- Your liver can hog your antioxidants when working hard—this can weaken your ligaments, tendons, cartilage, discs, blood vessels, eyes, nails, and other connective tissue.
- Your immune system can generate tremendous quantities of free radicals.
- Your immune system is well armed and determined to kill any invaders—this means big trouble for you if your body is mistakenly identified as "the enemy."

- Your kidneys control your mineral levels and change your activation of vitamin D with the seasons—and your kidneys judge what season it must be by the food that you're eating.
- A few days of low calcium can allow your good bacteria to stampede into your small intestine where they can steal precious nutrients like tryptophan and vitamin B_{12}.
- Overloaded kidneys can dump toxins into your bladder or out through your skin.

- Your liver breaks down your steroid hormones. If this action isn't done quickly, these hormones can overstimulate your reproductive organs—which can lead to their development of cancer.
- Thyroid hormones are crucial—yet problems with them are secondary to digestion, liver, and immune system problems.

ACKNOWLEDGEMENTS

A belated thanks to **Beverly Straight** for her help and support with my previous book, *Eating Alive — Prevention Thru Good Digestion*.

And thanks to **Daniel Voll** of New York for believing in the **Nine Liver Dwarves**.

Many thanks to **Scott Clack** for all the hours he spent finding research articles.

I wish to acknowledge these sources for their help with the research articles: **Barry Sears, Karen Rasmussen, Great Smokies Diagnostic Laboratory, Vibrant Health, Thorne Research, Healthcomm International,** *Clinical Pearls, American Journal of Natural Medicine, Townsend Letter for Doctors,* and *Alternative Medical Review.*

My appreciation to **Barbara Aldritt, Barrie Anderson,** and **Casey Martell** for proofreading the manuscript; to **Drew Welsh** for the initial cover designs; and **Michele Ibraham** for his input on how to make yogurt.

A big round of thanks to **Val Wilson, Ink,** for her endless diligence in editing.

I am most grateful to **Irene Hayton** for her keen eye and expertise in technical editing. Thanks to Irene's family for their patience and support during this lengthy project.

INTRODUCTION

In 1986, I wrote the book *Eating Alive—Prevention Thru Good Digestion*, which stated that the mysterious source of disease had been discovered. Disease was an overloading of the liver's detoxification ability, which could result in a vast array of physical, mental, and emotional symptoms. That book was based primarily on clinical experience with thousands of successfully treated patients. This new book, *The Secrets to Great Health*, verifies the direct connection between your liver function and your health. And, with the advantage of years of worldwide scientific research in this field, this book can go into much more depth on the subject. But before we get to that, let me explain that my knowledge wasn't founded on a brilliant, intuitive insight. My understanding that health, once lost, can be regained through improvement of digestion, was learned by my deciphering a program used by Naturopathic Physicians for many decades in Spokane, Washington.

Permit me to give you some background. My first experience with natural healing was with a renowned herbalist, to whom I'll introduce you later. In that brief exposure, I saw "the incurable" cured. From this experience, it became apparent to me that there were many shortcomings in the way Western medicine approached disease. I took further training in herbal medicine, practised briefly as a herbalist, but found I wanted a more scientific foundation and went back to college. I picked up two years of Sciences to augment my two years of Arts at university, and then applied to a college of naturopathic medicine.

In the first two years, I studied basic medical sciences— identical to those taught at any medical school. The course I loved most was Physiology, and the poet laureate of physiology was Arthur C. Guyton, author of our medical physiology text. Guyton simplified the complexity of the human body by demonstrating that your body adjusts your thermostat to 98.6 degrees F. and knows how to keep your temperature there. Your body also knows how to maintain your blood pressure at 120 over 80. In fact, your body knows a lot of other clever responses, too, such as how to digest food, detoxify poisons, regulate fuel consumption, maintain blood sugar levels, fight off invaders, repair damage, and keep your body running like the proverbial Swiss clock—and I'm not referring to a cuckoo clock!

You are a well-designed and beautiful piece of equipment, built to succeed on a planet that can be demanding. The rhythms of the solar system can subject you to extremes of light and dark, hot and cold, rain and drought, feast and famine, peace and pestilence. Yet you are designed to adjust and adapt to survive all that, and be healthy enough to give birth to or sire children and raise a family. This ability of your body to keep itself running smoothly and efficiently in constantly changing conditions is called homeostasis.

Following Physiology class came cadaver dissection. We examined eight bodies that had failed miserably to live up to the ideal of homeostatic harmony. It wasn't the fact that they were dead that made them so physiologically disappointing; it was that they were so filled with <u>pathology</u>—the evil nemesis of perfect physiology.

One of the bodies had belonged to "Billy the Sailor," so named by the students because of the anchor tattooed on his forearm. His stomach walls were so thickened with cancer, it's likely that only liquid could have passed through its narrow passageway. One of his kidneys was a big, bloated cyst that when punctured, oozed a vile fluid no one dared touch. The lungs were severely blackened and were likely also cancerous. It took little imagination to picture "Billy" as a heavy drinker and smoker for most of his life.

Then there was the "China Doll," a lean lady whose connective tissue was hardened with calcium, which made her body rigid as porcelain. Her diaphragm was the size of a dinner plate and of the same texture. Tapping it, you would expect to hear a ring as if it were high-quality bone china. One ovary was the size of a large baseball but with the density of a bowling ball. It was easy to picture her shuffling along very slowly on her walker for many decades, unable to even step up onto a curb or stair.

Then there was "Adipose Annie" from whom we had to strip off many inches of sticky, yellow fat—perhaps a hundred pounds of it—to find, underneath, the body frame of a thin person.

Throughout the eight bodies, there were numerous gallstones; artery "gravel"; thickened intestinal walls; damaged hearts, lungs, and brains; tumours; enlarged livers; etc. The presence of so much pathology could have been the reason these people had died; as their ultimate cause of death, most of them could have had any number of diseases written on their death certificates. And if a stroke hadn't actually killed some of them, surely their cancer or a heart attack would have.

The fact that they were old could also be an explanation, except that most of their pathology was many decades—if not a whole lifetime—in the making.

Anyway, there existed a giant gap between the ideal physiology of Guyton's text and the gross pathology we saw daily in cadaver dissection class. I expected that the whats and whys of this discrepancy between health and disease would be clarified during second year classes. No such class was taught in second year—nor in third.

By fourth year, I could see that a scientific education couldn't bridge that gap between health and illness because scientific research hadn't invested much effort in that direction. Research was usually concerned with identifying specific pathologies and focusing treatment—usually drugs or surgery—at reducing the major symptoms of that condition. In some research, there was a small shift toward replacing the drugs with vitamins or herbs, but the focus was still on pathology—not the *cause* or the *correction* of it.

That fourth year, in 1983, there was a lot of excitement about the recent discovery of prostaglandins, which looked promising because prostaglandins seemed to be at the root of most diseases, and studies showed that these strong hormones could be influenced by diet. So in my little black notebook that we students were encouraged to keep to record remedies to be used for certain diseases, I would add "flax seed oil" beside my notation of vitamin B_6, zinc, and vitamin C—which seemed to be the panacea for all ailments because of their effects on prostaglandins. In student clinic, however, the results from using these treatments weren't very spectacular. Oh sure, there were improvements in some people—if they were already reasonably healthy. The more serious problems showed little improvement.

The naturopathic college was aware of the limitations of science and had recently begun a search to locate older doctors with time-proven methods so that the students could learn directly from them. Soon I was visiting a doctor who had been recently "discovered" in Spokane, Washington—where he had been practising for many years. His name was Dr. Harold Dick; his program was being carried out exactly as it had been shown to him by Dr. O. G. Carroll, 40 years previously.

Dr. Dick's wife had been cured of severe rheumatoid arthritis in 18 months by O. G. Carroll's treatments and this motivated Dr. Dick to get his doctorate in Naturopathic Medicine in Portland, Oregon. After graduation in 1955, Dr. Dick worked with O. G. Carroll until he started his own practice.

O. G. Carroll had had his arthritis reversed in the 1890s under the care of Alex LeDoux, who had studied in Europe under Father Sebastian Kneipp. LeDoux, along with the other Ls—Lane, Lust, and Lindlahr—brought naturopathic principles of healing to North America from Europe. After Dr. Carroll's arthritis was reversed, he studied with LeDoux and Lindlahr in Chicago until 1908, when he moved to Spokane and started his own practice.

Dr. Carroll's interest in electronics enabled him to add electrical stimulation to Father Kneipp's hot and cold packs to shorten the three-hour treatment to 45 minutes. Even though the treatments took a lot less time, he felt they were twice as effective. Dr. Carroll called these shorter treatments "constitutional" hydrotherapy treatments because the goal was to raise the patient's overall vitality. In fact, at one point in his long career, *Life* magazine declared that O. G. Carroll was the busiest doctor in the US.

Dr. Dick's program, which was based on O. G. Carroll's approach, consisted of food-sensitivity testing, "constitutional" hydrotherapy treatments—alternating hot and cold body-wraps, interspersed with electric stimulation of the abdominal organs, especially the stomach—and various herbs and homeopathic medicines. Little consideration was given to the patient's specific "pathology." The hydrotherapy treatments were designed to "jump-start" the person's digestive system—which Dr. Carroll and Dr. Dick felt was at the root of all chronic disease—whether or not the person complained of digestive problems.

By listening to the patient's heart sounds, these doctors were able to monitor the individual's digestive organ function and adjust the treatments accordingly to improve the digestion. As a patient's organs regained function, the person's various diseases would disappear as if by magic. I was amazed at the results I saw at Dr. Dick's office. Arthritis, colitis, psoriasis, asthma, and even MS would often disappear after only three to 12 weeks of treatment.

I certainly never saw results like this at student clinic, and it definitely wasn't placebo effect due to doctor's charm, as Dr. Dick's bedside manners were gruff—to say the least. What he lacked in diplomatic skills, however, he more than made up in the confidence department. He would actually tell patients to throw their drugs into the garbage can—right then and there—or he would not treat them. No other doctor I know would dare to do such an audacious thing today, myself included.

When I set up my practice as the Northshore Naturopathic Clinic in North Vancouver in 1983, I modelled it after Dr. Dick's program—with one variation. I used *muscle-testing* to determine which organs in a patient were the weakest, rather than listening for heart sounds as the doctor had done. I found that in patients with chronic disease, the stomach, intestines, and liver were universally weak.

After one or two weeks of dietary changes, hydrotherapy treatments, and herbs or homeopathic medicines, testing might show a strong stomach and intestine, but often the liver was still weak, and the patient didn't feel much better—or was only partially improved.

When all three weak areas—digestion, intestines, and finally the liver—tested healthy after a period of time on the program, complaints of gas, bloating, heartburn, and diarrhea would disappear. Even more serious digestive problems like irritable bowel, Crohn's disease, and ulcerative colitis would fade away a little later. Fatigue would usually lift, along with depression, irritability, moodiness, and cloudy thinking.

Other results were more difficult to explain.

There was the young girl with chronic "tummyaches" and teeth so transparent, you could almost see through them. Shortly after we changed her diet, her stomach aches were gone, and her teeth became pearly white for the first time in her life.

And the child who kept banging his head against the wall— until we changed his diet and his digestion improved, then he stopped banging his head.

And the woman who had consistently pulled her hair out by the roots for 30 years—she finally stopped doing so after only a few months on our program.

And the lady with life-threatening peanut allergies who returned to my office six months later, nonchalantly eating a handful of peanuts.

I've kept a notebook on my desk in which I've jotted down many of the ailments I've seen reversed by simply improving the trio of digestion, intestines, and liver. Here are a few examples.(The patients' initials are in capital letters.)

BB: indigestion, sinusitis, chronic fatigue, concentration problems
RM: indigestion, fatigue, fibromyalgia
NA: indigestion, fatigue, headaches
CA: indigestion, fatigue, Crohn's disease
AR: chronic tonsillitis, headaches, chronic otitis with speech and learning problems
DM: indigestion, headaches, dermatitis, snoring
WH: nausea, headaches, joint pain, chronic cough
MR: irritable bowel, diarrhea, fatigue
CB: irritable bowel, diarrhea, anxiety/panic attacks
NT: indigestion, colitis, psoriasis, hot flushes
MJ: indigestion, diarrhea, PMS

RC: indigestion, diarrhea, fatigue, migraines
JM: irritable bowel, arthritis, hyperthyroid
JJ: colitis, hyperthyroid
AB: indigestion, chronic cough, fatigue, depression
JP: indigestion, headaches, vaginitis, geographic tongue
DD: Crohn's disease, infertility
VR: asthma, chronic cough, edema, arthritis
CN: indigestion, headaches, epilepsy
NM: colitis, polymyalgia rheumatica
SC: indigestion, fatigue, headaches, acne, eczema
SW: irritable bowel, diarrhea, carpal tunnel syndrome
MP: indigestion, acne
CH: indigestion, asthma, sinusitis,
CP: Crohn's, ankylosing spondylitis

Just this morning, I received a call from a 72-year-old patient from northern British Columbia whose recent medical checkup showed that his prostate swelling has disappeared, his blood pressure is now normal, and his severe asthma is virtually gone. All his indigestion and hiatal hernia symptoms have disappeared since he has been following the food program we worked out for him at the Clinic six months ago.

I could go on and on to describe the changes in hundreds more individuals, but the point is that many, many symptoms and diseases—seemingly unrelated and mysterious—can be corrected by improving our diets and digestion. **But since the feeling of well-being will only occur <u>after</u> the liver is working properly, it seems obvious that the liver is the junction box from which nearly all symptoms of illness—physical or emotional and sometimes even mental—must originate.**

While it's always gratifying to have patients' chronic health problems disappear quickly and effortlessly, there's little to be learned from this. It only reaffirms what I already believe. There are other patients where the results weren't quick, weren't easy, and weren't complete. Or where the results seemed complete, but the symptoms soon returned. They're the patients with the unhappy faces and the frustrated voices. Patients with difficult problems help keep a doctor from becoming complacent; their needs motivate the doctor to constantly search and experiment—adding to and subtracting from both the diagnosis and the treatment—to create improvement in their conditions.

My testing of the patients who were very slow to respond to treatment revealed that **these individuals usually had lymph problems that were secondary to their liver problems and, invariably, lymph problems meant immune system problems.**

Even after their liver function had been improved, it might take two to six months or more before they would show any improvement in their symptoms. I had never heard of any direct connection between the liver and the lymph before, so this was quite a puzzle at the time.

This link between the liver and the lymph—and therefore, the immune system—as well as the *slow* improvement in some patients, became the focus of my digging through research documents for a number of years. This research became especially critical after I stopped the hydrotherapy treatments—after having done them routinely for five years. Since patients were by then travelling from further distances for a consultation with me, it became more difficult for them to come into my office several times a week for hydrotherapy treatments, for weeks or even months on end.

Since I had been counting on the hydrotherapy treatments to begin the improvement of the patient's digestion, I had to make sure that the diet and supplements I was now recommending would work as well as the hydrotherapy treatments had.

Two of my office staff members devoted one day per week to pulling research articles from medical libraries, and a naturopathic student in Seattle spent one day each week doing extensive research for me at the University of Washington Medical Library.

A big breakthrough in diagnosis came when I added a new electronic diagnostic technique from Germany to augment the muscle-testing. This helped—in theory—to separate the organ testing into smaller subunits; it isolated the "intestine health" readings into small and large intestine zones, and the "liver strength" readings into a number of different parts—such as gall bladder, bile ducts, and portal vein.

As expected, bile toxicity showed as a major issue in most everyone. Unexpected, however, was the fact that the portal vein showed as a liver problem almost as often.

The portal vein carries fluids from the digestive organs to the liver. Pathology texts say that portal vein problems are seen in people who have liver damage, such as cirrhosis of the liver. The damaged liver would block the flow of blood travelling from the digestive system to the liver via the portal vein. This damming of the portal vein could lead to back-pressure on the portal vein—called portal hypertension—which, in turn, could lead to serious medical problems, including coma. Since these portal vein problems originated from liver damage that was considered irreversible, the major treatment to relieve the portal pressure was surgery—to remove the obstacles in the liver.

But not only was I diagnosing portal hypertension in people who had <u>no indication</u> of liver damage, I was finding that after several weeks of treatment with diet and improved digestion, the indications of portal vein problems would be gone. Obviously there was something going on in the liver that could cause a blockage of the portal vein, and yet could disappear quickly with dietary treatment.

In a sense, these results weren't unusual because I often found that patients had early-stage undiagnosed thyroid problems that would usually disappear with improved digestion and liver function without any direct thyroid treatment. I wanted to know what there was in the liver that could cause reversible portal vein fluctuation in so many people, so I read all the research I could find that related to the portal vein.

Eventually, I came across research articles that gave an important clue to solving the portal vein mystery. (Please see #87 and #88 in the Research section.) This research clearly showed that the liver had **valves** that controlled the flow of fluids in and out of the liver—and that when these valves were closed, the portal vein would back up, creating bloating in the abdomen.

Shortly after this insight, I explained to a patient that her abdominal bloating was a result of her liver valves being closed. She immediately asked who had closed them without her permission. Spontaneously, I replied, "Why, **Bloaty**, the **Liver Dwarf**, of course." Thus was born the first of the **Nine Liver Dwarves** that I would create to help explain liver function to my patients. In a sense, these **Dwarves** *are* real because their personalities are composites of the thousands of patients I've seen.

Bloaty became the key to unravelling the intricate mysteries about how your liver is so closely linked to your portal vein, your bile, and your lymph system (and your immune system)—and therefore, to your overall health.

With my new insight about how a healthy but overworked liver can result in portal vein problems, I began to instigate a number of small changes in my Clinic program, to see how the body would respond. The two medical problems most frequently seen to recur in patients were ileocecal valve discomfort and low production of digestive enzymes by the pancreas. Adding more proteins solved the problem of low digestive enzyme production, and improving calcium absorption solved the problem of the ileocecal valve. I had mentioned in my previous book that ileocecal valve problems weren't very common and were, ironically, often seen in people who read the most health books. In the decade since I wrote *Eating Alive,* however, the ileocecal valve has become the major source of liver stress seen in my practice. The ways in which health-conscious people are actually able to worsen their health by weakening the ileocecal valve are now very clear—thanks to **Itchy**, the kidney **Liver Dwarf**, who helped me solve this riddle.

Shortly after making dietary adjustments to improve the ileocecal valve, some remarkable improvements occurred—much faster than expected. A 17-year-old patient with Crohn's disease who had been housebound, doubled over with excruciating abdominal pain for two years, was back in school, symptom-free, in five days. No more excruciating intestinal cramps, no more bloody stools—just a normal kid getting an education. A more typical timeframe for an improvement of that magnitude would have been two to six months.

Then, another patient with Crohn's disease became symptom-free in three days. At that same time, I saw two patients with breast cancer. Both women had had breast cancer years before; they had had very bad experiences from the conventional treatment and now refused to undergo it again. This was unusual since most women have such a fear of breast cancer that they'll agree to undergo any treatment, no matter how dire. These two women, however, both wanted to use my program as their primary treatment for their small, *early-stage* tumours that had been biopsied as malignant.

A few years earlier, I had seen two other female patients with *advanced* breast cancer fail miserably trying to do the same thing; at that time, I had been unable to help them.

The first was **Norma Meyers**, the renowned herbalist whom I had met at a Vancouver seminar on herbs. I had simply expected to learn which wild plants were edible. To my astonishment, this lady went on to describe how—as a young teacher many decades before—she had had breast cancer considered incurable. Norma had soon begun to take herbal treatment in Ontario from a native Indian medicine man. Since she had little money, she paid her way by working for this man. She made his herbal formula while he drove around in his Lincoln Continental, delivering it.

After Norma's breast cancer had gone into remission, she devoted herself to the study and practice of herbal medicine. When I met her, she was about to sponsor a seminar in Alert Bay, a small fishing village where her husband was a hereditary Kwakiutal chief. Cormorant Island, where Alert Bay is situated, was accessible by local ferry from northern Vancouver Island.

Of course, I was skeptical; I'd been raised on Marcus Welby and Ben Casey—popular medical TV shows of the Sixties. I believed that doctors knew *everything* and that this woman was probably crazy as a loon! I was, however, also young and curious—with some money in the bank—and the idea of spending a month of summer on a West Coast island sounded pretty good to me. I volunteered to help her set up the seminar. In my mind, I was going to spy on her and see just how cuckoo she really was.

And she was cuckoo, all right. A little bit, anyway; she hugged trees when she didn't feel well, and then her spirits seemed to soar again. When diagnosing patients, Norma used a rubber bathtub stopper—suspended on a piece of fishing line—

as a pendulum to locate the source of their problems. She offered to introduce me to my spirit guides, but I declined the offer. Spirits sounded too spooky to me!

Yes, she was a little strange, but there she was, treating people with herbs she knew they couldn't pay for. She took them into her house, fed them, gave them a warm place to sleep, and found free clothes for them. And while *she* was a bit unusual, some of the patients were *really* bizarre and, in my mind, more than a little dangerous. Some were strongly under the influence of alcohol. But her laugh—part giggle, part belly-laugh—would defuse the most tense situation and seemed to immediately sober the most hostile drunk.

One of my jobs was to go around the native reservation to make sure certain patients were taking their medicines. Several of them were in severe shape. They had more than a foot in the grave: they had a foot and a liver! They wouldn't have lasted long without the free herbal supplements Norma provided. I saw these individuals get better; they were soon up and around and very grateful for this reprieve. Their new-found health soon allowed them to go back to drinking, however, and within a week, they'd be back where they started—in terrible shape.

I left Alert Bay and Norma Meyers with a wider viewpoint on health and healing, which was strengthened when I saw my then-girlfriend's mother reverse her arthritis using herbs and diet—after cortisone had failed. This success eventually led to my registering at naturopathic college.

And now, 10 years later, here was Norma Meyers—an earth angel if ever there was one—coming to see me to help her reverse the breast cancer that had flared up again during a period of intense stress. The cancer wasn't responding to her own herbal treatments. I really had nothing much to offer her and, sadly, she passed away soon after.

I began to do more research. In a short while, the second patient came in to see me to have her late-stage breast cancer reversed. She was in her mid-30s, a single mother unable to work because of rheumatoid arthritis that forced her to use a cane. She had very advanced cancer in one breast and was told that if she had surgery, it might extend her life by a month. She had a high opinion of natural healing and was certain that the cancer would be easy to get rid of.

I had much less enthusiasm than she did, but reluctantly agreed to work up a program for her. Within a few months, she was bouncing around with no cane, no pain in the joints, and a slight decrease in the size of her swollen, cancerous breast. The improvements in the breast turned out to be temporary and the cancer soon began its growth again, not responding to anything we tried. Her family all turned against her and criticized her for not having the surgery.

One day she came into my office carrying a big box from which she pulled a pair of large, red boxing gloves. She asked me to put them on. She said she needed me to fight harder for her because no one else was on her side. I took the boxing gloves home and would occasionally jab away at the walls with them. I would like to say that from this I had a great insight that reversed her cancer, but that wouldn't be true. She died after a drawn-out, bedridden period on morphine.

I *did* start fighting harder, but not with boxing gloves. To the ongoing research I was already doing on the mysterious portal vein and its relationship to liver problems, I added a systematic research program—to learn everything I could about breast cancer.

Those are the stories of the two women whose breast cancer I failed to help reverse. The other two women who had come to see me also had great expectations for having their breast cancer reversed. For these two, I was able to integrate into their programs some of the results of the latest medical research. Also, unlike the two previous patients, these two had very early-stage breast cancer, and they still had time to change their minds if results weren't seen quickly. I worked up a diet program for them that included some of the new insights I had received through research and my consultation with the **Nine Liver Dwarves**.

A month later, one of the two women gave in to her fear, and had her tumour removed surgically. To everyone's surprise, including my own, her tumour now biopsied *negative* for malignancy. She was interviewed for an article by *The Vancouver Sun* newspaper, and the writer also asked me what had made her cancer disappear. All I could say was that her liver was now working better.

That's the same rather intangible explanation I've used over the last few years when treating more than 20 women with unexplained infertility. Once their livers were working better, they became pregnant and each had at least one child. "Their livers were working better"—a factual statement certainly, but far from insightful.

The second breast cancer patient had no conventional treatment for her cancer, and her breast tumour completely disappeared within six weeks. Her reasoning for its disappearance was that the prayers of her churchmates had made her cancer go away. While I'd seen other cancers, particularly lymphoma, go into remission before, this was the first time that I'd seen breast cancer go into remission.

During the same time period, I treated a number of early-to-middle-stage MS patients who achieved 80 to 90 percent improvement over several months—as opposed to the six to 12 months it usually took for improvement to be seen in previous MS patients. Similar startling results were seen in patients with atherosclerosis, scleroderma, sarcoidosis, lupus, eosinophilic fasciitis, and systemic mastocytosis—conditions generally considered difficult to treat and slow to respond.

That's not to say that all patients with these conditions received the same remarkable results, but it does show that the disease is not always the limiting factor. The ability to return to health can depend more upon the strength and determination of the patients' physiology—and their determination to follow a program—than on the label of the pathology.

The changes in diet that I prescribe are based on a better understanding of how the liver functions and malfunctions, and how to correct it if it's not working properly. The dietary changes and the subsequent "improved liver function" have helped patients with stubborn conditions to get well again.

My first book, *Eating Alive*, set forth the philosophical premise that good diet and good digestion are the keys to great health. *The Secrets to Great Health* goes into much more detail on the "hows" and "whys" that support that premise, and includes further suggestions on how to make your diet work for you, instead of against you. *The Secrets to Great Health* will show you why your liver is the key to your health, and why there's such a fine line between your liver's ability to save you from disease or to throw you into the bottomless pit of pathology.

I would like to take credit for solving some of the mysterious problems that create and cure ill health, but the real credit must go to the old doctors who struggled through hard years— convinced that diet was the key to health—while Medicine and Politics ridiculed and even persecuted them. Their only allies were the patients who had been helped by them.

Unfortunately, in spite of all the recent research that verifies the old doctors' insights into the benefit of diet therapy, the Politics of Big Medicine remain the same. Established medicine still prefers to modify pathology with drugs or surgery, although it's often mistakenly referred to as health care. Since the <u>*cause*</u> of disease is repeatedly ignored, disease continually resurfaces—and the cost of "health care" goes up.

While I received a good academic grounding in biochemistry at naturopathic college, I am not a biochemist. I've gone through as many medical journal research articles as I could find, and I've summarized that research at the end of this book.

The research is almost a book in itself, with well over 550 excerpts from leading medical researchers of the last century. It's especially interesting to see how much information is actually available about the cause of cancer, and which foods can stimulate or inhibit it.

I don't look at any of the information in *The Secrets to Great Health* as a guaranteed cure for any disease, especially cancer. Severe diseases will take time to reverse—if they are reversible—and cancer doesn't always leave you enough time to try things that are experimental. This book, however, does point out that many diseases—including cancer, long considered irreversible by many doctors—have been reversed in some people. This should at least increase hope for those who are ailing and in despair—and, **<u>most important,</u>** <u>should help the reader avoid developing these diseases.</u>

As you will see in this book, anything that improves liver function can also help prevent or improve **digestive problems; fatigue, anxiety,** and **depression; weight problems; allergies;**

hormonal imbalances; infertility; heart attacks; autoimmune diseases; and **cancer.**

So now I take great pleasure in introducing you to these somewhat reclusive—but universally loved—dwellers in your liver's cellar: the **Nine Liver Dwarves!**

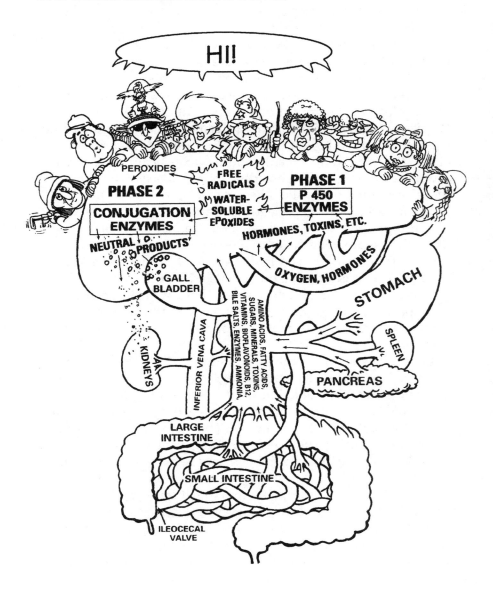

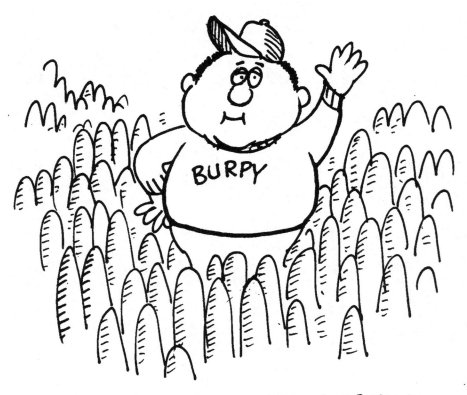

BURPY... IN THE GARDEN OF VILLI

CHAPTER 1

Burpy: Guide To Digestion

Hi! **I'm Burpy,** one of your **Nine Liver Dwarves**. In fact, I'm your **Digestive Liver Dwarf**.

Every time you eat, **toxins** are produced in your **digestive system**. Therefore, every drop of **digestive fluid** has to be picked up by your **portal vein** and delivered to your **liver** to be detoxified and then you feel great! If more **toxins** come in to your liver than I can detoxify, or if the **liver's detoxification enzymes** aren't working properly, then I just dump the toxins out into your **bile**—which gives you a mess of **digestive trouble**.

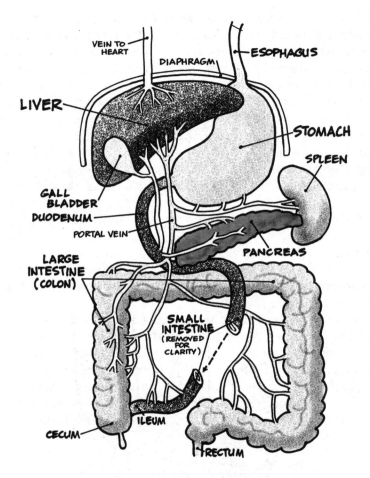

OVERVIEW OF THE DIGESTIVE SYSTEM

It's good to see that you're taking our complete tour of your body. We **Dwarves** are camped in your liver, trying to keep your whole body running as smoothly as we can. Work, work, work—that's all we have time for!

We each look after our own little part of your body, and my specialty is your digestive system. Later, you'll be meeting the other eight **Dwarves** and hearing about the important jobs they do.

You'll eventually see that *my* job is the most important, because good digestion is your key to great health. The other **Dwarves** think I'm too technical but that's just because they're jealous that I've got such a big, beautiful system to work with. If you find my words a little too big, just continue, because the other **Dwarves'** jobs are simpler than mine. In fact, I think the other **Liver Dwarves** themselves are a little simpler, too. You'll see soon enough, and you can judge for yourself.

And there's no quiz at the end of this book, so please don't try to memorize everything. We're supposed to be getting a replacement **Liver Dwarf**. He's a doctor and he's going to finish off the tour. I'm sure he'll be able to simplify a lot of the more challenging information when he arrives—if he gets here on time.

Let's start right here at your liver. Your liver has hundreds of jobs to do, but one of its most crucial tasks is to act as a great big filter for your digestive system.

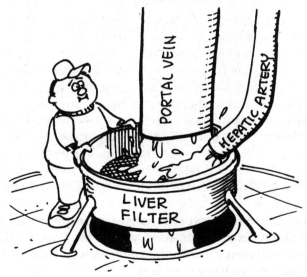

The purpose of your digestive system is to begin the breakdown of foods. It busts those luscious hunks of tasty delight—your meals—into small pieces that can be delivered through your blood system to your cells, which will then burn most of them as fuel.

Here I must give you a warning of the greatest importance: food is a like a double-edged sword—on one side, it's *absolutely necessary* for survival, but on the other, food can *severely injure or even kill you*, if used without the utmost caution.

Some foods have toxins in them. For example: plants often make poisons of different sorts just so they won't be eaten by predators. All kinds of germs in food—like bacteria, viruses, or parasites—can make poisons, too. You don't want all this mess sneaking past your hardworking **Liver Dwarves** and creating a whole lot of irritation, do you?

Sometimes you make us work extra hard when you have those late Saturday-night parties, where you intentionally dump in all kinds of poisons—like alcohol. I know it gives you a buzz, but it keeps us **Liver Dwarves** working overtime.

As if all this poison stuff coming from outside your body weren't bad enough, you've also got bacteria living "downstairs" in your **large intestine**. We call them "**The Boogy Boys**." They're messy little guys, especially when they invite all their ugly friends over—the **parasites**, **yeast**, and **viruses**—to share in the fun of all that food you're eating.

When they start fermenting and putrefying your food, it's a living nightmare for your faithful **Liver Dwarves**. Your **portal vein**, which is supposed to be delivering all the freshly digested nuggets of food to us at the liver, turns instead into a **toxic sewer line** for all those party animals. That's when I desperately try to filter out all those dangerous poisons with the liver so they won't enter your bloodstream! Imagine if all this stuff hit your brain—it'd be damaged in no time.

When I'm dealing with The Boogy Boys, it isn't a one-night-New-Year's bash I'm talking about. This can go on 24 hours a day, seven days a week, all year long—for decades! The Boogy Boys can create the same diseases in your body that alcoholics get—even if you don't drink—because they can actually make alcohol from all those sweet things that they like you to eat.

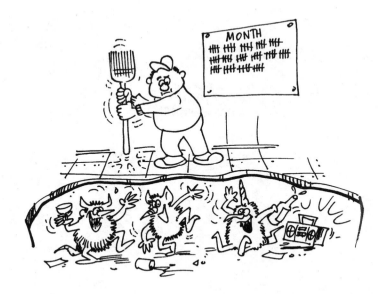

Now let me set you straight. We **Liver Dwarves** are not afraid of work. In fact, we love work; we thrive on it; we can't live without it! We're tough and we're fighters! As long as you've a breath left in your body, you can be sure we're still hard at work helping you. We just ask that you help us, that's all. The more you know about how hard we have to work to keep you healthy, the more you'll want to help us out.

So let's get started on your digestion. The most important thing about digestion is that you need to digest your food quickly. You want to get full absorption of the nutrients, instead of giving The Boogy Boys a chance to make party poisons and then dump them into your liver. Your mouth was invented to take in food, and it was designed to chew the food. The less yakking and the more chewing you do, the better your food digests. I believe I learned that as a freshman in **Liver Dwarf College**, from the renowned Professor Chewmore.

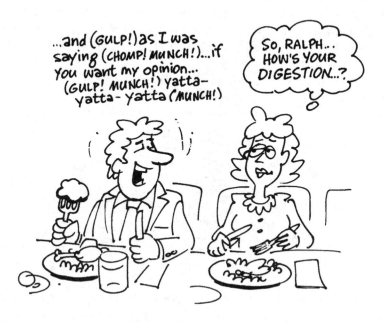

Also, the better your food smells and tastes, the more **saliva** you'll make. Saliva contains **enzymes**—such as **lingual lipase**, which begins **fat** digestion, and **salivary amylase**, which begins your digestion of **starches**. Your tongue likes to help out, so it secretes proteins that have **antibiotic** properties. Also, **Epidermal Growth Factor** from your mouth stimulates the development of gastrointestinal tissue, and maintains a thick, protective mucous layer that helps protect against ulceration. When you lick your skin, **nitrite** from your saliva reacts with the skin to create **nitric oxide**, which kills bacteria.

Saliva lubricates your **esophagus** and because saliva is alkaline, it further protects your esophagus from any acid that might sneak up into it from your **stomach**. As you know, your esophagus contracts rhythmically to push the food down toward your stomach. This is the beginning of **peristalsis**, the muscle action that will propel food through your digestive system—at a speed that will optimize absorption of nutrients and minimize the retention of toxins from The Boogy Boys.

At the bottom of your esophagus, the food passes through

the **cardiac valve** into your stomach. The cardiac valve isn't a true valve but, because the esophagus enters the stomach at such a sharp angle, it does prevent the stomach acid from going up into the esophagus, unless you get into bile trouble, which you'll learn about later.

The stomach walls are made of layers of tough muscle—the electrically powered "motor" of this mixmaster. As electrical nerve waves pass into your stomach muscles, they mix and "knead" the food mass with strong, rhythmic contractions.

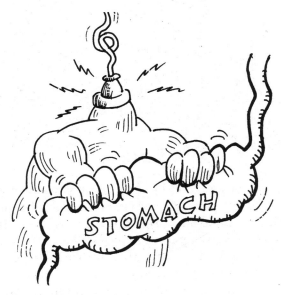

STOMACH MUSCLE AT WORK

Like your entire intestine, your stomach has **mucous** cells, which make mucous to lubricate and protect. Your stomach also has two very special types of glands: the **oxyntic (gastric) glands** and the **pyloric glands**.

The first 80 percent of your stomach is mainly made up of oxyntic glands that secrete three things in addition to mucous: **intrinsic factor**, **pepsinogen**, and **hydrochloric acid**. Intrinsic factor binds with **vitamin B_{12}**, precious to your **bone marrow** for the formation of red blood cells. And since B_{12} doesn't get absorbed until the end section of your small intestine, the intrinsic factor not only helps in the absorption of B_{12} through your intestinal wall, it also helps protect B_{12} from The Boogy Boys, should they happen to sneak into your lower small intestine—if you could imagine such a ghastly event.

As you'll learn from **Itchy**, one of The Boogy Boys' most sacred ancient dreams is to one day sneak into the small intestine, where they can regain possession of that hallowed symbol of the power of the light—which they feel was so unjustly taken from them many centuries ago—vitamin B_{12}! It's their Holy Grail. Just another of the many silly myths these primitive creatures believe in.

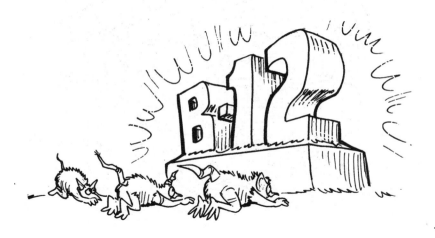

When secreted, the various types of pepsinogen are inactive until they are activated by hydrochloric acid to form **pepsin**. Pepsin has strong protein-digesting abilities—as long as your stomach maintains its acidity. The powerful combination of acid and pepsin can easily kill most **microorganisms** and parasites that might be in your food. It takes a pH of about 2 to 3.5, however, to turn inactive pepsinogens into active pepsin that can shatter your protein foods into smaller protein chains (**polypeptides**) and kill any bacteria, yeast, or parasites that might come into your stomach or upper small intestine.

Hydrochloric acid (**HCl**) contains three million times more hydrogen ions than your blood does, and it takes a lot of energy to produce this very strong acidity. In fact, according to my latest stomach-meter reading, it takes over 1,500 calories to make just one litre of gastric juice, which contains mainly HCl. You see now that my work can get technical at times. You can also see that digestion is very hard work, which indubitably makes *me* your most important **Liver Dwarf**.

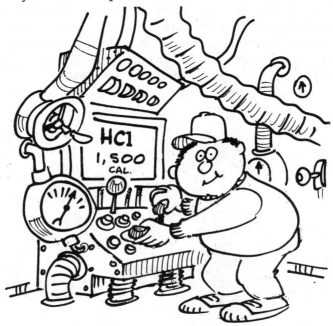

If the pH of your stomach should ever get as high as 5, your pepsinogens won't get activated into pepsin and therefore, your proteins won't get fully digested. As your immune system struggles to clean up these hunks of incompletely digested proteins, this can lead to a dramatic increase in **allergies** and other immune system problems.

Even scarier is the wide assortment of bug-eyed parasites, yeast, and bacteria that can turn your intestine into a zoo if your stomach pH were to get that high.

Stomach acid is not only important for your digestion of protein, it's crucial for the absorption of some minerals. Low pH in your stomach allows proteins to bind to your minerals so that they'll be able to get through the tough intestinal wall to where you can use them. This is called **chelation**. Your stomach also secretes small amounts of other enzymes that help digest **butterfat**, starches, and **gelatin**.

The bottom portion of your stomach contains mainly pyloric glands, which secrete mucous, some pepsinogens, and the **hormone gastrin**. Gastrin and two other substances, **histamine** and **acetylcholine**, increase hydrochloric acid production by the oxyntic glands. As your stomach churns, it kneads the food and mixes it with the strong digestive juices to begin to form a fluid mass called **chyme**. I keep the bottom valve of your stomach— the **pyloric valve**—open slightly, to allow water out into your small intestine so that water won't dilute the effect of your stomach's digestive juices.

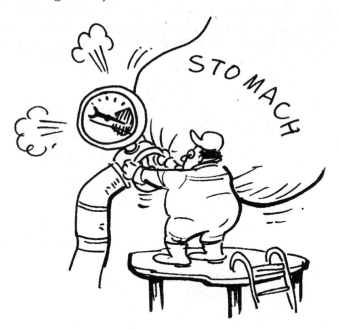

The intense contractions of your stomach gradually pump small amounts of chyme through your narrow pyloric valve into the **duodenum**—the first section of your small intestine— where things get even more interesting. The small intestine continues the **peristaltic action** of your stomach—mixing, kneading, and slowly moving the chyme down from your duodenum, through the **jejunum**, and finally to your **ileocecal valve** at the end of your **ileum**.

I think the small intestine should be renamed the *long* intestine, since it's about 10 feet long! Certainly, it's far more important than the stubby and much shorter large intestine—also called the **colon**—because it's in your small intestine that most of your digestion and the absorption of nutrients takes place. The large intestine is the sleazy hangout of that disreputable crowd of troublemakers—The Boogy Boys. That's why I normally keep your ileocecal valve tightly closed to keep those messy scum out of your treasure-laden small intestine.

As lengthy as your small intestine is, it doesn't provide nearly enough room to do all the digestion and absorption I'm responsible for, so I've added some folds that increase the surface area by three times. Then on these folds, I've added millions of **villi**, which add 10 times *more* surface area.

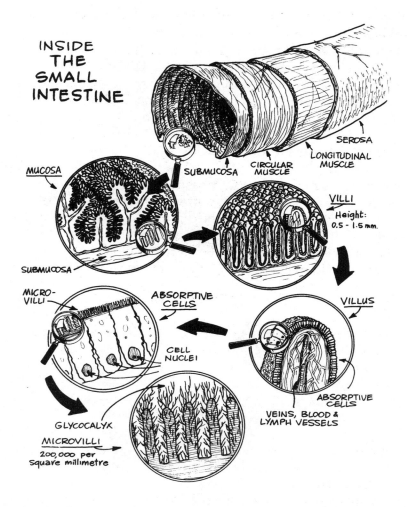

INSIDE THE SMALL INTESTINE

MUCOSA

SUBMUCOSA

SEROSA
LONGITUDINAL MUSCLE

SUBMUCOSA   CIRCULAR MUSCLE

VILLI
Height: 0.5 - 1.5 mm.

MICRO-VILLI   ABSORPTIVE CELLS

CELL NUCLEI

VILLUS

ABSORPTIVE CELLS

VEINS, BLOOD & LYMPH VESSELS

GLYCOCALYX

MICROVILLI
200,000 per square millimetre

I learned these tricks in sophomore year at **Liver Dwarf College**, from Professor Stretchmore. There is one more special trick she taught me that allows even more absorption to take place in such a narrow, crowded space.

You see, there are two types of cells on the surface of the villi. The **goblet cells** make mucous, and the **absorptive cells** absorb. To increase the surface area 20 times more, I've erected about 600 **microvilli** on the top of *each* of the millions of absorptive cells. Called the **brush border**, this forest of microvilli is soft and fuzzy, like velvet. When I get bored with the **Liver Dwarf** work, I go for a slide down the brush border. It tickles my tush in a nice kind of way.

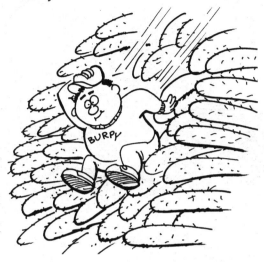

The microvilli are powered by interlinked protein fibres that can make the forest wave and dance when happy, or shrink away when irritated. Extending from the membrane of each microvillus is a wave of tentacle-like enzymes called the **glycocalyx**, which digest primarily **disaccharides** and polypeptides.

The disaccharide enzymes are less deeply rooted in the membranes of your microvilli than are the protein-digesting enzymes, and that makes them much more fragile and more easily damaged.

Since many of these enzymes self-destruct with each meal you digest, or they are broken down by enzymes from your **pancreas**, it's a constant struggle for me to keep a replenished stock of enzymes on hand in the glycocalyx. I have to constantly renew them, which means I have to make a new absorptive cell on the **villus**, plant 600 microvilli on it, and then start growing glycocalyx.

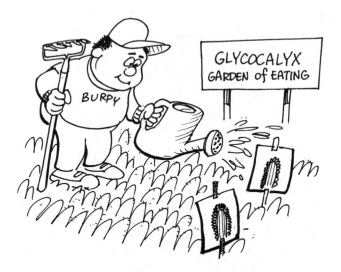

These enzymes will gladly die the next time you eat, just to help digest your food. Now there's dedication! An absorptive cell might have been born, produced microvilli and enzymes, then broken off from the tip of the villus into your bowel, all in a few days, and all to help you digest and absorb your food. It makes me darn proud to be the **Liver Dwarf** in charge of your digestion—when I have so many heroic helpers.

The beginning section of your small intestine, the duodenum, makes two hormones: **secretin** and **cholecystokinin**. Secretin is stimulated by hydrochloric acid and it activates your pancreas and **bile ducts** to secrete alkaline juices to neutralize the acid chyme. Proteins and fats in the chyme stimulate the small intestine to make cholecystokinin and it, in turn, activates the production and secretion of digestive enzymes from your pancreas and the secretion of bile from your gallbladder.

Cholecystokinin stimulates your pancreas to make up to 10 times the required amount of digestive enzymes. This is extremely important because it's in your small intestine that the enzymes work their magic, breaking the large "chunks" of protein, starch, and fat into smaller "bits" of polypeptides, disaccharides, and fatty acids.

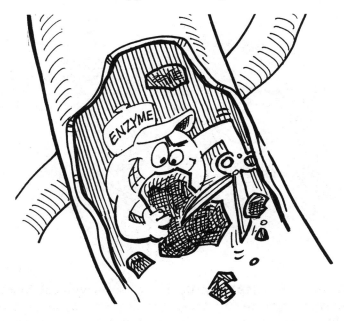

    As powerful as these tiny enzymes are in carrying out their
mighty work—chopping gigantic Goliaths into small pieces—
they perform best when their working conditions are
favourable. Enzymes need the right temperature, maintained by
your **thyroid gland**—and they need the right pH, too, set by the
alkaline secretions of your pancreas and bile ducts, which
counterbalance the acid pH of your stomach secretions. Slight
fluctuations in temperature or pH in your small intestine can
make the enzymes much less effective.

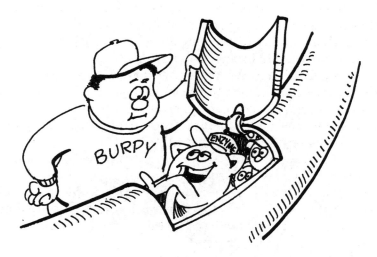

... A nice, warm day like this... surely
you don't expect a 100% effort...

I secrete **picolinic acid** into the pancreatic juices to bind to
zinc and improve its absorption. I also put picolinic acid into
breast milk; I add about three times more picolinic acid than I
do zinc. This gives a nursing baby a good start with zinc, which
is so important for growth. I'm sure **Bitchy** will tell you more
about the importance of zinc.

Picolinic acid is one of the many important products that
Liver Dwarves make from the amino acid **tryptophan**, one of
the 10 amino acids you must get from the proteins in your diet.
From these amino acids, I can make 10 others. We won't have
time to explain *all* the things we **Liver Dwarves** make from all
the amino acids, but we'll go into more detail on tryptophan
throughout the tour, so that you'll realize how crucial a single
nutrient can be to your overall health.

Also, I mix a little special **Liver Dwarf** formula (that I learned
in junior year at **Liver Dwarf College**, from Professor Kilmore)
into your pancreatic juice to annihilate any Boogy Boys that
might try to sneak into your pancreatic duct.

The digestion of carbohydrates proceeds rapidly with the addition of the pancreatic enzymes. **Pancreatic amylase** is stronger than amylase from your mouth, and within 30 minutes, starches are broken down from complex sugars—mostly into **disaccharides**. Disaccharides are two sugar molecules joined together. **Maltose**, from starch, consists of two **glucose** molecules; **lactose**, from milk, is a glucose joined to a **galactose** molecule; and **sucrose**, from plant sugars, is a glucose and a **fructose** molecule bonded together.

As these disaccharides pass close to your intestinal wall, they're embraced by the wavy enzyme tentacles of the glycocalyx, where they're split into single or simple sugars like glucose, galactose, and fructose. These simple sugars are then absorbed into the microvilli, where they're transported via blood vessels to your portal vein.

Protein digestion starts with pepsin in your stomach—if your stomach acid pH is low enough to activate the pepsin. Pepsin is particularly important to break down the tough **collagen fibres** of meat so that your pancreatic enzymes can get access to the proteins. Your pancreatic enzymes that are responsible for breaking down proteins are converted in your small intestine into their active forms, namely **trypsin, chymotrypsin**, and **carboxypolypeptidase**. These enzymes break the peptide chains of amino acids into smaller and smaller pieces, until they're reduced to chains of a few amino acids, called **dipeptides** and **tripeptides**.

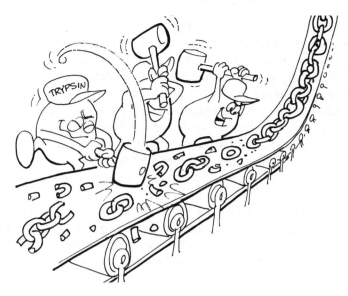

Further digestion takes place through the action of the enzymes of the glycocalyx, outside of your intestinal membrane, and digestion is completed by enzymes inside the membrane. I don't digest all the proteins completely; there are some proteins—such as pancreatic enzymes and **glutathione**—that are better absorbed intact so that they can continue their good work.

One of the amino acids that's obtained from your diet is **methionine**. I convert it into **homocysteine** for transport to the liver. Homocysteine is a bit toxic, but in the liver it's converted back into methionine or into cysteine, which are both used in liver detoxification.

The reason that your pancreatic digestive enzymes are so effective at breaking down starches and proteins is because they work best in a water-soluble medium. Fats, however, aren't water-soluble, so extra effort must be made to digest them. If there's a tough job to do, you need a tough helper, and that's where I come in again. You see, your liver is not only a filter for your digestive system, it also has hundreds of other jobs to do—including the digestion of fats through the production of **bile**, which I personally supervise, to make sure it gets done right.

Cholecystokinin stimulates the release of bile from your gallbladder, especially if you have eaten fats recently. It's the responsibility of the bile to make fats more water-soluble so that the enzymes can get to work on them. Specifically, it's the job of the **bile salts** and **lecithin** secreted in the bile. These ingredients weaken the tension of the fat globules so that the kneading action of your intestine can knock them down into smaller particles. The **pancreatic lipase** enzymes can then break these particles into **fatty acids** and **monoglycerides** that are then carried by the **bile salt micelles** to the microvilli. Here, they separate from the bile salts, and because of their fatty nature, diffuse through the membrane of your small intestine into the absorptive cells. The bile salts then return to the chyme, where they pick up more fatty acids and monoglycerides.

I recycle over 90 percent of the bile salts by absorbing them from your small intestine and bringing them back to your liver. In fact, I once broke the **Liver Dwarf** record by recycling a single bile salt more than 20 times before I finally lost it in a bowel movement. Nearly broke my heart when it swirled away that day. It was like losing an old friend.

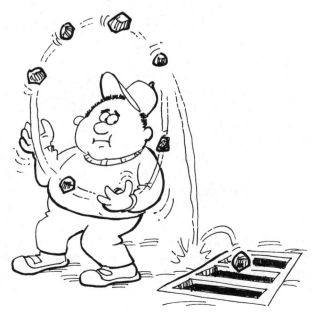

Inside the absorptive cells, the fatty acids and monoglycerides are formed into **chylomicrons** that then enter the centre of the villus, where they're absorbed into the **lacteal**, the entrance to your **lymphatic system**. Short-chain fatty acids, such as butterfat, are more water-soluble so they are absorbed directly into your portal vein as are the amino acids from protein digestion and the simple sugars, like glucose and fructose.

If I'm a little short on bile salts, I just whip up some more by converting **cholesterol** to an acid form, and then I add amino acids. It's another simple but effective recipe I learned many centuries ago at **Liver Dwarf College**.

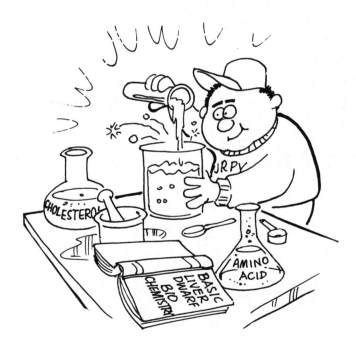

Bile salts can be sent directly to your duodenum from your liver, or they can be stored in your **gallbladder**. To store a large amount of bile in the gallbladder, it's necessary to concentrate it by removing water and minerals and returning them to the liver through your gallbladder's portal vein connection.

Concentrating the bile for storage in the gallbladder turns the bile from a light yellow-brown colour to a darker brown, or even a dark green colour, and it turns your stool those same colours. When the secretin hormone tells me that a lot of stomach acid is being dumped into your small intestine, I have to add **bicarbonate** into the bile to help your pancreas neutralize the pH, so that your pancreatic enzymes will work best.

Of course, your digestive juices kill off most of The Boogy Boys that come in with your food. If any of The Boys get past the digestive juices, I roll them up in balls of mucous and send them down through your ileocecal valve into your large intestine where they belong!

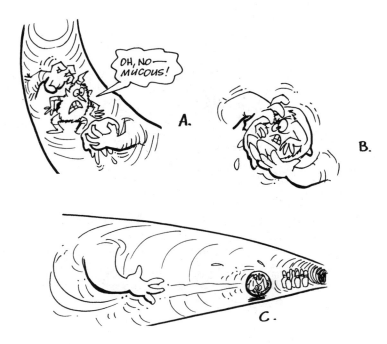

I can put up with The Boogy Boys as long as they stay on the other side of your ileocecal valve!

Throughout your small intestine, the active absorption of vitamins and minerals also takes place. All these little goodies—

amino acids, simple sugars, short-chain fatty acids, vitamins and minerals—get sucked up, almost as if I vacuumed them, and they get blown into your portal vein for delivery to your liver.

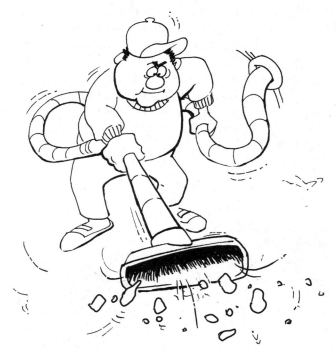

We **Liver Dwarves** like to throw The Boogy Boys the hard-to-digest scraps, like **cellulose**, fibre, or some of the starches or incompletely digested lactose. We just shove it through the trap door to your large intestine and then quickly slam the door shut before they can sneak up into your small intestine.

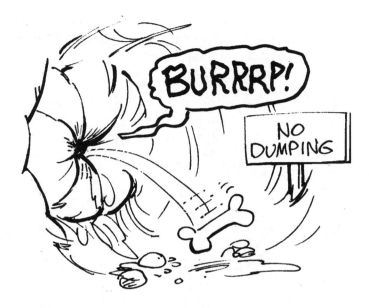

I hear rumours that The Boogy Boys make a few good things out of these tough fibres, like **vitamin K** and short-chain fatty acids, and they draw the water out of the chyme, leaving a harder substance that becomes a bowel movement. I don't trust them much, though. A lot of them are fermenters, which means they're messy eaters. Oh, I don't mind absorbing the short-chain fatty acids they make from fermenting starches but generally, I don't absorb nearly as enthusiastically from your large intestine as I do from your small intestine. I shudder at the thought of absorbing any alcohol or other swill that they might be brewing up.

To help keep them out of your small intestine, I hire a few mercenary bacteria as guards to lurk just above your ileocecal valve. Their job is to take bile salts out of the chyme and **deconjugate** them. This deconjugated bile becomes slippery and irritating to any Boogy Boys that might attempt to sneak up into your small intestine. They slip and slide their way right back into your large intestine where they belong.

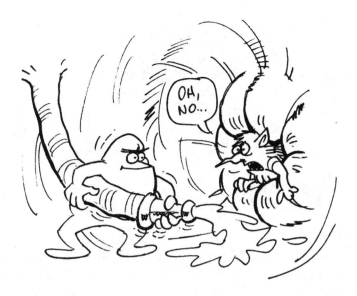

Because I do such a good job of keeping your small intestine tidy, I don't need to make much **melatonin** in your small intestine. Oh, didn't I tell you about melatonin yet, and its ability to protect against **free radicals**? Didn't I tell you about free radicals, either!? Well, excuuuuse me!

The foods we eat are a concentrated form of energy that originated in a nuclear explosion in the sun. The **chlorophyll** in plants manages to grab this energy and store it in many forms that we eventually take in as food. The purpose of digesting the food is to transform it back into energy that your cells can use. Of course, energy is good, but like anything powerful, it can also be very dangerous.

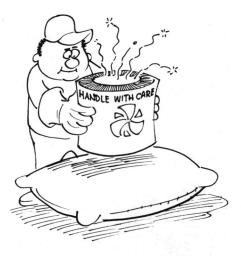

Oxygen, for example, is the single most important nutrient that your body needs, yet in the form of **oxygen free radicals**, it can also be extremely harmful. Oxygen needs two paired electrons in its outer ring to be fairly stable, which is why oxygen is often found as O_2. That is: two oxygen molecules—each with two electrons—joined together to gain the stability that comes with sharing a pair of electrons.

When these happy couples are split apart, however, sometimes one oxygen will end up with only one electron that will desperately try to rip another electron out of the surrounding area. If it rips the electron from a **cell membrane** or from **DNA**, *that* can cause damage, as **Sluggy** will describe to you in more detail later.

Because the digestive process handles such tremendous amounts of energy in the foods it breaks down, it can be the source of free radicals—which can cause direct damage to your digestive organs. As the **Liver Dwarf** in charge of digestion, I have to do everything I can to protect your intestines and digestive organs!

Among the many hormones I use to regulate the flow of food along your digestive system are two called **serotonin** and **melatonin**. Serotonin is made from the amino acid tryptophan, and serotonin generally has a stimulating effect throughout your digestive system. For example, serotonin stimulates stomach secretions and mucous membranes and too much serotonin can make some people experience nausea and even vomiting.

I make melatonin from serotonin. Melatonin is generally calming, as opposed to the stimulating effect that serotonin has. What I'm most proud of is that I've managed to combine two jobs in one substance because melatonin is not only a **neurohormone**, it's also a very strong **neutralizer of free radicals**, or **antioxidant**.

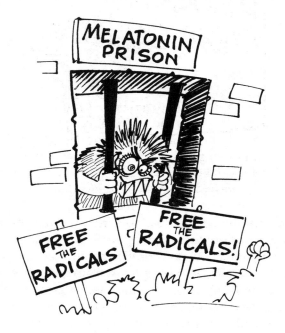

I learned this little trick in senior year at **Liver Dwarf College**, from Professor Quenchmore, who has lived longer than any **Liver Dwarf** in history, and who is still going strong! I make quite a bit of melatonin in your upper digestive system because the large amount of oxygen in your esophagus, stomach, and duodenum—reacting with the food and digestive juices—can create a large number of free radicals that must be quickly quenched by melatonin.

The large intestine—or colon, if you prefer—doesn't have much oxygen, which is why most of The Boogy Boys in there are called **anaerobic**—that means they don't like oxygen. Yet I still have to make large amounts of melatonin in your large intestine because The Boogy Boys are such sloppy eaters that your intestine needs a lot of protection from the toxins that they make.

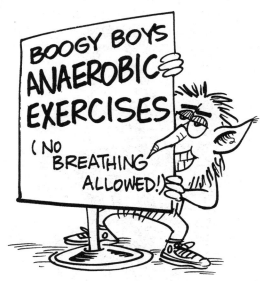

Serotonin and melatonin are also made in much smaller amounts in your brain. **Spacey** will explain later how this can have a powerful effect on your physical and emotional health.

Note that I didn't say I make a *lot* of melatonin in your small intestine, and the reason I didn't say that is that I don't. Hmmmmm, I'm starting to talk like **Spacey**. Don't worry; you'll meet her later. Did you understand what I said? I don't make *much* melatonin in your small intestine and the reason is because I've got a backup system in place throughout your digestive system—throughout your body, actually—but it's especially effective in the small intestine so that melatonin isn't so necessary there. This system consists of two enzymes: **glutathione peroxidase** and **glutathione transferase**, which use a common "fuel," **glutathione**.

The glutathione peroxidase enzyme, with a simple swipe of its mighty **selenium** sword, can slash deadly **peroxides** into harmless water.

The glutathione transferase enzyme also uses glutathione, but in this case, to quench any larger electron-hungry molecules before they can do damage. Glutathione is my gladiator, my single-handed slayer of evil-doers.

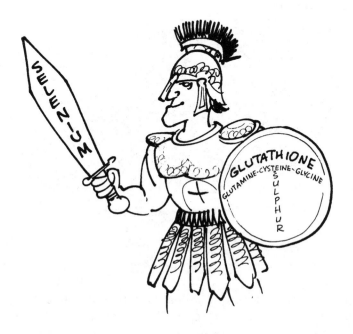

It's so important that I must make sure there's plenty of glutathione for these two important enzymes to operate. Glutathione is a protein, which means it's made of amino acids linked together, like a train. It's a short train, however, as it contains only three amino acids. The **sulphur**-carrying amino acid **cysteine**—really the workhorse of glutathione—is sandwiched between the amino acids **glycine** and **glutamine**.

Glutathione has to be assembled in your body from these three amino acids to meet the needs of the two enzymes, glutathione peroxidase and glutathione transferase—with the exception of one specific area: the small intestine. Glutamine and the small intestine are secret lovers so whenever the small intestine sees glutamine, it gives it a big hug and a kiss, and invites it in.

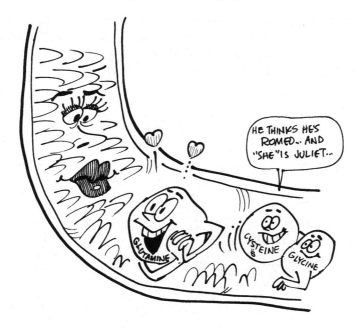

The cysteine and glycine attached to the glutamine, of course, get invited in along with it. So this is how glutathione slips into the small intestine intact, without being broken up by digestive enzymes.

The small intestine thus has ready access to glutathione from the food that's entering the body during digestion, so I just run the glutathione straight into glutathione peroxidase and glutathione transferase enzymes, and they get right to work protecting you from nasty fatty peroxides that might be trying to sneak in with your food. Then you and I can rest peacefully at night, knowing that everything is safe because **Gladiator Glutathione** is guarding the gate!

Digestion is a complex process but, like most systems of your body, it pretty much runs itself if you treat it right. For the most part, the billions of Boogy Boys in your large intestine keep themselves under control with their own style of vigilante justice! They compete with each other for food and make chemicals that inhibit their competitors so that of the hundreds of species of Boogy Boys, just one usually won't get the upper hand. **Candida yeast**, for example, hide in the deepest nooks and crannies where they won't have much to do until you and your Boogy Boys have died. Then, they'll quickly recycle you by turning you into plant food. Yes, it's true—yeast and fungus are graduates of Composter College.

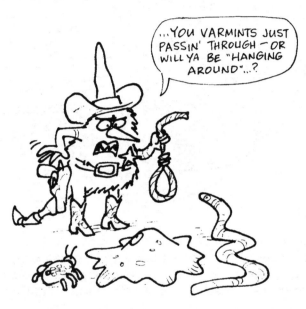

They do cooperate with each other as well, though. Most of The Boogy Boys are anaerobic, which means they can't *stand* oxygen, so they allow a few **facultative bacteria** to hang around. Facultative bacteria can live with or without oxygen so if oxygen does enter the large intestine, they quickly use it up before it harms their anaerobic (oxygen-hating) Boogy Boy buddies.

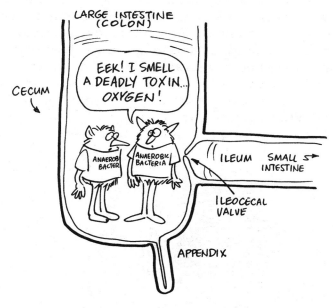

Antibiotics can kill off some of the intestinal bacteria, allowing others—like **Clostridium difficile** or Candida yeast—to multiply quickly and take over the vacancy, sometimes creating obvious problems such as **diarrhea** and **colitis**. They can also create a wide range of more subtle symptoms, as the famous **General Achy** will describe later.

The barriers that I put up—like hydrochloric acid, digestive enzymes, and bile—will keep most foreigners like **amoebas**, **protozoa**, "outsider" bacteria, and even **worms** from getting established in the intestine.

Glutathione and I personally assure that your small intestine stays strong and tidy so that I can absorb everything from there like a vacuum cleaner. In fact, the other **Liver Dwarves** used to call me Hoover, until they built the dam by the same name. Then **Spacey** got confused and started calling me "That Dam Dwarf," so I switched my name from Hoover to **Burpy**.

Now, I'm going to tell you about the image that makes **Liver Dwarves** wake up with a start at 3 A.M. in a cold sweat, a blood-curdling scream hurling from our lips. Behind this nightmare is the scary scenario that The Boogy Boys are running loose in your small intestine. They're eating the sugars, from which they make alcohol; eating the fats and the minerals; stealing your vitamin B_{12} and tryptophan and other amino acids; and overwhelming your glutathione enzymes. They deconjugate the bile salts in your upper small intestine, which further disrupts your amino acid absorption. And then, they smash the enzymes of your (sob) beautiful glycocalyx so you can't digest lactose or maltose or **gluten** any more.

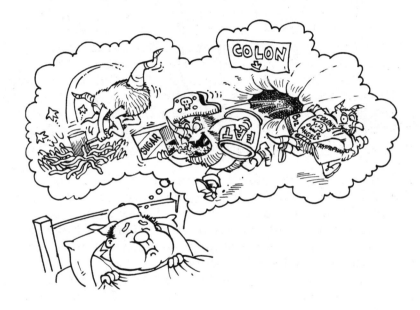

As their nasty party rolls on, *every* drop of their waste products is quickly absorbed from your small intestine into your portal vein and sent directly to your liver. We **Liver Dwarves** then must work overtime to deal with the situation. This isn't just a transient bad dream from eating too much spicy food before bedtime; this is the reality that **Liver Dwarves** have to deal with from day to day—a flood of toxins pouring into your liver from your portal vein.

If The Boogy Boys get through your ileocecal valve and into your small intestine only a foot or so, the problem may be manageable, if we **Liver Dwarves** work long and hard to minimize the damage. The small intestine, however, is about 10 feet long. The further up into the small intestine they go, the more they can steal your nutrients and make toxins—which means more work for us **Liver Dwarves** to do!

Maybe **Itchy** can tell you later what *you* can do to help keep The Boogy Boys on the large intestine side of the ileocecal valve because he's in charge of the plumbing—and that includes the ileocecal valve. In the meantime, I'll keep on telling you more about my job, and how painful and heartbreaking it can be when *you* are working *against* me instead of *with* me.

Since the digestive juice is potentially toxic, I run every drop of digestive fluid through your portal vein into your liver, to be carefully inspected and certified as safe, or to be promptly detoxified by your liver. I take the portal vein fluid inside the liver where the vein branches off into millions of **sinusoids**.

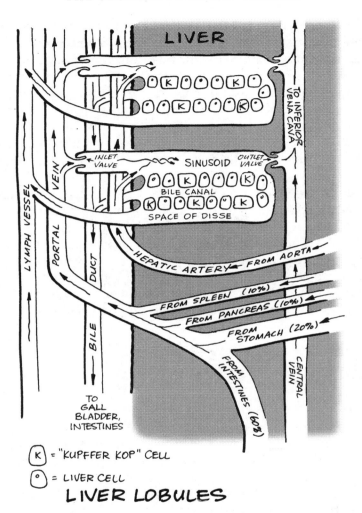

LIVER LOBULES

The entrance to each sinusoid is guarded by an **inlet valve** operated by **Bloaty**, your next **Liver Dwarf** guide. If the toxins in the portal vein fluid are mild enough that they're not likely to directly damage your liver cells, **Bloaty** lets the portal vein fluid into the sinusoid. Thirty per cent of the cells lining the sinusoid are **Kupffer Kops**—**macrophages** fixed in position under the stern leadership of the famous **Liver Dwarf, General Achy**. The first priority of sinusoidal security is for The Kupffer Kops to gobble up anything "foreign"—including Boogy Boys and other microorganisms, as well as **antigen-antibody complexes**—that may be trying to sneak into your liver through your portal vein.

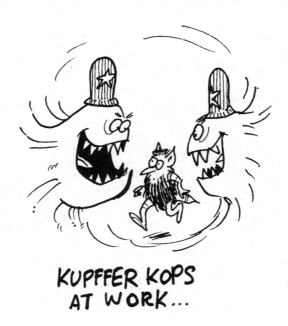

KUPFFER KOPS
AT WORK...

There are always some toxins coming in every time you eat, even if The Boogy Boys are behaving themselves, so the second priority in the sinusoids is to neutralize any incoming toxins.

Your liver cells have two sets of enzymes that I use for detoxification—the **Phase 1 P450 enzymes** and the **Phase 2 conjugation enzymes**. These enzymes are found throughout your body, but by far the greatest concentration is found in your liver—which certainly shows how incredibly important I am! It's the Phase 2 enzymes that do the actual detoxification—but since they can only neutralize water-soluble substances, any chemicals or hormones that are fat-soluble must first go through Phase 1 of liver detoxification to be made water-soluble.

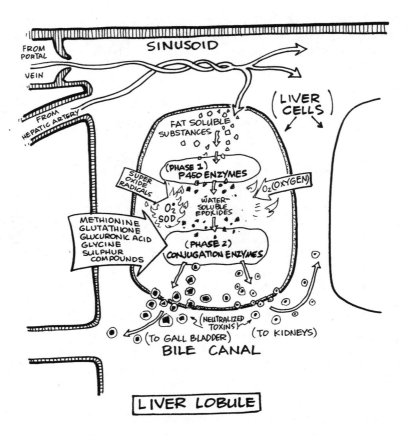

LIVER LOBULE

There are more than 100 Phase 1 P450 enzymes. Each one specializes in making one or two fatty substances water-soluble by adding oxygen to them. These water-soluble intermediaries are called **epoxides** and they can be as much as 60 times *more* toxic than their fat-soluble precursors—they can even damage your DNA and cause cancer, as **Sluggy** will explain later. Yes, that's what I said—your liver's Phase 1 P450 enzymes make epoxides that can be carcinogenic.

When oxygen is added by the P450 enzymes to make an epoxide, a free radical called **superoxide radical** is spun off to the side. These free radicals must be immediately quenched by *super*oxide dismutase enzyme (SOD)—I call it **Super OD**—which needs **manganese, copper,** or zinc for its super strength.

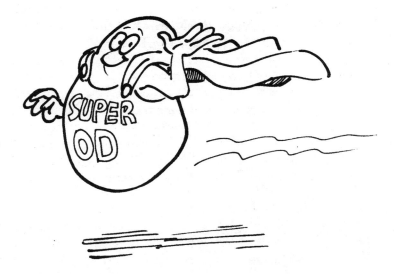

Superoxide radicals being spun off by your P450 enzymes are supposed to be caught and neutralized by Super OD. Superoxide radicals aren't as dangerous as you might think. All Super OD has to do is say "Boo" and throw some hydrogen at them, and they quickly turn into oxygen and **hydrogen peroxide**.

So you can see that fatty toxins entering your liver through the portal vein can have their toxicity *amplified* when your P450 enzymes make them water-soluble and, at the same time, superoxide radicals and hydrogen peroxide are produced during this Phase 1 step. Since toxic water-soluble epoxides can create cancer, and hydrogen peroxide can spin off the deadly hydroxyl radical, which can create *any* disease, you're in immense danger!

Fortunately for you, your Phase 2 conjugation enzymes quickly bind water-soluble toxins with **glutathione**, **methionine**, **glycine**, **glucuronic acid**, and **sulphur compounds**. And then there's **catalase**, which helps to break up peroxides. I'm especially proud of glutathione. It's a very strong free-radical scavenger and continues the good work that it has done earlier in your intestine: nabbing pesky peroxides, epoxides, and other toxic troublemakers.

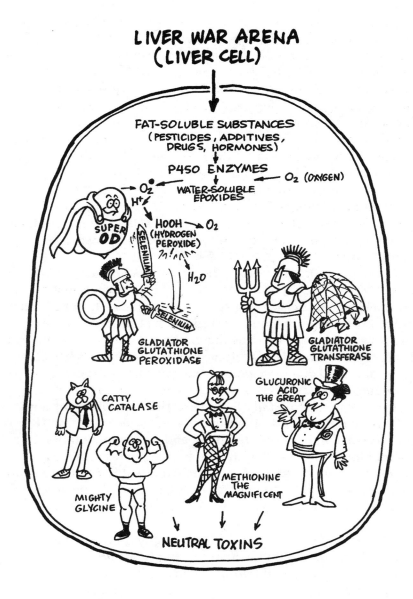

I count so much on glutathione peroxidase, which has been waiting so patiently in your Phase 2 liver conjugation system, anticipating this opportunity to show its mettle at deactivating peroxides—or should I say metal, because this enzyme gets its super powers from *selenium*. One slash of glutathione peroxidase's magic selenium sword quickly turns Super OD's peroxide product into harmless H_2O: water.

When your conjugation enzymes are finished their skilled work, toxins are no more, as they are now bound up and neutralized. The smaller ones are eliminated through your kidneys; the larger ones, I eliminate through the bile into your duodenum and they're eventually removed in the stool. As long as your liver can keep up with neutralizing the toxin load, there are no symptoms or problems—no matter how many toxins pour in through your portal vein. It's only when your conjugation enzymes can't neutralize all the free radicals, peroxides, and water-soluble toxins as fast as they are produced by your P450 enzymes, that my job as a **Liver Dwarf** gets complicated.

I'm hoping that the doctor, the new **Liver Dwarf**, will be able to explain why sometimes the conjugation enzymes just don't seem motivated to get to work after some foods are eaten. They get sleepy and want to just lie around, ignoring the buildup of hydrogen peroxide made by Super OD.

Hydrogen peroxide then binds to your fatty acids and cholesterol as they come in from the portal vein, creating **fatty acid peroxides** and **cholesterol peroxides** that together are called **lipid peroxides**. If a lipid peroxide contacted one of your cell membranes, a powerful **hydroxyl radical** could be released into the membrane—which could lead to destruction of the membrane.

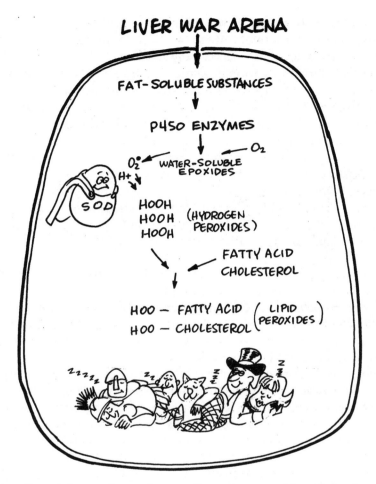

A cell membrane is made up of two layers of fats linked together. Each fat consists of a head that's attracted to water and a tail that's repelled from water. The fats in one layer are facing in the opposite direction to the fats in the other layer—with the heads facing outward and the tails lined up with the tails of the fat in the opposite layer. Along the membrane are found many of the proteins—including enzymes—that are crucial for a cell to do its work.

A hydroxyl radical set adrift in this sea of delicately linked fats can have the effect of a bowling ball knocking over bowling pins. The fats that get knocked askew by this deadly free radical force can generate even *more* hydroxyl radicals, and, as they race down the membrane, they can rip holes in nearby enzymes as well. If that enzyme—such as a P450—were to leak out some **iron** or copper particles, any peroxides with which the iron or copper came into contact could release an *explosion* of hydroxyl radicals, and that could create tremendous damage to your cells!

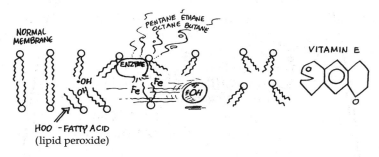

HOO –FATTY ACID
(lipid peroxide)

I keep vitamin E ready at about every 1,000 fats to nab any free radical that might come ripping down the membrane. This is like one cop catching a burglar. It could work out fine, but can one cop stop a riot? Not very likely.

Selenium-powered glutathione peroxidase is the greatest of your Super Hero Super Enzymes because it grabs hydrogen peroxide made by Super OD—*before* it binds to your fats—and slashes it into water. Water! What a deal. Water, instead of lipid peroxides. How I *love* glutathione peroxidase. (*Smooch, smooch!*) Of course, if lipid peroxides were to be formed, glutathione peroxidase could return things to normal by reducing the lipid peroxides to harmless fatty acids. Glutathione also recycles vitamin E, which provides further protection to your membranes.

Believe me, once you've experienced a **major hydroxyl-radical explosion**, you'll never want to have it happen again. It's the smell that I always remember—the smell of decaying fatty membranes. Maybe *you* wouldn't smell it, but we **Liver Dwarves** have to put up with all the **hydrocarbon gases** that are given off in the process: **pentane, ethane, butane**, and **octane**, to name a few of them. Sounds like a gas station! Thank goodness you've got glutathione peroxidase to prevent all that.

If you've been contaminated with heavy metals—like **mercury** from your dental fillings or **cadmium** from smoking— these metals might have replaced your selenium, leaving your glutathione peroxidase weak and ineffective. These same heavy metals can also interfere with Super OD by affecting its copper/zinc levels. Glutathione peroxidase is especially important because it's the only enzyme that can stop the formation of hydroxyl radicals before they start "bowling" your membranes to oblivion. With glutathione peroxidase on duty, those hydroxyl radicals have little chance of scoring a strike as they bowl down your membranes.

A buildup of free radicals from the P450 enzymes and the resulting rise in fatty peroxides can put your precious liver cells in extreme danger. If the peroxides build up, I try a little trick I learned on my own, after graduation. I throw some water-soluble **bioflavonoids** or other **antioxidants** into the liver cells to help the enzymes neutralize the peroxides and free radicals.

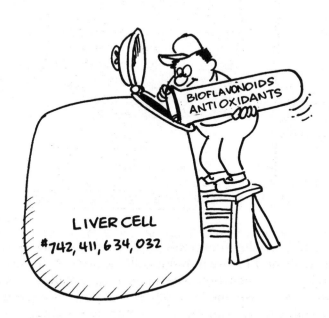

If the Phase 2 conjugation enzymes—especially glutathione peroxidase—still can't neutralize the peroxides, and if these toxins start flooding out of the liver cells into the sinusoids, that's when I have to make a simple but crucial decision. Simple, because I don't really have any alternative. There's really only one thing I can do with excess toxins: I just dump them into the bile!

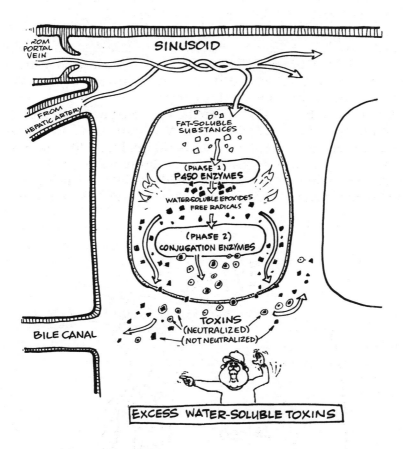

That's all I can do! This creates a problem because now your bile gets toxic and I store it in the gallbladder, which can get irritated by this concoction. Then, every time cholecystokinin stimulates its release, the toxic bile enters your duodenum where it will irritate your bile ducts, **pancreatic duct**, and especially your duodenum—as well as disrupt your fat metabolism.

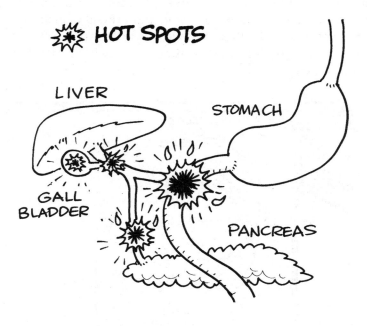

Your esophagus, stomach, and duodenum—and in fact, your entire intestinal tract from mouth to rectum—are really the same muscle, and a muscle can react to irritation in only one way: it **SPASMS**. Food entering a spasmed digestive system may find it easier to come back up, rather than go down. This can result in burping, belching, nausea, and even vomiting. I suppose you can see now how I got my name: **Burpy, The Digestive Liver Dwarf. Burpy—the Bile Guy!**

When a muscle spasms, it also shortens. As a toxic bile-irritated stomach/esophagus muscle shortens, it pulls up into the diaphragm. This can force open the top valve of the stomach—the cardiac valve—allowing hydrochloric acid to reflux up from your stomach into your esophagus. There, it can generate heartburn, a burning sensation under your breastbone, and even chronic sore throats.

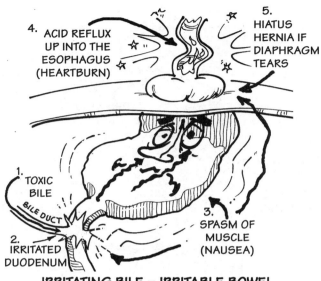

4. ACID REFLUX UP INTO THE ESOPHAGUS (HEARTBURN)

5. HIATUS HERNIA IF DIAPHRAGM TEARS

1. TOXIC BILE

BILE DUCT

2. IRRITATED DUODENUM

3. SPASM OF MUSCLE (NAUSEA)

IRRITATING BILE = IRRITABLE BOWEL

It's not necessarily true that your stomach is making too much acid. When you have acid reflux or heartburn, it's because your bile is irritating your stomach so much that acid is leaking up out of your stomach into your esophagus. The new **Liver Dwarf**, the doctor, will try to help you with that. I certainly hope he can help me with my digestion (*burp*).

If your diaphragm should tear, the spasmed stomach can pop up through the diaphragm into your chest cavity. This is called **hiatal hernia** and it can interfere with breathing and cause heart attack symptoms. A hiatal hernia can allow even more acid to escape from your stomach, especially when you are lying down or bending over.

The secretion of toxic bile can weaken the **duodenal membrane**, allowing The Boogy Boy bacteria, **Helicobacter pylori**, to penetrate it.

Let me tell you that of all the low-down, no-good Boogy Boys, Helicobacter pylori is probably one of the sneakiest. It's an airborne Boogy Boy that flies in on common houseflies—and if it gets inside you, it makes **ammonia** to neutralize your stomach acid enough to give itself a foothold in your stomach.

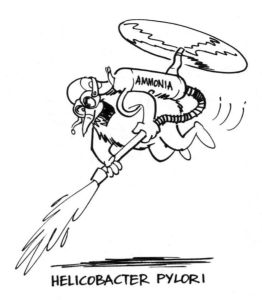

HELICOBACTER PYLORI

If Helicobacter manages to slip in under your mucous membrane because of low stomach acid or toxic bile irritation, your immune system attacks it and that can create **gastritis** and **ulceration**.

Spasming of the stomach and small intestine can interfere with their production of digestive juices and enzymes and give The Boogy Boys more opportunity to do more fermenting of your food. So, as if burping and belching and heartburn weren't enough, now you get g-a-s. Yes, those little bubbles of olfactory offence are my work, too. If I have to dump an overload of toxins into the bile, it can contribute to more gaseous passings. Of course, your other **Dwarves** have found different ways to deal with liver overload, and they'll be telling you about that soon. No matter what the other **Dwarves** might tell you, remember that **Burpy, the Bile Guy**, is the most important. Ah, I see **Bloaty**'s getting ready to continue your tour, so I'll slip back into your liver and check your bile ducts! So long, and have fun.

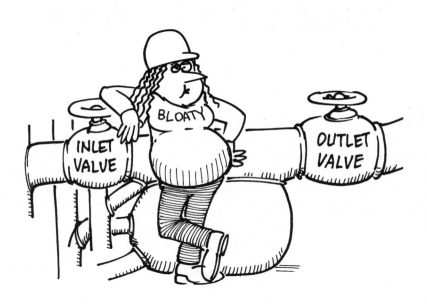

CHAPTER 2

Bloaty: Guide to Your Portal Vein

Hullo, I'm Bloaty, the Portal Vein Liver Dwarf.

If **toxins, rancid fats,** or **peroxides** overload your **liver's detoxification system,** I have to close the **valves going into or out of your liver. Closing the inlet valves** causes **bloating in the abdomen,** which can cause **problems anywhere in the digestive system, pelvic area,** and/or **spleen.** Closing the **outlet valves** causes your liver to **swell up** and **spill fluid, toxins,** and **proteins** into your **lymph system.**

My job in your liver overlaps with **Burpy**'s job, so some of what I tell you at the start might be similar to what he told you. But stick with me, because you'll soon know why *I'm* your most important **Liver Dwarf**.

After every meal, there's going to be some toxins entering the portal vein. Some toxins come directly from the food. The rest of the toxins are made by The Boogy Boys in your large intestine. The portal vein's job is to pick up every drop of blood from your digestive system and deliver it to your liver to be detoxified. And it's my job to monitor and control the flow of the portal vein so that the liver can do its many important jobs as well as possible.

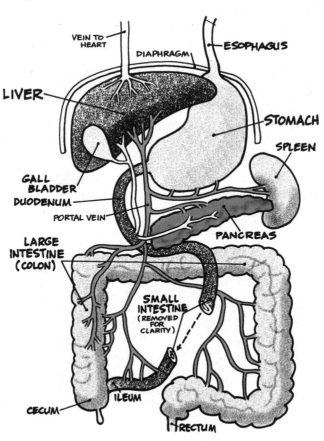

Did you know that almost 30 percent of your body's blood goes through your liver every minute? So you could say that in less than four minutes, your liver handles every drop of blood in your body. Some enters your liver through your **hepatic artery**, but most comes in through your portal vein. **Burpy** told you that your liver cells detoxify things, but before your blood can be detoxified by your liver cells, it has to get there. That's my job, and that's why *I'm* your most important **Liver Dwarf**.

Your liver's workforce is made of millions of hardworking and multitalented liver cells that contain a wide range of enzymes, including your detoxification enzymes—both Phase 1 and Phase 2. The liver cells are arranged in units called **lobules**, which are surrounded by your body's circulation pipes and ducts—portal vein, hepatic artery, bile ducts, lymphatics—and your **central vein**, which is at the hub of the lobules.

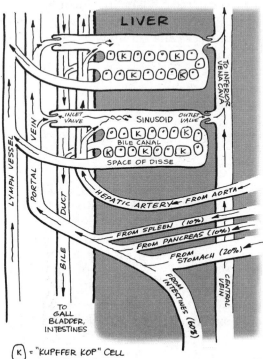

LIVER LOBULES

Portal vein blood enters your liver lobules through the sinusoids, where it mixes with the freshly oxygenated blood arriving via your hepatic artery. Lining the sinusoids are two types of cells. The bigger ones are the **Kupffer cells**. We call them The Kupffer Kops because they're part of the immune system. Their main job is to arrest any of The Boogy Boys that might have somehow snuck through your intestinal membrane into your portal vein and had an easy ride to your liver. The Kupffer Kops quickly put the grab on them and—get this—they munch, munch, and eat 'em all up. How I love those Kupffer Kops! They make life much more enjoyable for an old, overworked **Liver Dwarf**.

The other cells lining your sinusoids—the smaller ones—are the liver cells, loosely packed so that fluids can pass between them into the narrow **space of Disse**. The liver cells that line the space of Disse can now readily absorb nutrients and toxins from your portal blood. And so, charged with oxygen from your hepatic artery, your liver cells get on with their work.

These are a few of the jobs a liver cell has to do.

- Neutralize toxins
- Make bile salts
- Deactivate hormones
- Lower or raise the sugar levels of your blood by listening to the commands of your pancreas to make and store glycogen, or release it
- Oxidize fats for energy
- Produce cholesterol, **phospholipids**, and **lipoproteins**
- Change sugars and amino acids into fats such as **triglycerides**
- Remove ammonia by the formation of **urea**
- Produce amino acids and **plasma proteins**
- Use vitamin K to make blood coagulation products
- Store iron and vitamins A, D, and B_{12}
- Activate **vitamin D**
- Make **CoQ_{10}** and many other products crucial to your health

Oh, those millions of liver cells are the hardest working and the most versatile of all your cells.

The storage of **iron** and the making of bile reminds me of something that **Burpy** neglected to tell you. He said that your portal vein drains your *digestive system*. Now this is true, but he always forgets to say that it also drains your **spleen**, which isn't really a part of your digestive system. But indirectly, your spleen plays an important role in bile production which, as **Burpy** told you, is crucial for efficient digestion.

Your spleen, located on the left side of your abdomen, across from your liver, is also a filter of your blood. Your liver and portal vein are mainly concerned with filtering toxins that come from *outside* your body. (Remember, anything inside of your intestine is still *outside* your body. Things aren't *officially* in your body until they've been screened and certified safe by the liver.) Your spleen is focused on filtering **internal blood**. Its job is to deal with infections and get rid of old and weak red blood cells. In a sense, your spleen is an incinerator for removing the old, the bad, and the ugly from your blood.

When a young **red blood cell** is released from your bone marrow, its job is to be a packhorse for iron in the form of **hemoglobin**, which can pick up oxygen or carbon dioxide. The red blood cell carries oxygen from your lungs to the cells, then reverses the trip carrying a load of carbon dioxide, all the time nibbling on glucose from your blood.

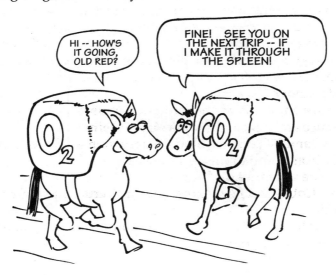

The transfer of oxygen and carbon dioxide on and off that young red blood cell takes place in the **capillaries**, which are slightly smaller than the eight-micrometer-in-diameter red blood cells. The discoid shape of a healthy red blood cell allows it to contort through the narrow capillaries, which in effect "wring" the oxygen out of it and substitute carbon dioxide. In the lungs, the capillaries there reverse the process by removing carbon dioxide and adding oxygen to the hemoglobin of your red blood cell workhorses! As oxygen is *so* essential to your cells, it's important that your red blood cells do their job well, so your spleen puts them through a little test to see how young and flexible they *really* are.

As your red blood cells go deep into your spleen, the passageway becomes narrower. The eight-micrometer-in-diameter red blood cells have to squeeze down to three micrometers in size to get through.

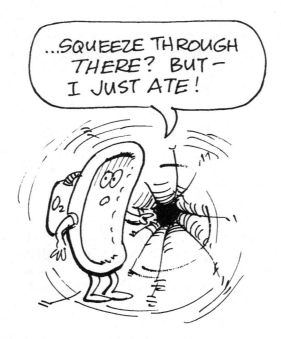

If your blood cells are weakened due to old age or infection, they burst and the surrounding **macrophages** gobble up their remains. This takes place in many parts of the body, but particularly in the liver (by The Kupffer Kops), bone marrow, and spleen.

The iron that the hemoglobin was carrying is either stored in your liver where it might be used in the P450 enzymes, or sent to your bone marrow to be recycled in new red blood cells. The **porphyrin** of the hemoglobin is converted into **bilirubin**, and becomes an important part of bile. So your spleen plays an indirect role in digestion by supplying raw materials for bile production; it also has the very important job of maintaining a clean and effective blood and oxygen system. Spleen blood provides 10 percent of your portal vein supply to your liver, and your pancreas provides another 10 percent; and 20 percent of your portal vein blood originates in your stomach, and 60 percent, the biggest portion, comes from your intestine, by far the largest tributary of the portal vein stream.

My job as controller of your portal vein flow is normally simple. I have two sets of valves to control. One set controls the blood going into each of your millions of liver sinusoids, and the other set controls blood going out. Usually, I just leave the valves pretty much wide open. The large amount of blood flow coming through your liver means that there should be little resistance to the flow as the next destination for your blood is your heart, which is always desperate for a large blood supply.

The trouble arises when there are more toxins coming into your liver than the detoxification enzymes in your liver cells can deal with, or when the P450 enzymes in your liver are making free radicals, toxic peroxides, and epoxides faster than your conjugation enzymes can neutralize them. These two situations are dealt with in two different ways: by closing the valves *going into* the liver sinusoids (**the inlet valves**) or by closing the valves *leaving* the liver sinusoids (**the outlet valves**).

First, I have to guard against very strong toxins that may try to enter your liver from the portal vein as these toxins could damage your liver cells. In this case, I must tighten down your inlet liver valves to block this toxic portal blood from entering your liver.

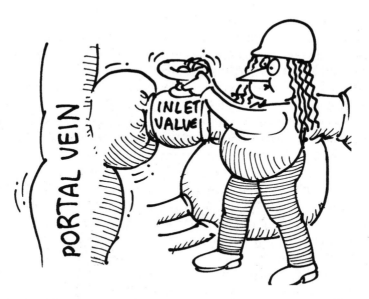

This is like building a dam in a river—you're going to get a pool of fluid backing up behind the dam. In a badly damaged liver—as in **cirrhosis** or severe **hepatitis**—this backup can be somewhat permanent. If there's just a short-term supply of portal vein toxins, then I shut down your inlet liver valves for a short while, until things settle down.

After your liver catches up with the detoxification, I open up the valves again and things quickly go back to normal. About all you might see is a little bloating in your abdomen. If toxins continue to overload your liver so that I have to keep your inlet valves tightened down even longer, then your portal vein will back up even more. This can create back-pressure on your whole portal vein system, although different parts may be under more pressure than others. There's going to be more bloating in your abdomen, as well. Oh, I guess you've figured out by now that that's how I got my name—**Bloaty**.

If your portal vein backup lingers very long, not only can a considerable bay window be developing on you, but the membranes of your intestine can be left simmering in their own toxins. This can contribute to a breakdown of the intestinal membrane strength and result in even more toxins and Boogy Boys getting into your portal vein.

Continued back-pressure in the portal vein is like pumping your bicycle tire up, but not stopping. Something's going to blow—eventually. This back-pressure contributes to **Crohn's disease, colitis, irritable bowel, ulcers, fistulas, fissures, pruritis ani, proctitis, gastritis, duodenitis, diverticulitis,** and **esophagitis**.

When I have to tighten down your inlet liver valves, the *most common* vein to become engorged is your **hemorrhoidal vein**.

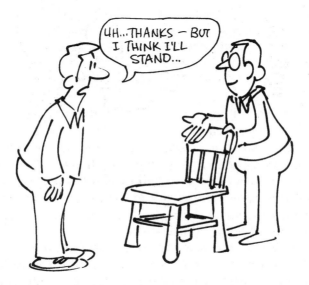

While many people—even doctors—look at hemorrhoids as a localized problem, it's actually one of the many signs that I, **Bloaty the Liver Dwarf**, am hard at work tightening up the valves going into your liver, to save you from an even worse fate. If your veins are weak due to low nutrient levels, they're going to be less able to stand the back-pressure I subject them to when I close the liver valves. That can make a vein bulge out quite remarkably and once stretched like that, it is sometimes difficult for it to regain its original shape.

The *most dangerous* enlarged vein is the **esophageal vein**, because if it becomes engorged with blood and then ruptures, it can cause severe bleeding that's difficult to stop. Increased back-pressure on your portal vein can also cause your spleen to swell considerably as it tries to compensate for the increased fluid. This can result in poor incineration of old red blood cells.

The pancreas is partially protected from increased portal vein pressure by the enlarging of your spleen, but it, too, can suffer damage to either its digestive enzyme portion or its much smaller part that makes the **blood-sugar-regulating hormones: insulin** and **glucagon**.

As the backup below the liver continues in your portal vein, the increasing pressure starts to force open other veins, some of which have been dormant since your birth.

During the nine months you spent in your mother's womb, all your food and oxygen were supplied via the umbilical cord from your mother's placenta. Since your lungs weren't needed, they were filled with amniotic fluid. The right ventricle of the heart wasn't required to pump to the lungs so it was used instead to pump old blood back through the umbilical cord, to be detoxified by your mother's liver. This shunting of blood back and forth from your mother to you required some special pregnancy plumbing. Blood coming in from your mother needed the umbilical vein and **ductus venosus**, while blood going back to your mother required the umbilical artery and **ductus arteriosus**.

The cutting of the umbilical cord brings an abrupt end of blood circulation to the baby, and its supply of vital oxygen suddenly disappears; within minutes, serious damage could be done. Fortunately, the body is designed to deal with these changes.

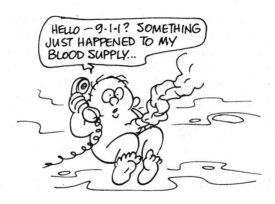

In the newborn babe, the sudden change in blood pressure in his or her heart causes a flap to close between the two atriums, forcing blood from the right atrium into the right ventricle. At the same time, the loss of fluid in the lungs allows them to expand, decreasing the resistance to blood flow.

Now, the blood from the right ventricle begins to pump through the lungs, picking up the precious oxygen and returning it to the heart. The increased oxygen in the ductus arteriosus causes it to slowly close off. The circulation and oxygenation of the cells has now begun.

The cutting of the umbilical cord also results in gradual closure of the ductus venosus, which increases the pressure in the portal vein enough so that portal blood can force its way into the sinusoids of the liver, thus beginning the process of detoxification.

So, in a very short time after birth, dramatic shifts in circulation patterns result in fully functioning circulation, oxygenation, and detoxification systems in the baby. The residues of the old circulation system, now obsolete, lie dormant as discarded and forgotten dried-up channels. When I have to shut down the valves going into your liver, however, the increased back-pressure in the portal vein can open up some of these long-dormant alternate routes. These veins can expand and start to carry portal blood in unexpected directions. These openings are called **collateral veins**. Toxins from the intestine—like ammonia—that get past the liver's detoxification enzymes into the main circulation, can create severe havoc with the **nervous system**, as **Spacey** will describe later.

Meanwhile, back at your liver, I'm constantly adjusting your valves, trying to minimize the problems. Eventually, I have to open up the inlet valves so your liver can get back to work. When I open up your inlet valves, portal blood starts to flow into the sinusoids and then into the liver cells, which immediately start running them through the two phases of enzyme detoxification.

My second goal is to minimize any peroxides and toxins going *out* of your liver into your main bloodstream, where they could cause direct damage to your nervous system, including your brain. **Burpy** deals with extra toxins by dumping them into the bile, which can cause some digestive discomfort; but when I shut down your liver valves, much more serious problems can result.

The Phase 1 P450 enzymes make the toxins water-soluble by turning them into epoxides, which can make them even more toxic. During this oxygenation process, they spit out free radicals, which become peroxides that can make deadly fatty peroxides. The Phase 2 enzymes are supposed to then conjugate the epoxides and peroxides to make them neutral. Of course, in someone with *any kind of health problem at all*, you can be sure the P450 enzymes are amplifying toxins much faster than the conjugation enzymes can neutralize them. In fact, it's very rare these days for me to see the conjugation enzymes keeping up to the P450 enzymes. Even in people who appear 100 percent healthy, often their conjugation enzymes aren't keeping pace with their P450s.

Free radicals made by the P450 enzymes are very short-lived, and will have been turned into peroxides long before they get to me at your outlet liver valves. If the conjugation enzymes— glutathione, in particular—are unable to completely neutralize hydrogen peroxide and it becomes bound to fats to form lipid peroxide, I have to work at breakneck speed to stop these toxic fats from getting past your liver into your main bloodstream. They could travel throughout your body, spewing hydroxyl radicals and creating tremendous irritation or even damage to the membranes and enzymes of your arteries, brain, heart, and other organs. So I must close the outlet valves, and fast! Sorry, but I have to do it—it's for your own good. Closing them will also give your liver cells more time to try to complete their detoxification process.

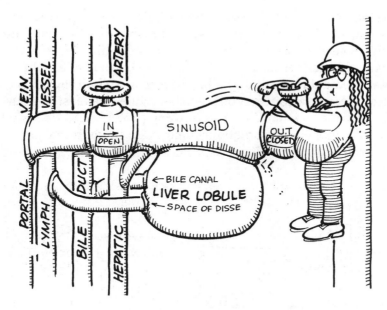

I've already explained that if I have to close the *inlet* valves to your liver, then the backup in your portal vein can affect your digestive organs and spleen function. When I close your *outlet* liver valves, the back-pressure in your liver sinusoids interferes with your liver cells' ability to do their hundreds of jobs effectively. The back-pressure in the liver sinusoids will allow proteins to be dumped directly into the bile, which makes the bile much thicker. This can lead to the formation of *bile sludge*—a mixture of **cholesterol crystals** and granules of **calcium bilirubinate** in a bile thickened with protein and mucous—which is like fine sand. Of course, if you improve your diet and liver enzyme function and I can open your outlet liver valves again, the sludge will soon "melt" away.

If I continue to keep your outlet liver valves closed because your conjugation enzymes are unable to completely neutralize all of the free radicals, peroxides, and epoxides produced by your P450 enzymes, then the bile sludge can go on to crystalize and form stones. Stones can also form in your bile ducts and even in your liver.

Sometimes the gallbladder gets into such rough shape from stones and toxic bile that it has to be removed surgically. The surgery, however, can't correct the imbalance in your liver's detoxification enzymes, so the symptoms of toxic bile and bile sludge—such as digestive troubles—may continue even after the gallbladder has been removed, since the toxic bile is *still* irritating the duodenum. The key to removing bile sludge is to get your conjugation enzymes working at least as fast as your P450 enzymes so that I'll stop dumping proteins and toxins into your bile. Stones can sometimes melt away if you really get your liver working well.

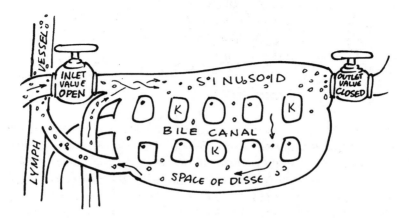

The other thing that can happen when I shut the outlet valves is that your liver can swell up with tremendous amounts of fluid. Behind your liver runs your **inferior vena cava**, which drains blood from your **leg veins, pelvic area**, and **kidneys**. This is the vein into which the central vein of your liver lobules also drains. Swelling of the liver due to closing of the outlet valves can push the inferior vena cava against the spine, thus interfering with its ability to drain your lower body, especially your kidneys.

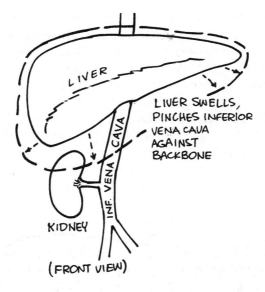

(FRONT VIEW)

The liver in most people would have to enlarge a lot to pinch this vein against your spine (**cirrhosis** of the liver can cause this type of swelling). Some people, however, have a groove in the back of the **caudate lobe** of their liver that the inferior vena cava runs through so that the liver almost completely surrounds the inferior vena cava. In these folks, the slightest swelling of the caudate lobe of the liver can pinch off the inferior vena cava.

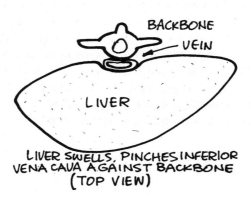

LIVER SWELLS, PINCHES INFERIOR
VENA CAVA AGAINST BACKBONE
(TOP VIEW)

This pinching of the inferior vena cava results in a backup of fluid, which can cause **varicose veins** in your legs. This can lead to the blueing and swelling of your feet and ankles, and even ulceration of your lower leg.

Congestion of your pelvic area—due to a swollen liver impinging on your inferior vena cava—can lead to a number of problems for your **reproductive organs**. For example, congestion of your **vaginal** area can result in your immune system not being able to control normal local organisms such as yeast, and the result is an overgrowth of yeast. This is not a vaginal yeast infection, as the yeast have always been there. It's an overgrowth of the yeast due to a swollen liver blocking the drainage from the pelvic area. Blockage of the inferior vena cava due to liver enlargement can also lead to any number of kidney problems. But it's **Itchy**'s job to look after your kidneys, so he'll tell you all about it.

The increased back-pressure also opens the gaps between the liver cells leading to the space of Disse. It's *extremely important* to note that each of your liver's millions of spaces of Disse have a direct connection to your lymph system, so that any excess fluid in the liver can be returned to your circulation. Closing your outlet liver valves will not only allow more *fluid* to drain into your lymph; now, even digested food particles from your portal vein, toxic peroxides plus epoxides made by your liver enzymes, and plasma proteins, neurotransmitters, and hormones from your hepatic artery can pour directly into the space of Disse and from there, into your lymph system. This dramatic increase in debris in your lymph can set the stage for a whole series of immune system problems—from colds to cancer, from allergies to arthritis, both acute and chronic—as **Achy**, the renowned General, will tell you later.

As you can see, I—**Bloaty**—am the most important **Liver Dwarf** because I must adjust your liver valves just right, or you're in _big trouble_! Enjoy your tour with **Gaspy**. She's got a little heart problem—and lung problems and liver problems. In fact, her whole body is a problem. She'll be along in a minute or so, if she makes it. She's a little slow.

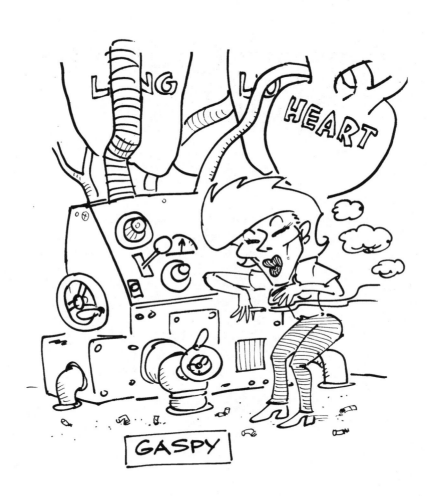

CHAPTER 3

Gaspy: Guide to Your Heart

Sigh, **I'm Gaspy, the Circulation Liver Dwarf**.

I'm the **Liver Dwarf** in charge of your **heart**. Wow, can things get in trouble when **Bloaty** shuts down those valves and blocks the blood flow to me. If I don't get enough **blood**, then I don't get enough **oxygen**, and without oxygen, there's no more me—or you! Oh, my!

I'm supposed to give you a tour of your **heart and lungs**. Since I had to walk a couple of steps to get here, I'm all out of wind. Just give me a minute to catch my breath, and I'll be okay. I guess you've already figured out how I got my name.

I need a cigarette—bad. This is the last one I'm going to have. Give me a light, will you, please? Ahhhhh, that feels a little better (*cough, cough*). I used to hate smoking till the last liver that I worked in. Heavy smoker—lots of nicotine floating around in the blood. All of us **Liver Dwarves** got hooked. The rest of the **Dwarves** managed to kick it, but I haven't had to because I'm still in great shape! (*Cough, cough, cough!*) Hey: Tell you what! You hold me up, and I'll tell you about my job. Thank you, I feel a little better already. Here we go!

The liver acts as a regulatory valve for your **circulation system**. You see, your heart is the pump that propels your blood around your body. Actually, your heart is a bunch of pumps all joined together. The right side pumps blood to your lungs, and the left side pumps your blood to every cell in your body.

Each side of your heart has two parts. The top part is called the **atrium** or **auricle**, and it receives your blood and then pumps it into the bottom part, called the **ventricle**, which is much stronger and is the actual pump part. Since the left side has to pump blood to the whole body, the muscles of the **left ventricle** are much thicker and stronger than the muscles of the **right ventricle**.

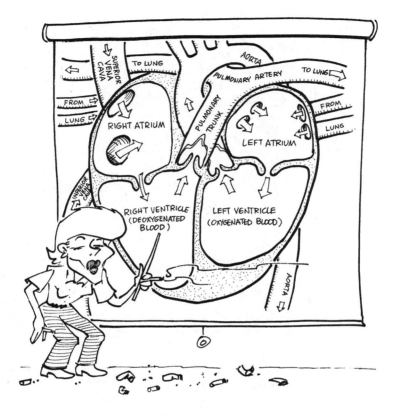

The **right atrium** sets the beat for the rest of your heart. You see, your right atrium controls the electrical wiring of your heart, so it gets to call the shots. It has an activator called the **SA node**—located at the top of the atrium—that I fire when the right atrium fills up with blood. When I activate your SA node, it causes the muscles of the right and left atria to contract, and your blood is quickly pumped into your right and left ventricles.

At the bottom of the right atrium is the **AV node**, which picks up the beat from your SA node, and then blasts the electrical impulse down through a bundle of fibres—the **Purkinje plexus**—between and around your ventricles. That makes your two ventricles fire in rhythm. As your right ventricle contracts, blood is pumped to your lungs.

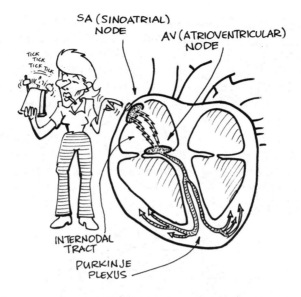

In the lungs, enzymes that contain zinc stimulate the iron in your red blood cells to dump the dull burden of carbon dioxide and pick up a batch of rosy, invigorating oxygen. This fresh blood then enters your left atrium and is pumped into your massively muscled left ventricle, which then whooshes it out your **aorta** to feed oxygen to every needy cell in your body.

Because your heart is working so hard, it has a tremendous need for fresh oxygen. The first arteries to branch off the aorta as it leaves the heart are the **left** and **right coronary arteries**, which feed oxygen back to your heart to meet its urgent demands.

As you probably know, you can go without food for weeks or without water for days, but you can only go without oxygen for a few minutes before cells start to get into serious trouble. Since I'm in charge of your circulation of oxygen, that makes ME, **Gaspy**, your most important **Liver Dwarf**. Actually, I'm feeling a little nervous and sweaty, so I'd better sit down here on the floor. On second thought, I won't, as I might not be able to get up again. I think I'd better quit smoking. Maybe next New Year's.

Your heart is the toughest muscle in your whole body, and it could go on forever if it could get enough oxygen. Even when it's resting, your heart uses up about 70 percent of the oxygen brought in by your coronary arteries. If a person is low in iron or zinc, he or she could be low in oxygen. If your lungs are damaged, there may not be enough oxygen in your blood. If your red blood cells have lost their discoid shape, they may not be able to load and unload oxygen and carbon dioxide properly in your capillaries.

In your sinuses, I brew up **nitric oxide**—partly to kill off any invaders that might try to sneak in there, but also to mix with the air breathed in through your nose. This diluted nitric oxide enters your lungs and dilates the blood vessels of the lungs and heart, and helps me do my job delivering oxygen.

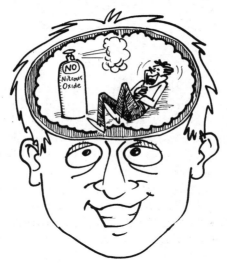

IT'S BEEN A LAUGH A MINUTE SINCE
WE STARTED GETTING NITROUS OXIDE
...INSTEAD OF *NITRIC OXIDE*...

If **Bloaty** shuts down your outlet liver valves and shunts toxins and fluid and proteins into your lymph, you can get all congested. And if you can't breathe through your nose, you're going to run low on nitric oxide and feel short of wind. Sometimes—maybe in the dead of night—you might run short of oxygen and you might feel like you're going to die. In fact, you might. Light me up another cigarette, will you? I'm feeling a little faint! This is *definitely* the last one!

Whatever the reason for their lack of oxygen, the cells start screaming at me to increase your circulation. But first, I have to fill up your right atrium with blood before I can hit the SA node to activate your heart's pumping action. The right atrium is always growling at me: "Give me your best shot. Give me more blood; I can take it! I can take all you can give me!"

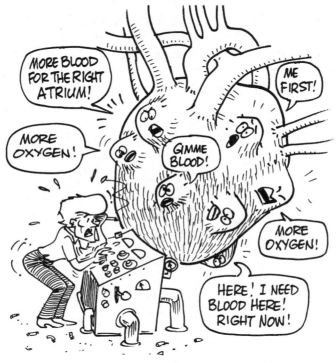

And I suppose it can, but the problem is, where do I get that blood from? There are only two places. One is the **superior vena cava**, which drains your upper body. Problem is, there's not a whole lot of blood there. The only other choice is the **inferior vena cava**, which has far more blood; it has 70 percent of the blood returning to the heart, compared to 30 percent in the superior vena cava. So the inferior vena cava is much bigger than the superior, so I think they should switch names. Ha! Ha! Ha! (*Cough, cough, cough. Retch!*) Oh, excuse me, I shouldn't have laughed; now I'm going to be hawking up phlegm for hours!

Normally, your inferior vena cava gives me all the blood I need, and I just keep hitting that SA node and your heart pumps, and that fresh, red blood zooms off to the rescue. The liver's central vein, however, is a major contributor to the inferior vena cava, and if **Bloaty** has your liver's *inlet* valves tightened down, that can result in a lot less blood being available for me to pump. Even bigger trouble can start when **Bloaty** tightens down your *outlet* liver valves. This not only blocks the main tributary of the inferior vena cava, the portal vein, but—if your liver swells up enough—it can also pinch your inferior vena cava against your spine. That effectively blocks the drainage of the rest of your abdomen, as well.

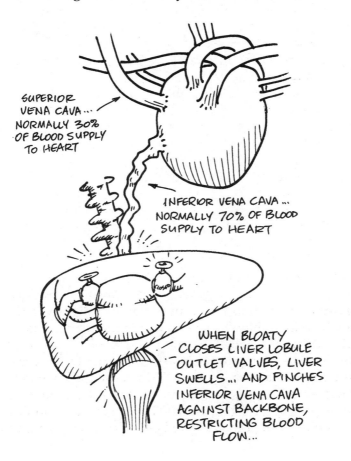

SUPERIOR VENA CAVA... NORMALLY 30% OF BLOOD SUPPLY TO HEART

INFERIOR VENA CAVA... NORMALLY 70% OF BLOOD SUPPLY TO HEART

WHEN BLOATY CLOSES LIVER LOBULE OUTLET VALVES, LIVER SWELLS... AND PINCHES INFERIOR VENA CAVA AGAINST BACKBONE, RESTRICTING BLOOD FLOW...

Seventy percent of the blood returning to your heart can get trapped below your liver if **Bloaty** starts fooling around with those liver valves! This can kill your heart and, obviously, you. Now, everybody's running low on oxygen and they're all hollering at me to get your circulation going. But what am I supposed to do? How can I increase the circulation if I don't have enough blood coming into the right atrium?

The heart itself can be the first to be affected because it needs more oxygen than most of your organs. And it's not just your heart muscle that needs oxygen. The SA node, the AV node, and the bundle of fibres that deliver the electrical messages throughout your heart also need oxygen. Without oxygen, they can start to fire erratically and your heart can sputter erratically. **Palpitations**, I think they call it. Or **fibrillation**. Damnation is what *I* call all those $25 words. All I know is, if there's not enough blood coming in, I can't fire the SA node as I'm supposed to do and as I'd like to, and then there's not enough oxygen—and everyone's blaming *me* when they should be blaming **Bloaty**, that old pot-bellied **Dwarf**.

To make things worse, when **Bloaty** backs up your blood in your portal vein and/or your inferior vena cava, your blood gets much more prone to throwing clots. Now *that's* all I need: to have a big, fat clot blocking the blood flow to your brain or heart.

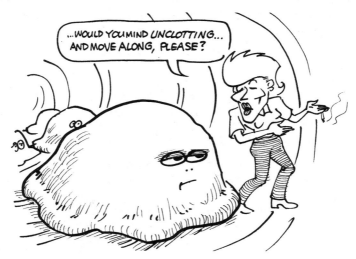

...WOULD YOU MIND *UNCLOTTING*... AND MOVE ALONG, PLEASE?

Of course, if your heart muscles don't get enough oxygen, they can die and create a really big problem.

Oh, I feel a pain in my left chest. Just sit me down on the floor; I can't stand up anymore. I need to lie down. Oh, Lord, if I make it through this, I'll quit smoking. I promise! Let me just take a couple more puffs. Whew! For a moment there, I thought I was going to have a heart attack! I wasn't getting enough oxygen to the heart.

People always think that to have a heart problem, you have to have plugged-up coronary arteries blocking the blood flow to your heart, but that's not the only way heart problems can happen. If you eat something that forces **Bloaty** to shut down your liver valves—like rancid pork—or if you have a strong emotional experience that does the same thing, you can reduce the blood and oxygen flow to your heart. If the oxygen supply to your heart becomes low enough, that can cause **angina, heart palpitations, irregular beats**, or even a **heart attack**.

Of course, if you have plugged-up coronary arteries already, the last thing you want to do is decrease your circulation even more by shutting down your liver. As the other **Liver Dwarves** will probably tell you, coronary artery blockage arises from the presence of lipid peroxides. Cadmium from cigarette and cigar smoking has something to do with increasing the production of lipid peroxides. But I've no time for that now; I've got a heart I have to keep running. So I'll be running along. Or walking. Or maybe crawling.

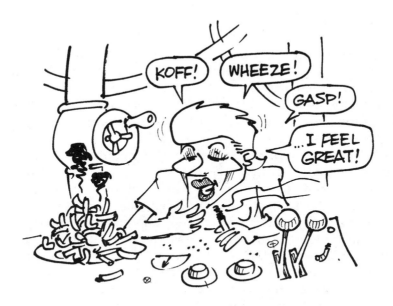

So you can see that your heart is important for your life, and your liver and lungs are important for your heart. Now, some people will try to convince you that smoking is bad for your lungs and heart, but that can't be true. I've been smoking for years and there's nothing wrong with me! (*Cough! Cough!*) I hope.

Say, if you'll just give me a lift up onto my feet, I think I had better shuffle back to your heart and see what kind of trouble **Bloaty**'s gotten me into. Keep breathing, or else you're in trouble! Could you give me a light for my *very last cigarette*? I hope I make it. By the way, do you know the emergency number for 9-1-1?

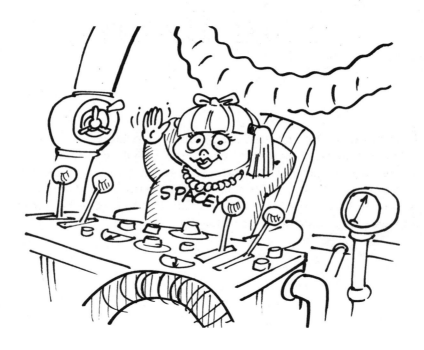

CHAPTER 4

Spacey: Guide to Your Brain

Is it my turn? I'm Spacey, the Brain's Liver Dwarf.

When you muck up your liver, you can reduce the flow of **oxygen** and **sugar** to your **brain**, which can give you "fuzzy thinking." If you muck up your small intestine, you can get low **serotonin** levels in your brain that can lead to **low self-esteem**, **depression**, **anxiety**, and/or **insomnia**.

My name's . . . um . . . (*tee hee*) . . . oh, yes, **Spacey**! I'm your **Liver Dwarf** guide to your brain. **Gaspy** has already told you how dependent your heart is on having a steady supply of oxygen delivered by your blood. Well, your brain is even more dependent. If muscle runs out of oxygen, it can still switch over to **anaerobic metabolism**, which means no oxygen is necessary. The anaerobic system is far less efficient, but at least it can keep things working for a short while without oxygen.

The brain is made of **nerve tissue**, which burns energy about seven times faster than muscle under resting conditions, but without oxygen it has little ability to burn glucose. What happens to me when I don't get delivered enough oxygen is my . . . uh . . . what's that thing I'm supposed to look after? . . . the gray, wrinkled thing . . . the drain ??? . . . oh, yeah . . . the brain! When the brain doesn't get enough oxygen, it starts to act strangely and forgets little things and even some bigger things. You didn't see where I put that chocolate bar, did you? I'm sure I had it just a minute ago. Somebody must have eaten it. Hmmmmm. Maybe it was me.

If the brain gets really low in oxygen, I'll have to lie you down. In an emergency, I have to shut down your whole nervous system. Then your body lies down quickly—usually with a big thud. Fainting, some people call it. When your body is horizontal, your heart doesn't have to pump uphill to get oxygen to your brain. Usually, putting your brain and heart at the same level will be enough to get your brain oxygen levels up. Other times, one part of your brain is especially low in oxygen and it throws a little tantrum, which some people call a **seizure**. So I shut everything down, and lay your body flat out.

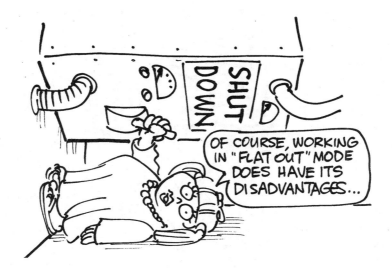

There's a little trick that I do to increase your oxygen flow more quickly: I put all your muscles into convulsions, and that usually gets things flowing again pretty fast.

Of course, if a blood vessel in your brain should break or get blocked with a clot, this can shut off oxygen *pronto*, and brain cells can start to die. We **Liver Dwarves** call this a stroke of misfortune, but you folks have shortened it down to **stroke**.

Your brain is capable of functioning at low temperatures but it's extremely vulnerable to temperatures that are more than six degrees above normal body temperature—so I've developed an air conditioning system for the brain that uses the **emissary veins** to keep things cool. I didn't put any valves in these veins so that blood can flow up through the brain to warm it up and then excess heat is discharged from your head into the air. If your head gets too hot during exercise or work, I reverse the flow so that the blood comes down the veins, bringing the cooler air temperature into the brain. This is why it feels so good to pour cool water on your head when you're hot, because it quickly cools down your brain.

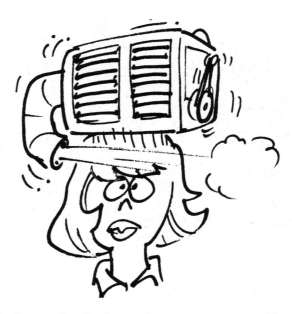

Not only is your brain dependent on oxygen and low temperatures, it's also dependent on glucose sugar delivered by your blood. **Glycogen** is the storage form of glucose in the body. Your brain only has about a two-minute supply of glycogen in storage, and can't burn fatty acids the way the muscles can, so I keep a large supply of glycogen stored away in your liver—to guarantee that a constant supply is always available to be fed into your blood for delivery to your brain. Say, I'm sure I didn't eat that chocolate bar—did *you* eat it?

Your pancreas is mainly a digestive enzyme producer but 2 to 3 percent of your pancreas also makes hormones. The **alpha cells** of your pancreas secrete the hormone **glucagon**; when it's needed, glucagon acts as a message to your liver that your blood sugar is getting too low. When your liver sees the glucagon, my job is to activate **cyclic AMP** in your liver cells, which in turn activates the enzyme **phosphorylase**. Phosphorylase breaks up stored glycogen and releases it into your blood so that your brain can get quick relief.

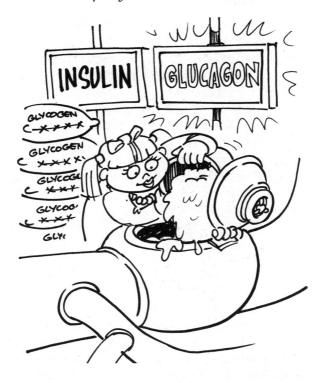

If I'm too slow, your brain starts to malfunction. Low blood sugar, or **hypoglycemia**, can feel like a dark veil is being pulled down over your eyes because your brain is getting less glucose than it needs. This can be quickly followed by physical weakness—your knees, especially, can get weak and wobbly.

If your blood sugar level starts to rise too high, then the **beta cells** of your pancreas secrete **insulin**. Your brain itself doesn't need insulin to directly absorb blood sugar because it soaks up glucose like a sponge.

About 80 percent of all cells in your body—including muscle cells, fat cells, and many others—absorb glucose when they bind insulin. These cells have hormonal receptors, consisting of four separate subunits, on which insulin can deliver its hormonal message. On the outside of the membrane are two alpha subunits where the insulin can dock. Zinc and **glucose tolerance factor** (GTF) help bind the insulin into the two alpha subunits, which then activate two beta units inside the membrane to turn on the cell machinery that opens the gates to let glucose flow into your cells.

Your liver readily responds to insulin, especially right after a meal when it's being flooded with sugars arriving via your portal vein. Insulin tells the liver to make and store glycogen. As much as two-thirds of the glucose in a meal can be dried out into glycogen by your liver and kept on hand. If insulin levels are still high, then I'll start converting the rest of the glucose into fatty acids, which I package into triglycerides—the shipping form of fat—and send off via the blood to the fat tissues for storage. So basically, I'll store any excess glucose as fat between your chin and your butt, or in your arteries. Look at all that fat *I* have. Hey, maybe I did eat that chocolate bar!

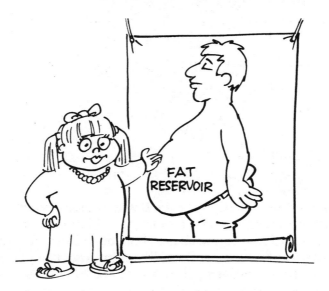

High triglycerides and cholesterol in the blood can "gum" up the connective tissue, making you feel stiff and creating things like **frozen shoulder,** and **Dupuytren's contracture of the tendons** of the palm of your hand—sure signs that your liver's struggling with your fat metabolism. If you find you're getting a lot of fat deposits, you're probably making too much insulin or you're short of the minerals—zinc or **chromium**—necessary for insulin to bind to the receptors.

Insulin tells the body to store fat in two ways: by causing the liver to convert excess glucose into fat and by telling the fat cells to store more fat. Not only does insulin tell the body to *store* fat, it also inhibits the *breakdown* of fat already being stored in the fat cells. So when I'm putting fat into cell storage, it's a bit of a one-way street. I can't easily take it *out* of storage at the same time.

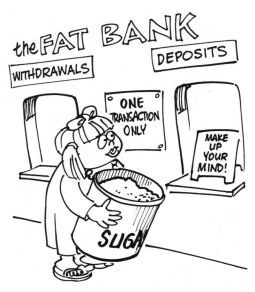

If you're not doing hard physical work or exercise, your muscles prefer to burn fat. In times of sudden danger, however, it's my job to supply your muscles with instant energy for fight or flight from a great fright. **Epinephrine**, also known as **adrenalin**, is a hormone secreted by your **adrenal glands**. It's designed for short-term use in extreme emergencies. In other words: fight or flight or lose your life—such as when you're being charged by an angry grizzly bear with froth dripping from its gaping jaws. Epinephrine gives incredible power to all the muscles of your body—especially your heart, so that it can pound blood, oxygen, and nutrients to your cells to meet the threat of the bellowing grizzly. Epinephrine is a dramatic hormone for dramatic moments, but it's only designed for short-term use, like to help you climb a tree fast.

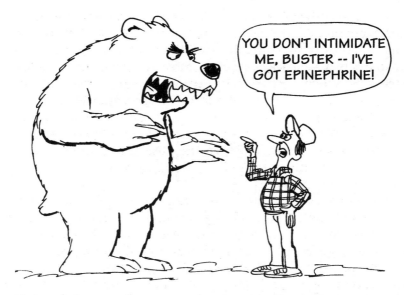

Epinephrine produces muscle power in the same way as glucagon hormone—by activating cyclic AMP and phosphorylase to release glucose from muscle glycogen into the blood. This extra hit of sugar is to provide energy for whatever extreme muscular escape mechanisms are appropriate.

I split the glucose into two **pyruvic acids** plus some hydrogens and get two **ATP** for energy. Do you know about ATP yet? **Sluggy** is going to tell you more about it later. Anyway, ATP is the fuel that your cells burn to run just about everything. ATP (**adenosine triphosphate**) is **adenosine** with three **phosphates** attached to it. When the third phosphate is split off, tremendous energy is released and **ADP (adenosine diphosphate)** remains. This energy is especially good for running—after opportunity or away from danger. **Sluggy** likes to blather on and on about how he's using glucose more efficiently than me because by using oxygen, he can get a few more ATP out of glucose than I can. That may be true, but his system is so slow that we'd all be dead long ago waiting for his energy output to kick in. I may only get two ATP out of a molecule of glucose but I can do it without oxygen and I can do it almost three times faster than **Sluggy**.

Since it takes several seconds for epinephrine to get glucose rolling out of muscle glycogen storage, I keep a few spare ATP available in your muscle cells at all times. In an emergency, they can do incredible feats fast, for a few seconds. Of course, a few seconds isn't long enough for phosphorylase enzymes to release glycogen, so I have another trick up my sleeve called the **phosphagen system** that's even faster and is also anaerobic (doesn't need oxygen). I keep some backup energy stored in your muscles in the form of **creatine phosphate**. I immediately recharge ADP with a phosphate stored in the creatine phosphate to reproduce ATP.

By the time creatine phosphate runs out, eight to 10 seconds have passed and glucose released from glycogen is pouring into the system to release two more ATP each. So I've just saved your life by giving you instant energy, first through your phosphagen system and secondly through glycogen release. Now you can see that I'm obviously your most important **Liver Dwarf**.

With training, an athlete can get the phosphagen anaerobic system to last up to 10 seconds and the glycogen anaerobic system to last up to one-and-a-half minutes—both systems providing fast energy without needing oxygen, and both sugar-powered. Oh, how I love sugar. I could bathe in it, swim in it, snort it up my nostrils. Sugar gives me energy and makes me feel so gooood! I love sugar and sugar loves me.

There are a few complications using sugar as fuel. When I use glucose without oxygen, the pyruvic acids and hydrogens that are created combine to form lactic acid—which I just send over to **Gaspy**; she can burn it up in your heart. Any excess lactic acid, however, can make you stiff and tired, very tired. But that's not my problem—I've done my job to save you from danger. Now it's **Sluggy**'s job to deal with the excess lactic acid.

The **glycemic index** measures how quickly your digestion is breaking loose the sugars from the carbohydrates you're eating and releasing them into the bloodstream. This has something to do with whether the glucose gets used as a fuel or whether insulin will cause it to be stored as glycogen or fat. Hopefully, the new **Liver Dwarf**—the doctor who's supposed to be

arriving soon—will explain more about this. I sure don't
remember much about it because I think my blood sugar level
has dropped to below my kneecaps, and my brain is getting
fuzzier than a teddy bear that got hit by lightning.

Sometimes I just can't keep your blood sugar level stable. If
the beta cells of your pancreas become damaged by your
immune system, they don't work as well at making insulin.
And remember, for insulin to bind to a cell, it needs zinc and
glucose tolerance factor (GTF), which contains chromium and
two **nicotinic acids**. Nicotinic acid (**nicotinamide**) can, in fact,
sometimes halt and even reverse the damage to the beta cells of
your pancreas if used in the earliest stages of damage.
Remember, too, that nicotinic acid is made from the amino acid
tryptophan, as is picolinic acid.

Sometimes, I make plenty of insulin but the liver and fat cells
ignore it. This is called **insulin resistance**.

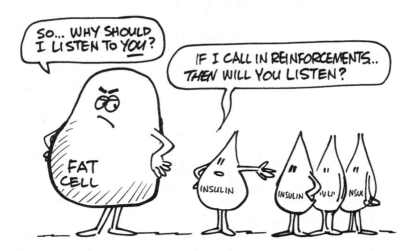

With insulin resistance, if I put out a lot more insulin than
normal, I can usually get the blood sugar levels back to where
they're supposed to be, but then I have high insulin levels. This
can result in more glucose being stored as fat, and also the
kidneys then dump out more **calcium**, as **Itchy** will tell you later.

Even when your pancreas is making glucagon and insulin
hormones properly, your liver might be having trouble

responding to them. The liver's trouble in responding to pancreatic hormones occurs when the P450 enzymes make more toxic peroxides than the conjugation enzymes can neutralize, forcing **Bloaty** to close the outlet valves of the sinusoids. The back-pressure that ensues in the sinusoids interferes with the liver cells' ability to quickly pull glucose out of your blood when your pancreas sends insulin, or to release glucose into your blood when your pancreas orders the raising of the blood sugar with glucagon hormone.

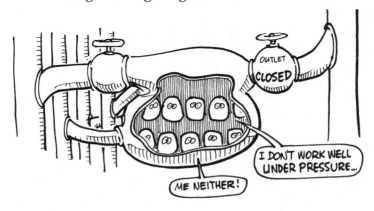

Poorly functioning liver cells can lead to an imbalanced blood sugar level that can affect your brain function—or high insulin levels that can reduce your body's calcium levels and increase your fat deposits, especially around your abdomen. This can greatly increase your susceptibility to heart attacks and diabetes.

Sometimes—during the night, usually when **Bloaty**'s taking her nap from 1 A.M. to 3 A.M.—toxins like homocysteine can sneak through the unattended outlet valves and cause irritation to your brain and heart. This can cause bad dreams, nightmares, restless sleep, early awakening, and fatigue on waking.

You can see that blood sugar is extremely important to your brain, and that your pancreas and liver work together—with the right nutrients—to keep a stable blood sugar level. The pancreas is the conductor of your blood sugar symphony, but it's your liver that has to dance, and dance well, to the tune of your pancreas, to create a successful show on the blood sugar stage.

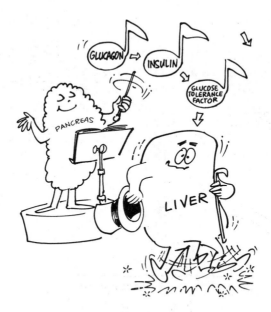

With inadequate liver detoxification enzyme function, chemicals, pesticides, and metals—like **lead**, cadmium, copper, and **aluminum**—which enter the body regularly from food, water, and air, can begin to accumulate in your body, especially in the brain and nervous system. These can contribute to **behavioural problems**, **learning disorders**, **autism**, **schizophrenia**, **Parkinson's disease**, and **Alzheimer's disease**.

Your nervous system also plays a role in proper brain function. Information is sent through your body via your nerves. One-way messages travel from one nerve to the next, across the **synaptic cleft**, which separates the two nerves.

The **sending nerve** prepackages hundreds of **neurotransmitters** in small **vesicles**. A signal travelling down the nerve causes an increase in calcium in the sending nerve, which causes the vesicles to rupture and release neurotransmitters into your synaptic cleft. On the other side of the cleft, the **receiving nerve** has **receptors** that are activated by the neurotransmitters.

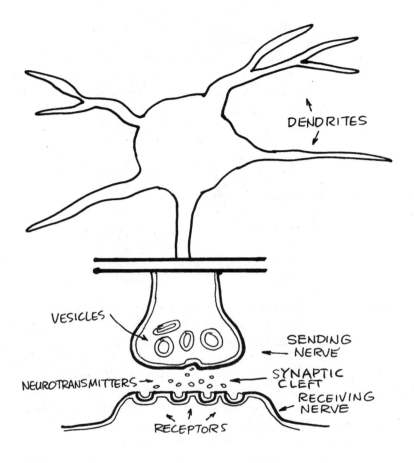

The receptors then open **potassium channels**—which act as a "red light" to stop the message—or open **sodium channels**—which act as a "green light" to send the message down the receiving nerve. Once the receptors have been activated, the neurotransmitters return to the sending nerve where they are reabsorbed or destroyed by **monoamine oxidase (MAO) enzyme**.

Each nerve system secretes a specific neurotransmitter, and while there are 40 neurotransmitters in your body, there are three important systems in your brain. Two of these use transmitters made from the amino acid **tyrosine**; they are the

dopamine and **norepinephrine systems**. The third—and perhaps most important for your mental and emotional well-being—uses **serotonin** as its neurotransmitter.

Burpy probably already told you that 99 percent of the serotonin in your body is made in your digestive tract. Of that, 10 percent ends up in platelets in your blood where it helps plug up any broken blood vessels. The *other* 1 percent of serotonin is made in your brain, under the stimulation of morning light. You see, brain serotonin is like an "on" switch in the morning. It turns you on early in the morning and brings you into the rhythm of life that has been so successful for the well-being of all your ancestors over thousands of years.

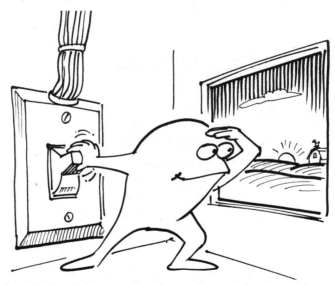

The first light of dawn stimulates the production of serotonin in the nerve cells of the **raphe nuclei**—in the deep cellar of your brain where the spinal cord and brain meet.

Serotonin is then sent from here up through the brain and down through the spinal cord. Thus, serotonin has a much *wider* range of effect than the other brain neurotransmitters. In addition, there are over a dozen different types of receptors for serotonin so that serotonin can have a much *broader* effect on your brain. Serotonin also bridges the gap from pure information-passing, into the world of emotion.

Accompanying the morning's rise of serotonin is an increase in **adrenal** and **thyroid hormones**, which altogether give you a surge of power to overcome the tremendous obstacles you might meet during the day while searching for food, shelter, and perhaps even a mate.

There will be physical struggles, emotional falls, and mental challenges. Nature can test you physically with extremes of climate and weather; struggling to pay mortgages and taxes can sap you mentally; love can be fickle and tweak at your heart. But serotonin and its accompanying adrenal and thyroid hormones give you the drive and the stamina and the confidence to leap over pitfalls and bounce back up when knocked down by rejection. When you succeed at finding the right food, then serotonin pats you on the back and tells you that you're a success. Your self-esteem soars and you're fulfilled and more confident. Most of your serotonin is made in your intestine, but serotonin's greatest impact is in your brain, through its effects on your emotions.

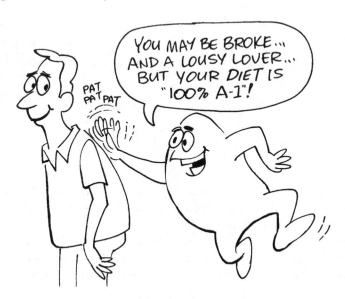

And it's not just serotonin that feeds back to your brain from your digestive system. Insulin and glucagon from your pancreas, while stabilizing your blood sugar, also go to your brain and help control weight. Gastrin and cholecystokinin from your stomach and small intestine also let your brain know how things are going. Cholecystokinin is formed when fat and protein—the hardest-to-find foods, and therefore the most precious—are eaten; it sharpens your memory to help your brain remember how the food was found and gives you a sense of satisfaction. You can't separate your brain from your gut: they are intimately linked.

You can have all the appearances of success: a satisfying job, a loving spouse and family, adequate income, respect from associates, yet something may not feel quite right. You sense a darkness, an emptiness, a dissatisfaction—perhaps an uneasiness, a feeling of inadequacy, maybe even anxiety—all of which can come from low levels of serotonin somewhere in your brain. Anxiety may be a result of low serotonin levels in the **amygdala**—the part of the brain associated with fear.

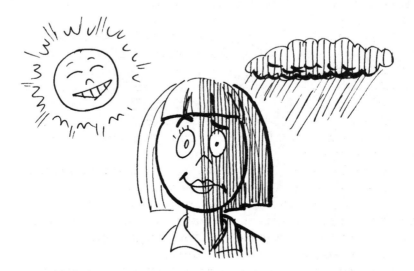

Low levels of serotonin and other neurotransmitters may be accompanied by inexplicable cravings—uncontrollable at times—for sweets, chocolate, refined starches, alcohol, tobacco, coffee, or even cocaine or heroin. Along with appetite disorders can come rapid mood swings, emotional instability, depression, anxiety, memory loss, learning disorders, physical weakness, and obsessive-compulsive disorders. Obsessive-compulsive disorders may be due to low serotonin levels in the **striatum**—the part of the brain that controls physical movements.

There can be an uncontrollable compulsion to bang your head against the wall or rip your hair out by the roots. Or shop for things you can't afford or gamble money you don't have. There might be a need for aggression or violence—often toward others, but maybe toward yourself. As your self-esteem crumbles without the reassuring support of serotonin, thoughts of suicide are possible. I know that when *my* serotonin is low, I feel like the least important **Dwarf**. I've often considered killing myself with chocolate.

You already know that nicotinic acid and picolinic acid are made from the amino acid tryptophan. Well, guess what serotonin is made from? You guessed it—serotonin is also made from tryptophan. An adult needs only one-quarter gram of tryptophan per day, but an average diet will have at least one gram, so tryptophan deficiencies *should* be rare.

If, however, The Boogy Boys get into your small intestine, they steal your amino acids. The disappearance of tryptophan will affect you before the absence of any of the other amino acids because tryptophan is the rarest amino acid. It's necessary for such crucial things as zinc absorption and self-esteem because it's normally converted into picolinic acid and serotonin. To make matters worse, Boogy Boys not only steal your tryptophan, those #!&%*$ Boys transform it into **indolepropionic acid**, **tryptamine**, **indoleacetic acid**, **skatole**, and **indole**—all of which can be very toxic to your nervous system, as well as to your kidneys, lungs, and intestinal membrane. Indoles made from tryptophan can contribute to constipation, sinus congestion, asthma, fatigue, and depression—to name just a few symptoms.

Tryptophan that does get absorbed from your intestine is processed by the liver enzyme **tryptophan pyrrolase**. Ninety percent of tryptophan is normally converted to nicotinic acid and picolinic acid by this enzyme, but **vitamin B_6** is necessary for these conversions to take place. Most of the other 10 percent of tryptophan is made into serotonin, but alcohol stimulates tryptophan pyrrolase to convert even more tryptophan to nicotinic acid. This is how drinking alcohol can result in less tryptophan being available to your brain to be made into serotonin.

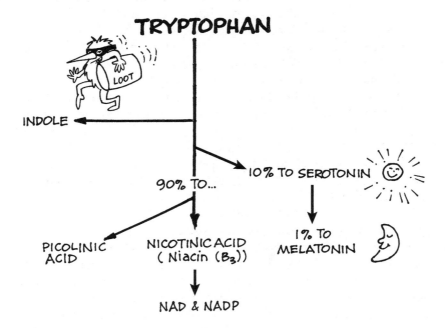

Burpy has told you that yeast and bacteria in the small intestine can produce considerable amounts of alcohol that have to be dealt with by your liver. So even the livers of nondrinkers can be affected by gut-made "home brew," and their levels of tryptophan—and therefore the brain's serotonin levels—can be lowered by the increased conversion of tryptophan into nicotinic acid.

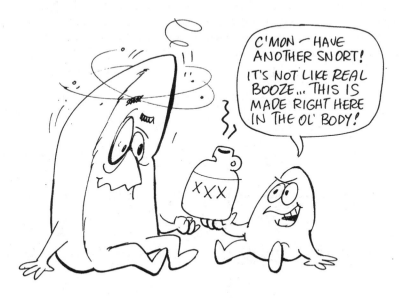

HOME BREW

The nicotinic acid made by your liver from tryptophan plays a role in the breakdown of alcohol. I convert it to **nicotinamide**. I then convert nicotinamide—with the help of vitamin B_6—into **nicotinamide adenine dinucleotide** (let's call it **NAD** for short) and **nicotinamide adenine dinucleotide phosphate** (**NADP**).

NAD and NADP have a special property (inherited from tryptophan) that makes them crucial to helping the function of hundreds of enzymes that carry on important energy reactions. Of all the 20 amino acids, tryptophan is not only the rarest, it's also the one that absorbs the most **ultraviolet (UV) wave energy**.

Only three amino acids absorb UV light, and tryptophan absorbs four times more than second-place tyrosine. NAD and NADP use this energy-absorbing gift from their not-too-distant common ancestor, tryptophan, to hold onto or give up energy in the form of **hydrogen**, while the enzymes are conducting their chemical wizardry. This gives them the status of **coenzymes**— official enzyme assistants! In effect, NAD and NADP are hydrogen-holders for the enzymes.

These two closely related coenzymes are so important for so many of the water-soluble enzymes—most are called **dehydrogenase enzymes**—formed within the cells that they tend to specialize. NADP prefers helping enzymes that **build things up**, while NAD prefers enzymes that **break things down**.

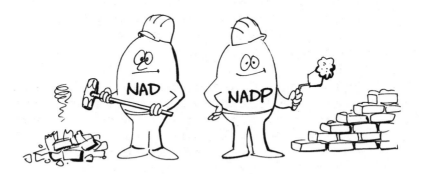

An example is the enzyme **alcohol dehydrogenase**, which begins the breakdown of alcohol by stripping one hydrogen off the alcohol and giving it to NAD to hold, thus forming **NADH** and **acetaldehyde**. This is the end of alcohol and the beginning of a **hangover**, as acetaldehyde is more toxic to the system than alcohol. If acetaldehyde isn't quickly broken down further, it can damage your liver and reduce its secretion of uric acid—which can lead to gouty arthritis, a fatty liver, and a buildup of lactic acid, which can create "stiffening" in your body. So while alcohol is only mildly toxic, acetaldehyde made from it by a poorly functioning liver can create damage to your liver and result in proteins and chemicals being dumped into your lymph, thereby triggering immune system allergies and/or immune reactions.

Chronic acetaldehyde poisoning can contribute to **multiple sclerosis (MS)** in those individuals whose intestinal flora ferment sugars into alcohol and acetaldehyde. Your immune system is bound to get excited trying to clean up this mess. As a result, your immune system cells can generate an incredible number of free radicals, so it's important that I keep them away from your delicate brain and central nervous system.

I coat the main nerves with a protective insulating coating called the **myelin sheath**. Then I establish a barrier between your bloodstream—which is full of patrolling trigger-happy immune cells—and your sensitive nerves. This **blood-brain barrier** is normally strong enough to keep your immune cells out. If they do get through the blood-brain barrier, they can damage your myelin sheath, thus "shorting out" your nerve signals. Intestinal fermentation is especially a problem if Candida yeast join the party, as they're the "biker gang" of intestinal fermenters, and can make much more of a mess than The Boogy Boys.

If all this fermentation is taking place in your small intestine, your liver is going to take a tremendous beating because your small intestine absorbs so much more actively than your large intestine. The Boogy Boys and Candida yeast in the small intestine may also be gobbling up your precious vitamin B_{12} since it's one of the last nutrients to be absorbed from your small intestine.

Vitamin B_{12} can be turned into a coenzyme, one that is crucial in strengthening and protecting your nervous system. **Coenzyme B_{12}** contains a very weak bond that may be broken easily by lightwaves, which is probably why plants do not contain vitamin B_{12}. Coenzyme B_{12} plays an important role in the breakdown of fatty acids that have an uneven number of carbons, such as **propionate**. First, **biotin** is used as a **cofactor**, then coenzyme B_{12} finishes the job.

Like NAD and NADP, coenzyme B_{12} helps to initiate energy transformations but in a much more complex way. While NAD merely holds hydrogen, coenzyme B_{12} isn't content to just hold it; coenzyme B_{12} tosses it around like a circus performer juggling flaming torches—thus generating a series of free radicals that it expertly spins around within itself without any damage being done.

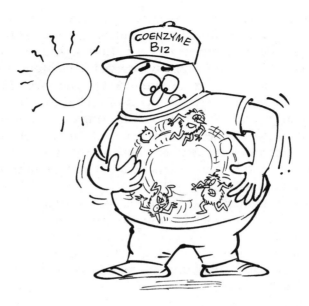

This is a masterful display of how we highly evolved **Liver Dwarves** have managed to use matter to manipulate energy for your benefit!

Of course, a shortage of coenzyme B_{12} can result in a lot of free radicals being released during the breakdown of propionate from fat, which can cause tremendous aggravation to your nervous system. Without vitamin B_{12} protection of your nervous system, you can experience memory loss, brain dysfunction, fatigue, lack of coordination, and neuropathies.

Numbness and tingling may be your first symptoms of vitamin B_{12} deficiency. When nerves are irritated due to low B_{12}, I sometimes try to "splint" them with a deposit of calcium. When this occurs in your shoulder, it's called **bursitis**. I know everybody *else* thinks that it's the calcium deposit that causes the irritation to the nerve, but now you know it's the irritated nerve from low B_{12} that forces me to slap on calcium to try to protect it.

Fortunately, at the end of its coenzyme duties, coenzyme B_{12} gets recycled, so only very small amounts of vitamin B_{12} need to come in through your diet.

You can see that NAD, NADP, and other coenzymes—like coenzyme B_{12}—play important roles in maintaining a healthy nervous system. All of this can fall apart with Boogy Boys in the small intestine disrupting tryptophan, vitamin B_{12}, biotin, and vitamin B_6 absorption. Low levels of NAD, NADP, and/or nicotinic acid are associated with diabetes, lupus, and other autoimmune diseases. The combination of low B_{12}—needed to protect your nerves—and high acetaldehyde can be the first step in the development of MS. The next step would be for your immune system to attack the myelin sheath that insulates your nerves. Since **Achy** is in charge of your immune system, maybe he can tell you what makes the immune system so crazy that it would attack your own nerves or your joints or the beta cells of your pancreas.

You can see how important it is for us **Liver Dwarves** to keep those messy Boogy Boys confined to the large intestine where they belong. You should be warned, however, that The Boogy Boys are fanatics! For generations, they have been brainwashed into believing that all vitamin B_{12} belongs to *them*.

There are still even more important steps left for tryptophan. Once tryptophan gets from your food, through your intestine, and past your liver into your bloodstream, it still has to get into your brain before it can be converted into serotonin. The obstacle in the way is the blood-brain barrier I erected to keep out irritants to your sensitive nerves. I need transporters to carry the amino acids across the blood-brain barrier but because of budgeting constraints, I was only given one transporter to carry the six largest amino acids, of which tryptophan is one. These six amino acids have to compete among themselves for that one taxi ride to the brain. Since tryptophan is the rarest of these six amino acids, its chances of getting across wouldn't be very high—if it weren't for a quirk of insulin.

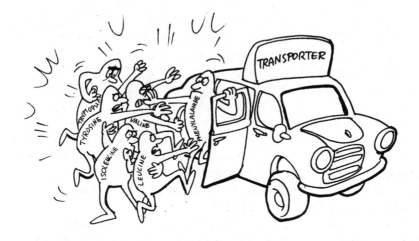

Insulin is secreted by your pancreas to stimulate your liver and other cells to pull excess glucose out of your blood. Amino acids, however, are also pulled from your blood under the stimulation of insulin. Tryptophan is the least affected by the insulin, so its ratio in your blood goes up as the insulin sweeps away its five competitors, making tryptophan most likely to become absorbed into your brain. Thus, people with low insulin levels can also have low delivery of tryptophan to the brain, and therefore, low serotonin.

Even when tryptophan gets into your brain, it must be converted by two enzymes into serotonin. This process requires vitamin B_{12}, **folic acid**, and/or the amino acid methionine. All of these can end up in deficient supply if The Boogy Boys get into your small intestine.

Since bright light—especially the bright light of sunrise—also stimulates your production of serotonin, and that light becomes rarer in the northern winter mornings, then low serotonin also becomes more common. This is one reason why depression is more common during seasons of low light.

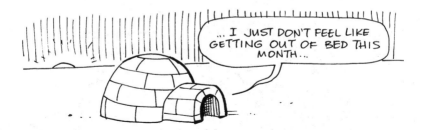

Why, I remember during World War II—when I was a **Liver Dwarf** stationed in Iceland—more than 120 soldiers killed themselves during the long, dark, frozen winters, some by trying to swim back to England!

Even in balmier climates, if people don't get outdoors enough, they can be more prone to low serotonin levels and depression and higher incidents of suicide. Of all the things that can create the mental, emotional, and behavioural problems associated with low serotonin levels, the most *obvious* is low light, but the most *overlooked* is low tryptophan levels due to Boogy Boys in the small intestine. Ironically, the low serotonin often leads to cravings for sweets, which can raise insulin levels and thereby increase tryptophan in the brain—and that high insulin can allow more Boogy Boys into your small intestine, as **Itchy** will explain later.

Serotonin starts the morning shift—usually along with the adrenal and thyroid glands—to stimulate your body to action. Both adrenal and thyroid hormones break down proteins. And prolonged action of these strong hormones can cause tremendous stress and damage to your body. As your adrenals become enlarged from prolonged stress, your **thymus gland** gets proportionately smaller—and the thymus gland controls your immune system.

Long-term high-adrenalin levels can cause severe damage to your heart because adrenalin's tremendous stimulation ability can "burn out" the heart muscle. The dangers to your heart muscle are greatly diminished by numerous enzyme systems that your body uses to quickly break down adrenalin into an **inactive oxidized hormone.** Later, NAD adds an **electron** to restore it back to regular adrenalin for reuse. If there's inadequate NAD, then the oxidized adrenalin instead becomes **adrenochrome**, which has free-radical-like properties.

While adrenochrome is less toxic to your heart than adrenalin, it can still cause **fibrillation** and **dysfunction**, particularly if antioxidant levels are low. More important to me—since I'm the **Liver Dwarf** in charge of your brain— adrenochrome and one of its breakdown products, **adrenolutin**, can pass through the blood-brain barrier and cause **psychotic ideas, paranoid delusions**, and even **hallucinations**. Together these symptoms are called **schizophrenia**.

So, a high level of stress, either physical, nutritional, or emotional—real or even imagined—can increase epinephrine. If combined with low levels of antioxidants and NAD, high epinephrine can lead to **severe mental imbalance**. Remember that NAD is made from nicotinamide, which I make from tryptophan; so many of the same things that cause low tryptophan/serotonin levels can also play a role in causing schizophrenia through low NAD levels.

There is a much quicker way that your central nervous system—and especially your brain—can get into big trouble. When **Bloaty** turns down your inlet liver valves really hard, or if there's major damage to your liver, there can be such a strong back-pressure on your portal vein that your collateral veins can open up wide. This can allow ammonia—made mainly by the intestinal bacteria eating amino acids in your intestine and spitting out the nitrogen residues—to spill out into your main bloodstream where it can cause mental delusions, hallucinations, and eventually, coma. This is one of the main problems from cirrhosis of the liver due to heavy drinking.

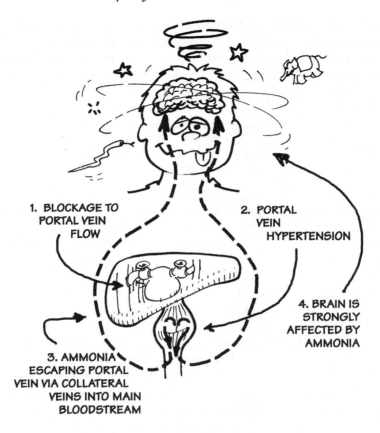

1. BLOCKAGE TO PORTAL VEIN FLOW

2. PORTAL VEIN HYPERTENSION

4. BRAIN IS STRONGLY AFFECTED BY AMMONIA

3. AMMONIA ESCAPING PORTAL VEIN VIA COLLATERAL VEINS INTO MAIN BLOODSTREAM

Of course, you can also get cirrhosis of the liver even if a drop of alcohol never passes your lips—if you have a sweet tooth and a bunch of fermenting yeast or bacteria in your intestine, especially your small intestine. Now, don't blame what's her name? Bluto? Bloato? Oh, yeah—**Bloaty**! She's just doing her best in a tough job, trying to adjust your liver valves.

As important as nicotinic acid, picolinic acid, and serotonin are, they're not necessarily the most important products of tryptophan metabolism to your overall health. Serotonin is your "on" switch, stimulated by the light of dawn, but **melatonin** is your "off" switch, activated by dusk; the rise in melatonin is your body's cue that it's time to repair and regenerate. As light decreases in the early evening, the **retina of your eye** begins to turn serotonin into melatonin. This begins a similar process deep within the centre of your brain where your pineal gland begins to convert serotonin into melatonin. By 9 P.M., your melatonin levels are getting high enough to make you a little sleepy, unless the pineal production is reduced by artificial light or by watching TV.

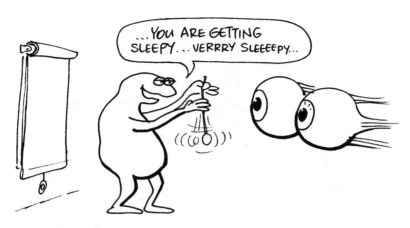

When melatonin increases at dusk, it gradually shuts down your adrenal glands, and brings sleep and the nightshift to repair the damage that might have occurred during the day. **Growth hormone** comes on to repair any proteins that might have been damaged. The deeper your sleep, the greater the repair.

While there are only two small differences in structure between serotonin and melatonin, the difference in function is dramatic. Unlike serotonin, melatonin can readily slip through any membrane, including the blood-brain barrier. Here in your **central nervous system**—with its high metabolic activity—a lot of free radicals are made and the nervous system's ability to regenerate is low. This is where melatonin performs the same powerful antioxidant role that it also carries out in your intestinal tract, neutralizing deadly free radicals.

Melatonin also stimulates your thymus gland to produce **thymus hormones**, which, when activated by zinc, motivate your immune system to get to work and repair your body and kill any invaders or **tumours**. By morning sunrise, after a full night of melatonin-inspired sleep, your body is rested and repaired, with regenerated organs, recharged with a ready supply of hormones, all eagerly awaiting another adventurous day in the sunny half of the cycle of life.

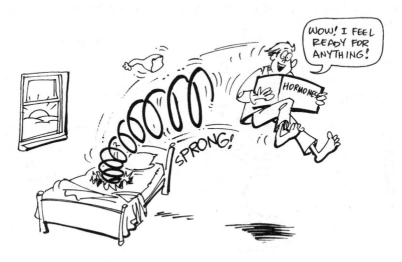

Nightly melatonin stimulates production of enough adrenal hormones to keep you active till about three in the afternoon. If you don't make enough melatonin—or are running under fear—you may run out of adrenal hormones, even before 3 P.M. Since adrenal hormones also help keep your brain supplied with a steady flow of glucose, you may get an early afternoon brain slump. Hopefully, the doctor, the new **Liver Dwarf**, can tell us what to do about that. In the meantime, I'll eat chocolate bars in the afternoon.

The cycle of life includes death, and your **pineal gland** plays a role here, as well. The pineal gland's capacity to make melatonin is limited. By 45 years of age, most people are making only one-half of the melatonin they made at 25 years of age. The gradual reduction of melatonin results in less buffering of free radicals, less nightly suppression of your adrenal hormones, and less immune-system regeneration of organs each night.

As melatonin decreases, the gradual loss of nightly repair is otherwise known as **ageing**. In other words, you're designed to be around and healthy long enough to raise your children, then you've got to really start looking after yourself if you want to stay healthy in old age. Of course, the earlier you start to do it, the better. Later, the doctor—the new **Liver Dwarf** we're expecting—will hopefully tell you about some things you can do to enjoy your spin at the wheel of life more, and how to make life easier for your hardworking **Liver Dwarves**!

So you've seen that there are many ways that your nervous system—especially your brain—can get into trouble, and that most of its problems stem from your intestine and the liver, the filter of the digestive system.

Well, I hope you've enjoyed your tour of the, um, gray thing. Oh yeah, the brain. I'm Stacey . . . or is it Tracey? I hope to see you soon, I guess. **Achy** is your next guide, but maybe you should call him **General**. Bye-bye. You didn't see my chocolate bar, did you? You're not sitting on it, are you? Please check. I desperately need chocolate! I'm **Spacey**!

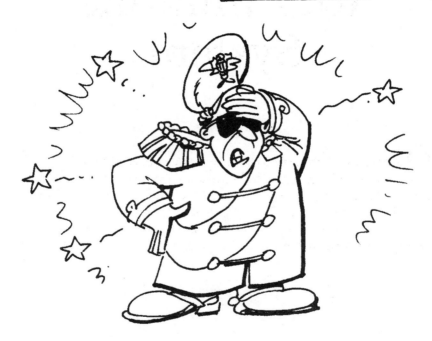

CHAPTER 5

Achy: Guide to Your Immune System

Owww! I'm Achy, the Immune System Liver Dwarf.

When **Bloaty** tightens down those liver valves, she dumps toxins, fluid, and proteins into your lymph that can screw up your **immune system**! Then you get **colds and the flu** galore, and if I let the immune system fight back too strongly, then **allergies** and **autoimmune diseases** can aggravate your body.

Some **Liver Dwarves** call me "General Achy" because I command such a large army of white blood cells, but it would be truer to say that I'm Generally Achy all over.

Just don't touch me, whatever you do. I hurt everywhere. My joints ache, my bones ache, my muscles, my tendons— sometimes even my eyebrows ache. I ache in the morning, I ache during the day, and I ache even more in the night. I ache worse when the weather changes for better, and I ache even more when the weather changes for worse.

Oh, I don't care what you call it—**arthritis, rheumatism, lumbago, polymyalgia rheumatica, gout, ankylosing spondylitis, fibromyalgia**. Who cares about fancy labels! All I know is I hurt, and I don't like it! Sometimes, I ache worse if I sit still. Then I know it's your liver that's the main problem. Other times, it hurts more if I move around, and then I know your kidneys are in trouble. Either way, it's all **Burpy**'s and **Bloaty**'s fault.

When **Burpy** hogs all the bioflavonoids and antioxidants— because he's trying to help the liver's conjugation enzymes to neutralize free radicals, hydrogen peroxides, lipid peroxides, and epoxides, made by your P450 enzymes—that can leave me without enough bioflavonoids and antioxidants to protect your **connective tissue**, and that causes **weak ligaments, tendons, cartilages, intervertebral discs, eyes, veins, capillaries, and even nails**.

Your nails break; your eyes get weak, sore, or blurry; your veins bulge; and as your ligaments and tendons get weaker, you start to sag. Arches start to fall; ankles start to turn—so your shoes don't wear evenly on the heels. Your discs start to bulge and protrude, giving you excruciating back pain that can extend down your legs. Then, your back starts going out. You just roll over in bed and "clunk"—out it goes again. Plus, you sprain things all the time, or with just a touch, you bruise! If you even sneeze, you can get nosebleeds.

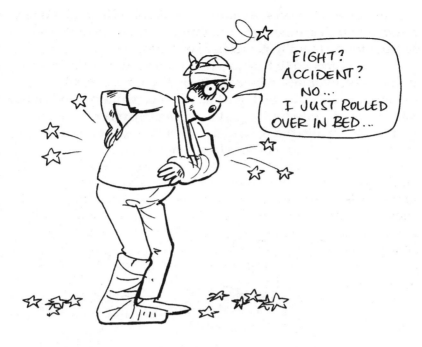

Now this isn't *anything* compared to what happens when your **immune system** turns against you; that's what really gets you aching, as I know too well.

I have immune-system-operated checkpoints in your small intestine at the entrances to your **lymph system**, called the **Peyer's patches**. While the rest of your intestine has a tough wall of cells stacked tightly together like bricks, the Peyer's patches have a dome-shaped "soft top," like a convertible, called **M cells**. I slide the top back once in a while and reach out into your small intestine to grab anything suspicious passing by, and drag it into the **villi** where it's given a thorough checkover by your **immune cells** to see if it's dangerous.

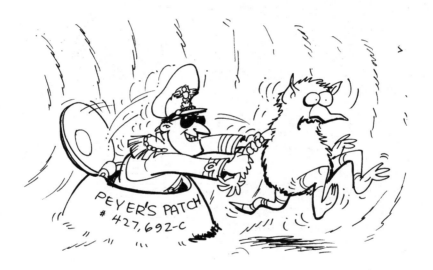

I've also got **dendritic cells,** starfish-shaped cells that link together to make an early detection web throughout your lymph nodes and the epidermis of your skin.

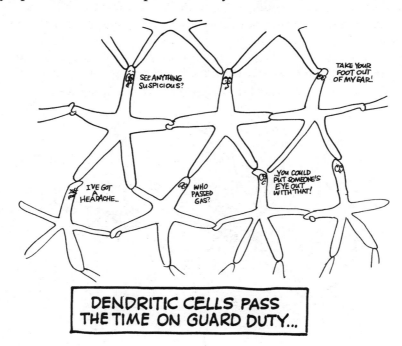

DENDRITIC CELLS PASS
THE TIME ON GUARD DUTY...

If a bacterium, an incompletely digested protein, or anything else suspiciously "foreign" is detected, one of my first-line troops—a macrophage I've affectionately nicknamed **Sergeant Mac**—will gulp it down. Sergeant Macs are brawny, alert, and tough as nails. Eating a hundred bacteria will hardly slow one down.

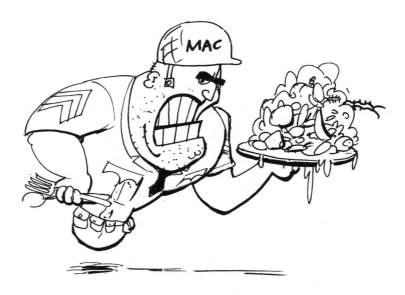

I keep them fixed in place in your spleen, bone marrow, lungs, and lymph nodes. And of course, I've got The Kupffer Kops stationed in your liver sinusoids. In addition, I have free macrophages roaming everywhere on field reconnaissance, looking for infiltrates that might be trying to slip through your fixed perimeter defences: your skin and membranes. I've got **monocytes** drifting around in your blood, ready to be activated into macrophages, if needed.

After a macrophage gulps down a bacterium, or even a much larger foreign particle, it releases **lysozyme** to digest the invader's fatty membrane and **proteolytic enzymes** to shatter its proteins. Tougher characters will be oxidized by producing superoxides, nitric oxide, and hydrogen peroxide, which as you know from **Burpy**, can generate the deadly hydroxyl radical. If that *still* doesn't kill them, I treat the hydrogen peroxide with

chlorine to form **hypochlorite**, which is extremely fatal to bacteria. If *excessive* superoxide and nitric oxide are produced, they spontaneously form **peroxynitrite**, a deadly generator of free radicals. Peroxynitrite is especially seen in smokers because smoking stimulates P450 enzymes to produce more superoxide radicals.

If the macrophage needs reinforcements, he sends out **tumour necrosis factor** (**TNF**) and **interleukin-1**. This brings nearby macrophages—even ones that have been working in fixed stations—rushing to the rescue. A net of **fibrin** is quickly set up around the invaders to keep them from getting away. This blocks the circulation into and out of the area, and causes the swelling associated with inflammation. We **Liver Dwarves** call this congestion.

At the same time, I'm sending in my second line of defence, the **neutrophils**. They're the Little Macs. They're **minimacrophages**, not as big or as tough as Sergeant Macs, but easier and quicker to make, which makes them plentiful, and also makes them—don't tell them I said this—disposable. I can get millions of neutrophils to the front lines within hours and they continue the good work that your magnificent macrophages have begun.

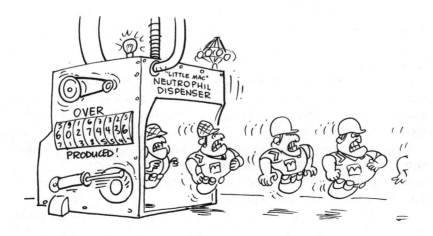

Neutrophils can suck in oxygen and then within seconds, can blow it back out in the form of oxygen free radicals such as superoxide radicals. The superoxide radicals can become peroxides, which can then generate the hydroxyl radicals that are so destructive to any would-be intruder.

The original macrophage, in the meantime, will have scurried over to the nearest lymph node to do an identity-check on what he's just eaten. He'll wear a fragment, such as a piece of cell wall on his chest—like a medal of honour—to show to the babyfaced and rather naïve **lymphocyte** reserves I keep stationed throughout your lymph system.

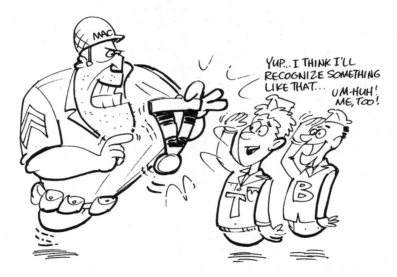

As the battle-hardened veteran macrophage displays his trophy, the rookie **B** and **T lymphocytes** take notes outlining the characteristics of the enemy displayed before them. In the background, the barrack speakers are blaring: "This is *not* a drill. I repeat, this is *not* a drill." If it's something that none of the **B cells** or **T cells** has seen before, they quickly sketch a particular feature that distinguishes this evil alien and this feature is now called an **antigen**.

Now that these cells know who the bad guy is, their leisurely days in the barracks are over. The enemy has been identified; war has been declared; there is a battle to be won!

The now-*sensitized* B cells quickly multiply and get promoted to **plasma cells** as they join the ranks of active fighters by releasing massive quantities of antibodies, also called **immunoglobulins (Ig)**—sometimes known as **gamma globulins**.

These antibodies are made from two heavy polypeptide chains and two smaller, light chains joined together to form a double-prong on one end and a single tail on the other end.

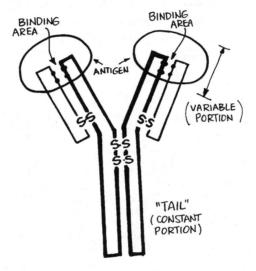

IgG ANTIBODY

Each of the prongs is specifically designed to attach to one enemy antigen so that all the antibodies made by clones from a certain B cell will have identical prongs. They will be different from prongs on antibodies made from B cells that are programmed to attack other enemies. I have to keep millions of different B cells on duty, each one programmed to make antibodies specific to one of the hordes of enemies previously identified.

Unlike the antibody prongs, the antibody tails remain somewhat the same on the various antibodies. Sometimes I join the tails of the antibodies together with what I call a J-chain, to make them bigger.

The antibodies are released into the slow-moving lymph system, which soon delivers them to the left collarbone area, where the lymph ducts empty into the **subclavian** vein where it joins the **jugular vein**. Now the antibodies are in the rapidly moving bloodstream, in search of the enemy—wherever it may be lurking.

If a bacterium or virus were to get in through a cut in your skin, crash through the dendritic cell early warning web, outflank the macrophage scouts, and get into your blood with the evil intention of doing you harm, this is when I enjoy ordering your B cells to roll out my biggest antibody surprise— **IgM**—to whom I lovingly refer as **Big Momma**!

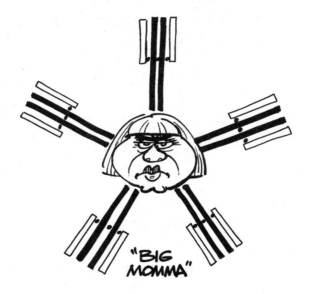

Big Momma is five antibody units joined together at their tails, with their five pairs of prongs protruding like the spokes of a wheel. When I send her rolling and rumbling through your blood vessels, you ought to see the desperate look those Boogy Boys have on their miserable mugs just before they get broadsided by Big Momma. (The Big Broad . . . Ha ha.) They barely have time to squeak out a plaintive cry of "Holy Cow— that's a Big Mother!" before they get squished.

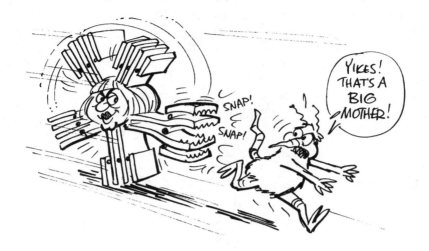

But Big Momma can't get them all every time. Perhaps there's a spy in our midst and, forewarned, some Boogy Boys manage to slip into the smaller nooks and crannies where Mama is just too big to go.

Of course, I'm well prepared for their little tricks, so after Big Momma has cleaned up all the easy stuff, I send in **IgG—the G-Men**. They're smaller antibodies and more adept at slipping into the dark little places where bacteria, viruses, and fungi might lurk.

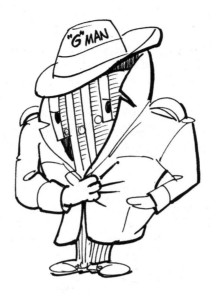

IgG comes in four subclasses—**IgG1, IgG2, IgG3, IgG4**—that consist of a variety of five different heavy chains and two different light chains that altogether make IgG the most versatile at digging away at those persistent intruders.

I make much smaller amounts of **immunoglobulin E (IgE)**, which sticks to either **mast cells**—which reside in tissues mainly near the respiratory system, intestines, and under the skin—or to **basophils**—a version of a mast cell that's adrift in the blood. If an antigen bumps into IgE bound to a basophil or mast cell, then that cell releases histamine, serotonin, **leukotrienes**, and other substances that strongly affect your circulation to help win the war against the invaders.

Most wars are won and lost in the trenches and the key battles to maintain your health are fought in the trenches surrounding your intestines. The delicate inner workings of your mind and body are separated from the billions of messy Boogy Boys only by the thin membrane of your intestine. Underlying the subfloor of the intestine is the **lamina propria**— the trenches, if you like—the thin line that defends you from disaster.

Here in this most volatile of danger zones is where IgM, IgG, and IgE have failed to stand up to the demands of combat. In the heat of pitched battle, my little B cell soldiers would see their weapons wilt and deform on the slightest contact with a protein-digesting enzyme, which—as you well know—are to be found throughout the digestive zone. Here, I have to keep very active patrols, yet how could I send my soldiers into such danger with faulty weapons? Stronger protection was obviously necessary to help them in this very dangerous situation.

They asked for—and I gladly provided them—their weapon of choice: the deadly **secretory IgA antibody**.

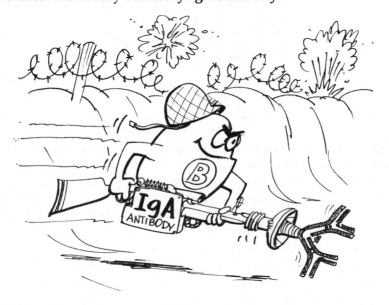

This antibody has two subclasses that together can readily mop up incoming bacteria, viruses, toxins, and food antigens. Yet, unlike the other antibodies, the IgA antibody can withstand the brutal conditions imposed on it by the extremely powerful digestive enzymes found along your gut. Because of its effectiveness in the trenches, IgA's services are in great demand for protecting membranes in other parts of your body. The IgA antibody accounts for about 70 percent of your total antibody production each day. An average-size adult secretes about three grams of IgA daily.

It's unique in appearance because it consists of two double-pronged antibodies joined together with a J-chain; its spectacular success is because I, **General Achy**—through my superb training at **Liver Dwarf Institute of Technology (LDIT)**—solved the problem of war in your trenches, once and for all!

I designed a **secretory component** that gives secretory IgA both its name and its ability to be secreted across any membrane without being damaged by enzymes. I personally install the secretory component inside the tail of every IgA antibody as it passes through the membrane so that it will *not* be broken down by digestive enzymes in the heat of battle. And I personally guarantee it will stand up throughout the toughest conditions of trench warfare. By prolonging the life of IgA, I'm also prolonging yours. No need to thank me—just your recognition of me as your most important **Liver Dwarf** is adequate. Thank you! Thank you again for your recognition. I would bow to your sincere appreciation of my work but I hurt so much, I don't think I could straighten up again!

There are those who say I should have patented secretory IgA. I suppose I'd have made millions of dollars by now and be living on Easy Street, but that's not the way of a **Liver Dwarf**. I volunteered for this **Liver Dwarves'** army and I volunteered to serve, not be served. There's a war to be won, thank God—for without a war, life wouldn't be worth living. It would be a damn bore, if you ask me.

Turning B cells into plasma cells and locking their antibodies onto invaders is a skirmish that has just begun—for the intruder is far from finished. As one antibody's prong attaches to a bad guy, the other prong might grab onto another bad guy—which might have other antibodies on it attached to other bad guys. Gradually, this whole mess of bad guys can get stuck together with antibodies; this is called an **immune complex**.

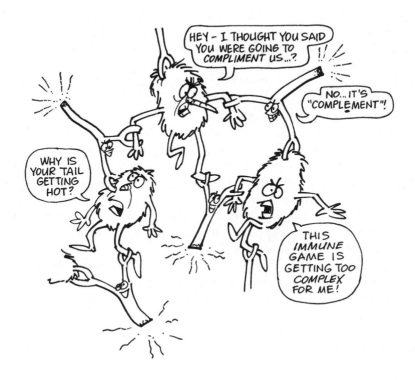

At the time of binding to the antigen, the tail of the antibody becomes "hot." That is, it begins to activate the **complement system**, a group of about 20 proteins that I keep floating around in the blood. The complement system continues the job of rendering justice. The "hot" antibody tail binds with the **C1** protein of the complement system, transforming it into an active enzyme and setting off a cascade of enzyme reactions. Many end products are formed, including **Membrane Attack Complex (MAC)**. These end products activate the inflammatory response, rupture bacterial membranes, neutralize viruses, and attract more macrophages and neutrophils—with their deadly bullets of superoxide, hydrogen peroxide, and hypochlorite— that could finish off these nasty invaders.

It brings a tear to my eye to see my little soldiers fighting and dying so valiantly in your trenches. God bless them all, those gallant fighters for your Freedom of Health. Yet I haven't finished my story, for there are still more of your heroes to introduce.

While the fuzzy-cheeked B cells have been turning into battle-ready plasma cells and preparing their armament of antibodies for full-scale defensive action, the T cells are going through a similar process of activation. As they become programmed against a specific enemy, they also begin to reproduce rapidly, with each offspring programmed to defend against that one "Bad Guy." Like the B cells, the T cells circulate throughout your body so that they'll find the "villain" wherever it may be. When an enemy antigen is spotted, the T cells quickly begin their deadly work.

Most of the T cells are **helper T cells**. They secrete **cytokines**, which include three types of **interferon, lymphotoxin**, and several different **interleukins**. **Interferons alpha** and **beta** warn neighbouring cells of approaching danger so they can make **antiviral** proteins. **Gamma interferon**—like the other interferons—warns cells and stimulates natural killer cells, but also further stimulates the B cells, T cells, and neutrophils to greater effort. Lymphotoxin is an even stronger stimulator of neutrophils.

Interleukins-4, 5, and **6** strongly stimulate B cells to transform into plasma cells and can get antibody production up to 2000 per second per plasma cell. **Interleukin-2**, gamma interferon, and lymphotoxin stimulate the **cytotoxic "killer" T cell** to bind tightly to the enemy cell where it can deliver its deadly one-two punch. First, it secretes **perforin**, a protein that pounds large, round holes in the invader's cell membrane through which it then pours enzymes called **granzymes** that react to blow the invader up.

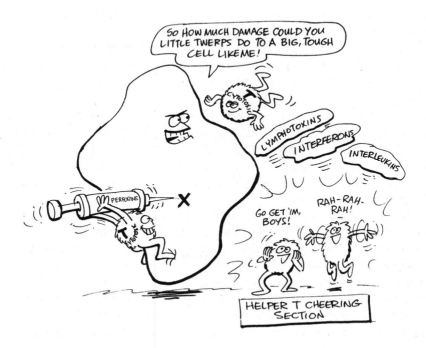

This is usually the end of the invader, yet the cytotoxic T cell can go on to kill many more virally infected cells or even cancer cells. The cytotoxic "killer" T cell is not to be confused with the **natural killer (NK) cell** that does a similar job but works steadily and quietly, more in the background shadows. It shuns the rah! rah! cheerleading that the macrophage/neutrophil/ B cell/T cell group require, although even natural killer cells will increase their attack if enough helper T cell cytokines are around.

The ultimate success of the whole immune system revolves around the sophisticated bag of tricks of the helper T cells stimulating and coordinating all the other soldiers of the immune system. This large group of T cells is so efficient at stimulating the B cells, macrophages, and neutrophils that I have to make **suppressor T cells** to "cool down" the helper T cells so they don't blow the whole body to pieces with their enthusiasm and effectiveness.

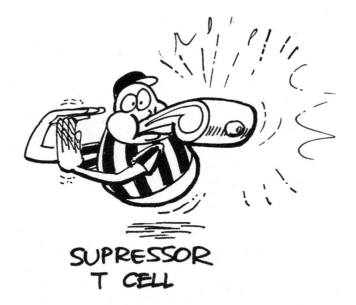

SUPRESSOR
T CELL

I've even trained all your cells to take their own lives rather than risk inadvertently supporting the enemy. All your cells know that if they're taken prisoner by viruses or cancer, the only honourable option is **apoptosis**—that is to blow themselves up! It's better to die honourably than to provide the enemy with your precious DNA.

The macrophages gobble up the mess—the final rendering of justice. Ah, the good old veteran macrophages: always the first to enter into battle and the last to leave. Both the B cells and T cells make **memory cells** that cruise the body long after the invader has been destroyed—in case the enemy should try again. A second invasion would be repelled faster because my soldiers are already armed and trained to deal with them.

The dangers that exist outside your body's borders of membrane and skin are real, but you can count on me to keep your multiple layers of defence well armed and ever vigilant. I stimulate your T cells with **thymulin hormone** from the **thymus gland**. It's inactive when first secreted so I quickly bind it with zinc to activate it to kick-start those helper T cells into action. Without the T cell **cytokine** stimulation, the B cells aren't very organized or motivated.

I've got your portals of entry guarded by fixed macrophages. **Tonsils** and **adenoids** are manned to guard the throat. Peyer's patches are aggressively checking the ID of suspicious characters in the intestine; and about 30 percent of the cells in your liver sinusoids are well-armed Kupffer Kops. Dendritic cells are on guard under the skin and throughout the lymph system.

The bloodstream is filtered and cleaned by the spleen. As the **splenic** artery brings blood into the spleen, it branches out into smaller arterioles. As the blood enters the **white pulp** of the spleen, it's thoroughly exposed to numerous T cells and a few macrophages, which begin immune reactions to any antigens in the blood.

As the blood makes its way through the white pulp, it's next exposed to hordes of B cells that hurl their antibodies at any antigens they might recognize. The blood cells then squeeze through the narrow **penicillar arterioles** as they leave the white pulp. Here, any weak, old, or infected red blood cells will break, spilling their contents. As the arterioles enter the **red pulp**, they dilate, becoming venous sinusoids surrounded by numerous macrophages and plasma cells that finish off any infections, antigens, or red blood cell remnants.

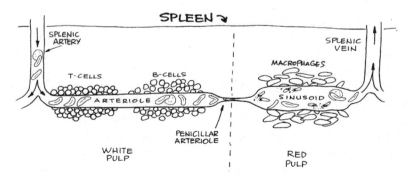

The spleen also secretes an antibacterial protein called **tuftsin**, which helps preserve Healthocracy and the **Liver Dwarf** way of life. Removal of your spleen can decrease your ability to fight bacteria. **Spleenopentin** is another immune stimulator that's produced by the spleen.

With a cast of billions of small—but inspired and deadly—
soldiers to help me, I have little trouble defending against
attack from outside. The real danger is from within and usually
starts in the intestine with The Boogy Boys running amok. I'd
given a lot of thought to that possibility when I designed my
defence plan. That's why I keep active patrols in the intestinal
trenches, armed to the teeth with my indomitable IgA—so that
when The Boogy Boys try to break out of the large intestine, we
can fight them fair and square, in a fight they'd surely lose.

Of course, when a child is being breast-fed, he or she receives
defensive antibodies—like IgA—from the mother's milk. If the
baby isn't breast-fed long enough and starts eating foods before
I have IgA fully developed in the infant's intestinal trenches,
some of the proteins from milk, eggs, soy, and wheat can get
into his or her lymph system before they're fully broken down
into amino acids. If that happens, the immune system will
attack the proteins as if they were invaders from Mars. The
battle results in allergies to foods like milk, eggs, soy, and
wheat. As the child gets older—and I get his or her IgA working
better so that fewer proteins get from the gut into the lymph—
these allergies will often fade away.

The LDIU—that stands for **Liver Dwarf Intelligence Unit**:
the secret crack team dedicated to protecting your precious
DNA from subterfuge—however, informs me that The Boogy
Boys have come up with a devious plot to crack your adult
intestinal defences. Not through headlong suicidal assault along
your intestinal trenches, for which I am well prepared, but
through a more insidious *sneaking* from your large intestine into
your small intestine by overcoming your ileocecal valve. If they
get into the small intestine, they can't defeat us in direct battle,
but neither can we defeat them because the intestinal
membrane will still separate us. They can't post a quick,
decisive win but they're relatively free to loot and plunder and
make life miserable for you by stealing your tryptophan,
vitamin B_{12}, and other nutrients and then fermenting some of
them into toxins.

We've always known that The Boogy Boys are fermenters
and that's why we keep them confined to your large intestine
where their work can be of benefit to you in breaking down

coarse fibres and converting them into short-chain fatty acids. Of course, **Burpy** doesn't absorb very actively from your large intestine because of the toxins they make during fermentation. If they manage to get into your small intestine, however, all of their mess gets absorbed and sent to your liver via the portal vein.

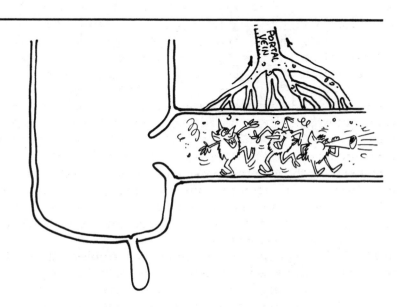

As long as your liver's detoxification enzymes—P450 and conjugation enzymes—are able to deal with it, there's no big problem for me—or, therefore, for you. The P450 enzymes, however, can *amplify* the toxicity by making free radicals, peroxides, and toxic epoxides.

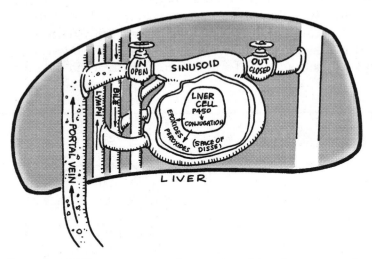

When the P450 enzymes make an **epoxide**, they can make four variations of each one. Some epoxide variations might be low in toxicity, but others can be deathly toxic to your DNA, as **Sluggy** will explain. If the conjugation enzymes are unable to quickly quench the rising tide of peroxides in your liver sinusoids, **Burpy** will try dumping bioflavonoids on them to simmer them down. If that doesn't work, he'll shunt some of the excess peroxides into the bile. If it looks as though the peroxides might get past the outlet valves into the main bloodstream where they could damage the brain and nervous system, then **Bloaty** has to close down the outlet valves.

When **Bloaty** tightens down your outlet valves, even a slight back-pressure into your liver sinusoids further opens up the already large gaps between the millions of **spaces of Disse**, allowing epoxides, peroxides, food bits, fluid, and proteins from your blood plasma to bypass all my regular defences and get dumped straight into your lymph system.

Your lymph system is designed to drain excess fluid from your cells and take it back into the circulation system. Fifty percent of your lymph system originates in your liver, while 25 percent of your lymph comes from your intestine and 25 percent comes from the rest of your body. The dumping of massive amounts of fluid, protein, and other stuff directly from your liver into your lymph system can put a tremendous burden on it.

Lymph system overload is most likely to show up where your lymph system is close to the surface, such as the neck, **inguinal** area (where your leg joins your pelvis), and underarm. The neck should be called the **bottleneck** because this is where the lymph creates the most obvious congestion.

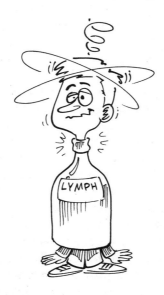

If the **liver lymph** is pouring an extra load of fluid, protein, peroxides, and epoxides into your main lymph system, it's my job as General of your immune system to get in there and clean it up!

Of course, I'll send in my little soldiers and they'll order a ring of fibrin to be strung around the invaders to seal off the area. This creates congestion and swelling in your lymph glands which can, in turn, block the **eustachian tubes** that drain your middle ears into your throat. Back-pressure in your eustachian tubes can lead to congestion, infection, and even rupture of your **eardrum**.

As well as being important for hearing, your **inner ear** plays an important role in maintaining your balance, by joining with visual input to send messages to your brain. Congestion of your inner ear can cause **dizziness, vertigo,** and **equilibrium and coordination imbalance**—and in some people, it can create reading, writing, and learning problems. The inner ear congestion can also contribute to **tinnitus**, which creates ringing and buzzing sounds inside your head.

Blockage in your **throat lymph glands** can also interfere with drainage of your **sinuses,** resulting in chronic aggravation there. Children, with their smaller throats and weaker immune systems, are especially prone to these kinds of problems. Of course, if their **calcium levels** are low, as **Itchy** will explain, then their membranes are going to be even more vulnerable to infections and irritants—like pollen and dust.

With all this congestion in your head, I sometimes have to use your nose as a safety valve so I get your nose running really well before your head blows up. Ha ha! That's a **Liver Dwarf** joke! Not bad for an old, underappreciated soldier **Liver Dwarf.** You should have seen me in my prime, when I could dance all night. Now, I can't even sleep all night because of the pain I'm in.

Swollen lymph glands in your throat are a sure sign that **Bloaty**'s tightening down your outlet liver valves. This is also where viruses and bacteria can get access to that large picnic basket of protein trapped in your neck's lymph nodes. They enter through your nose or mouth, and if they get into your throat, they might slip in through your **tonsils** into this smorgasbord of goodies.

As I send platoons, regiments, or even divisions of B cells and T cells into your lymph system to clean up the mess that **Bloaty** made by closing your outlet liver valves, they identify and attack each antigen they find. Antigens, like all living things, are mainly made from **carbon**.

Carbon is so important because it has four electrons with a tremendous drive to hold hands with four other electrons by **bonding**. This four-sided bonding ability of carbon makes it the building block of life, from which all the major structures crucial to living organisms are built.

While carbon has four hands to hold with, nitrogen has three, oxygen has two, and hydrogen has one.

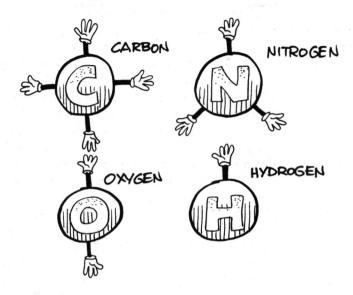

Notice that carbon, nitrogen, and oxygen can hold hands in two ways: using one hand or using two hands. **One-hand bonds**—called **single bonds**—are quite strong. **Two-hand bonds**—called **double bonds**—are even stronger bonds but they can be broken by powerful intruders, like oxygen or hydrogen. **Carbon-to-carbon double bonds** veer off at a 120 degree angle, creating a "kink" in the molecule.

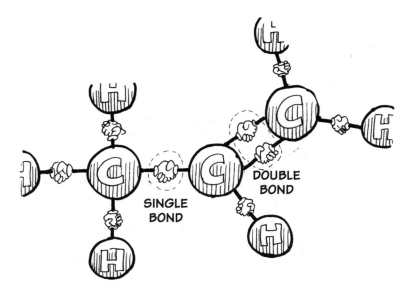

Sugars are **carbohydrates**—they're made from carbon, hydrogen, and oxygen. **Glucose** and **fructose** are **six-carbon** sugars. Sugars themselves can be bonded together to form **starch** or, by even stronger bonds, to form **cellulose**.

Fats are also composed of carbon, hydrogen, and oxygen but their energy is much more concentrated than that of sugars. **Glycerol** is an example of a small three-carbon fat.

A **protein** is made of a series of amino acids joined together like a train, and what separates proteins from carbohydrates or fats is that *every* amino acid has a nitrogen attached to it, and some amino acids also contain sulphur.

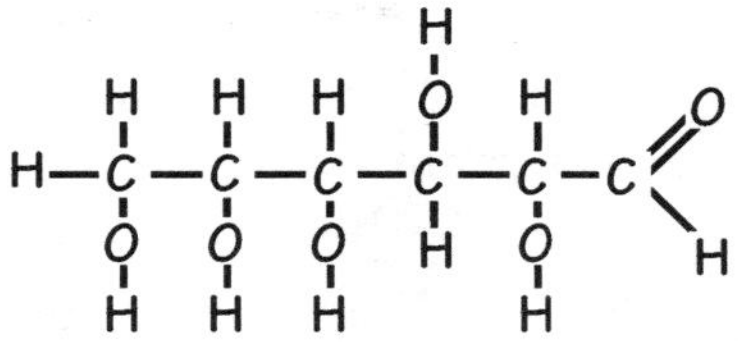

GLUCOSE
(A Carbohydrate)

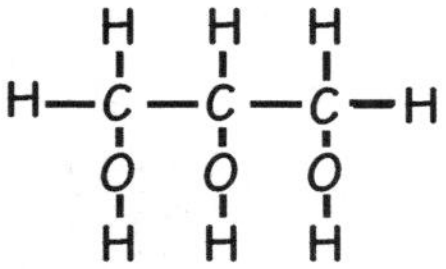

GLYCEROL
(A Fat)

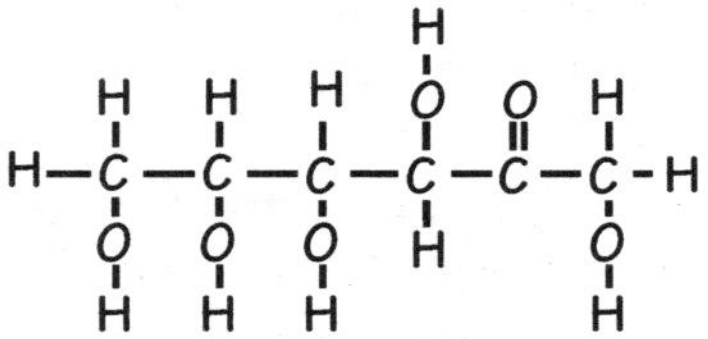

FRUCTOSE
(A Carbohydrate)

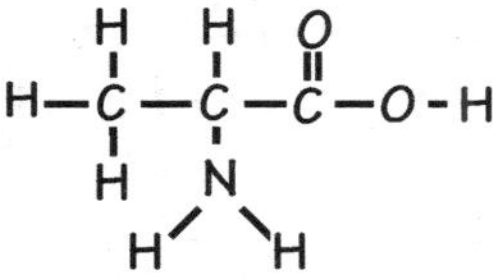

ALANINE
(An Amino Acid)

What's important to my little soldiers in their search for the enemy is that about 50 percent of a cell is made from protein, so that's basically what they're trained to search for when frisking a suspicious character for identification. And the antigens that trigger the activation of B cells and T cells are mainly proteins, although they may also have sugars or fats attached to them. Things that bind to a protein and make it more **antigenic** to your immune system are called **haptens**.

Since proteins are made from amino acids, when my B cell and T cell soldiers go into the lymph to clean up the mess that **Bloaty**'s dumped in there, they mainly use amino acids as their antigen template. While the B cells make IgA primarily to guard the membranes, IgG is their best ammunition in the lymph. Of the four subtypes of IgG antibodies, I keep IgG2 and IgG3 in reserve to fight **streptococci bacteria**, and I use IgG1 and IgG3 together to fight against viruses.

Against food antigens that get into your lymph, I let the B cells use IgG1 and IgG4 and sometimes IgE. The most common proteins that they use them against are **casein** in milk, **albumin** in eggs, and **gliadin** from the gluten in wheat. The IgE creates most of the dramatic symptoms associated with allergies.

The IgE antibody locks onto fixed mast cells or their floating free cousins, the basophils. If an antigen should then contact the IgE prongs, it would stimulate the mast cell (or basophil) to release histamine, cytokines, and **leukotrienes**. These substances, in excess, can cause **hayfever, asthma**, and **eczema** very quickly after exposure to an antigen, which is why this type of allergy is called **immediate hypersensitivity**. I should explain right now that histamine allergies are not the fault of my hardworking B cells—although they have long been blamed for making too much IgE. The large amounts of IgE in these strong allergies is not the fault of the B cells; they're only following orders from their supervisors.

Helper T cells make interleukin-4 to stimulate the B cells to make *more IgE* (and therefore more histamine) and helper T cells also make gamma interferon to get the B cells to make less IgE (and therefore, less histamine).

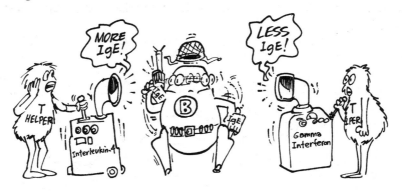

In the case of an infestation of worms and other large parasites, the helper T cells are following proper immune system protocol by increasing interleukin-4 production because the resulting high levels of IgE help—along with interleukin-5—to activate **eosinophils**. Eosinophils are white blood cells that carry a bomb called **major basic protein**, designed specifically to blow up the tough outer hide of worms. The problem is that it's not entirely selective and tends to blow up a little bit of you, too. But hey, war can be a messy business and I've got no time to worry about civilian casualties. My little soldiers have a job to do, and I say *Full Speed Ahead to Victory!*

Sometimes, it seems like the B cells are the bad guys because they're making too much IgE, but again, it's never their fault. The T cell helpers and suppressors are always the ones to blame. I remember one time—we had so much IgE and histamine that the mast cells were pumping out lots of **leukotriene C$_4$ (LTC$_4$**—the main thing that causes **anaphylactic shock**). Yes, there was so much LTC$_4$ that we were literally swimming in it, 'though drowning in it might be a better explanation.

Bloaty was slamming shut the liver valves, bronchioles were constricting, plasma was leaking, and the blood pressure was falling so fast, we almost died of anaphylactic shock. It was a close one!

I was so near to death, I saw my lives flashing before my eyes—General of your army, General of Napoleon's army, General of Attila the Hun's army, General of Genghis Khan's army . . . it makes my eyes moist knowing I could go on and on.

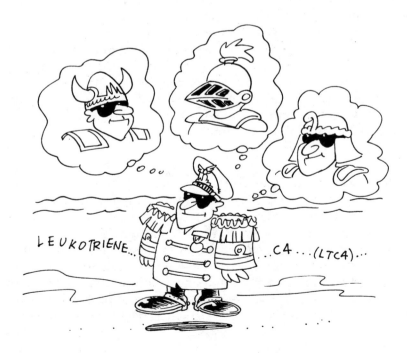

I was barely able to call a Code Blue Alert in time for the other **Liver Dwarves** to pull me out. Whew!

My investigation showed that the helper T cells hadn't been making enough gamma interferon to stop IgE production. I immediately put the helper T cells on court martial for dereliction of duty. The court martial let the helper T cells off. They were found Not Guilty because they hadn't received directions from their superior, the thymus gland. The thymus gland hadn't sent orders, not because it had run out of ink to issue them, but because it had run out of zinc! No zinc, no thymus hormone activation—so no directives to its helper T cells and no gamma interferon; the B cells kept pumping out IgE and the mast cells kept dumping histamine and LTC_4 kept building up. I almost died!

Well, you probably know by now what happened to the zinc. The Boogy Boys stole the tryptophan out of the small intestine so the pancreas couldn't make enough picolinic acid for zinc absorption. I'd like to put The Boogy Boys up on charges for war crimes, give them a fair trial and then the firing squad. Of course, I'd give them a choice of weapons to die by: Big Momma, the G-Men, or IgA. I wonder which one they'd pick?

When the B cells and T cells go into the lymph to clean up **Bloaty**'s mess, they make memory cells against all the "invaders" they identify there. Posters will be pinned up in the thymus gland with their antigen picture and the words **WANTED: DEAD!** printed underneath.

If any of them show up again, the second response will be faster than the first because their identities will be known and armed troops will be ready to attack them. This is the principle behind vaccination: give the immune system a little look at a potential invader so that it will, in future, be quickly recognized and destroyed. The problem is that immune reactions to vaccinations are generally more intense—though shorter-lived—than they are to an infection. This is because when a virus tries to sneak into your body along one of your membranes—such as those in your lungs—it's going to get hit hard by my famous secretory IgA, which of course I personally invented. Anyway, when a vaccine is injected through my perimeter defences by needle, it bypasses my front-line troops. This puts a tremendous strain on my reserve troops and they will sometimes overproduce interferon. The excess interferon can create problems, as **Sluggy** will explain.

The memory cells circulate throughout the body and, when they're mature, they seek to attack the antigen they're programmed to eliminate. They don't always get it right. They sometimes attack other antigens that *look* similar. For example, IgE programmed to attack a particular protein in **birch pollen** can be fooled into attacking a similar protein in celery, apples, peanuts, and kiwi fruit. This is called **cross-reactivity**.

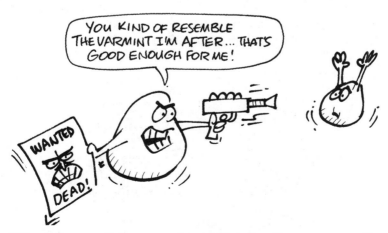

When the reactions occur immediately after exposure, it may be obvious what you're reacting to. There are, however, other reactions—like T cell reactions—that might take place several days after exposure. These are called **delayed reactions**, and it can be difficult to determine their origin.

This confusion can be increased if the antigen is a **phenol**. Of the 20 amino acids that make up the proteins that might get dumped into your lymph by **Bloaty**, most of them are relatively simple—made from straight carbon chains. Three amino acids, however, have a more complex structure involving six carbons holding hands in a diamond-shaped ring, and sharing six electrons that whiz around among them, giving them a unique electrical charge.

This six-sided carbon ring is called **benzene** and its six internally shared electrons are called the **aromatic cloud**, so things with aromatic clouds are often called **aromatics**.

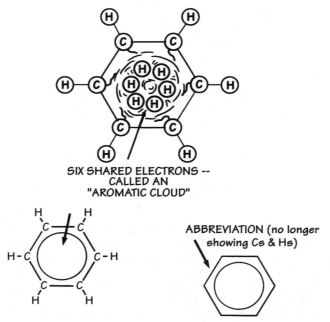

SIX SHARED ELECTRONS --
CALLED AN
"AROMATIC CLOUD"

ABBREVIATION (no longer showing Cs & Hs)

BENZENE — an aromatic molecule

The unique electron structure of benzene makes it highly reactive, which is why things with *aroma* certainly have an aromatic cloud. Our senses of smell and taste are highly sensitive to aromatics. In fact, neurotransmitters themselves are aromatics.

This reactivity is dramatically increased when benzene is bound to other molecules—in which case it is called a **phenyl**, sometimes referred to as **phenol**. The three amino acids that have phenols are **phenylalanine, tyrosine,** and **tryptophan**.

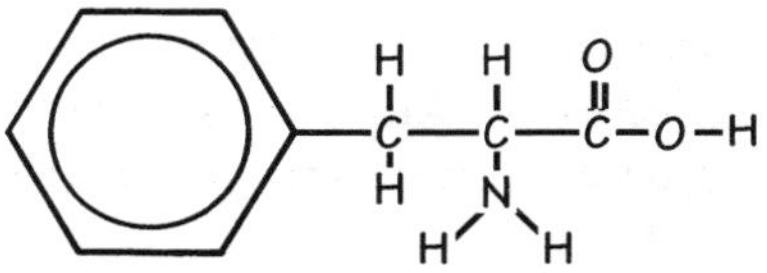

(BENZENE)   (ALANINE)
PHENYLANANINE

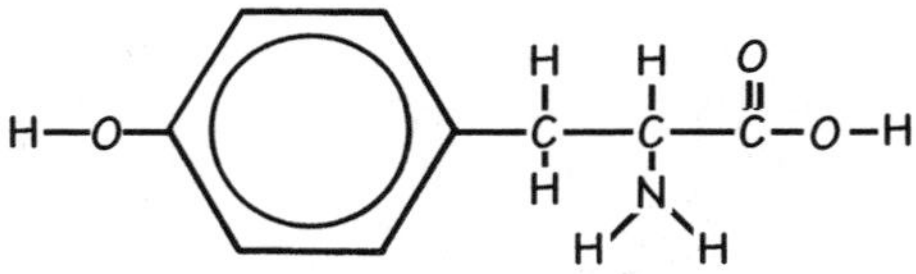

TYROSINE

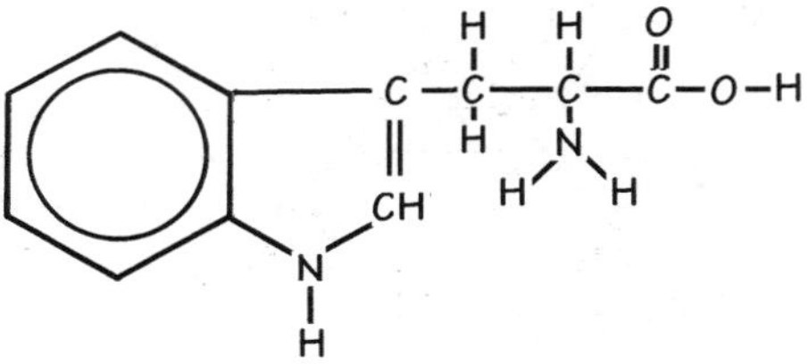

TRYPTOPHAN

If your immune system declares a phenol as an invader and attacks it with little or no IgE—and therefore less histamine— and more of the "quieter" IgG1 and IgG4, the symptoms may be much more subtle than those seen with a full-blown IgE-type allergy. The origin of the reaction may be difficult to trace because the phenols are found, in varying amounts, throughout the food chain, and phenols are also found in pollens. For example, **ragweed pollen** has a number of phenols like **caffeic acid, vanillic acid, coumaric acid, chlorogenic acid,** and **ferulic acid**—all of which are found in many foods. People allergic to ragweed will sometimes get cross-reactions to melons and bananas. People allergic to **latex** might also react to avocados. These subtle allergies are sometimes referred to as **hidden allergies**.

If the phenol **cinnamic acid**—formed from the aromatic amino acid phenylalanine—gets shunted from your liver sinusoids into your lymph system when **Bloaty** shuts down your outlet liver valves, your immune system attacks it as if it had detected an invader from Outer Space. Since your immune system may use IgG1 and IgG4 to attack, the symptoms of an allergy to cinnamic acid will likely be much more subdued than a full-blown IgE allergy.

Cinnamic acid, of course, was first found in cinnamon but can be found in many foods, especially fruits such as apples, grapes, and cherries—it's also found in carrots, chicken, and milk. Symptoms of an allergy to cinnamic acid can range from acne and eczema to bladder problems to spring hayfever, arthritis, and fatigue. As in many allergies, the person may crave what he or she is allergic to, and cinnamic acid allergies will often include **fruit cravings**. Another thing that can lead to *strong* cravings is **salsolinol**, a product of fermentation. High salsolinol levels can lead to extreme cravings for, and even addiction to, alcohol or chocolate.

Since Candida yeast are prolific producers of cinnamic acid and gallic acid when they're throwing a fermentation party in your intestine, they can produce a wide range of allergy symptoms. You might say that yeast are primitive organisms—but you can't say they're stupid. When they need more "goodies" to keep their party rocking and rolling, they know how to get *you* to fetch some more. So when you're gobbling down that booze, sugar, and chocolate that you *know* you shouldn't be eating, understand that *now you're working for them*—the fermenting Boogy Boys and yeast. Yeast use that sweet stuff to make more alcohols, like salsolinol, which gives you more cravings for alcohol and/or sweets. Yeast also make acetaldehyde, which is the main cause of petrochemical sensitivities.

Since chlorogenic acid and caffeic acid are phenols descended from cinnamic acid, cross-reaction can expand the symptoms to include congestion of the nose and ears, dizziness, headaches, and numbness and tingling of the extremities. People who are allergic to the chlorogenic acid in coffee may also react to the same substance in castor beans, apples, potatoes, and oranges and many other plants.

Individuals who are allergic to the bioflavonoid **quercetin** and its cousin **rutin** can react to some pollens, wheat, citrus, cherries, tea, apples, onions, and dozens of other things that contain these phenol bioflavonoids. Reactions can vary from mild to severe and can involve areas from digestive to respiratory. Even the thyroid and adrenals can be affected.

Those who react to the extremely common phenol **gallic acid** can suffer nose and sinus congestion, ringing in the ears, low-back pain, sugar cravings, hyperactivity, behavioural problems, and attention deficit. Another bioflavonoid that can generate similar allergy symptoms is **malvin**, although it can also be the trigger for immune system-related problems, such as **psoriasis**, and MS.

Fermentation by yeast in your small intestine can produce cinnamic acid, gallic acid, and acetaldehyde, which can create sensitivities to chemicals such as **perfumes** and **petroleum products**. Bacteria and yeast in your small intestine also have **decarboxylase enzymes**. These enzymes can convert your amino acids into **vasoactive amines**—such as turning **histadine** into histamine, or tyrosine into **tyramine**—which, along with the indoles from tryptophan, begin to weaken the walls of your intestine.

As if this weren't bad enough, immunoglobulins against these antigens can make your liver valves even more sensitive. As the valves become more sensitive, then **Bloaty** tightens them down even harder—which is going to dump even more protein into your lymph system, creating more antigen that your immune system has to attack.

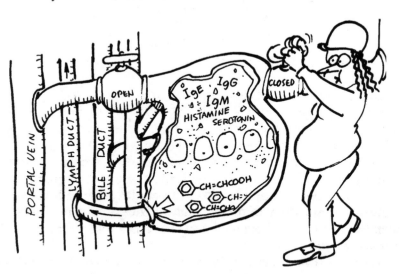

When **Bloaty** tightens down the valves going *into* your liver sinusoids, it causes backup on your portal vein. **Gaspy** and **Spacey** have already told you how this can reduce the blood flow to your heart and brain. The back-pressure on your portal vein can leave the membranes of your intestine "simmerin' in their own toxins." This can further weaken the "brickwork" of your intestinal wall, allowing toxins and partly digested food and even The Boogy Boys to slip between your intestinal cells and into your portal vein. This is called **"leaky gut syndrome."**

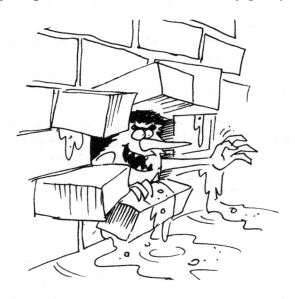

All this junk and debris can put more of a strain on The Kupffer Kops and increases the possibility of The Boogy Boys getting into your main bloodstream, which means your spleen will have to work harder trying to filter them out.

It's not only the digestive organs that drain into your portal vein. The spleen also plays an important role in feeding raw materials through your portal vein to your liver, as **Bloaty** has already explained. With the increase of back-pressure on your portal vein, your spleen swells up to act as a reservoir for the increased fluid.

While this heroic act may temporarily save your body from a lot of grief, it makes my job as immune-coordinator really tough! The intestines are leaking more stuff into your portal vein; the detoxification enzymes and The Kupffer Kops are struggling to keep up with the load; your lymph system is jamming up with fluid, toxins, and proteins; and now, as your spleen tries desperately to incinerate the antigens out of your blood, it can swell up like a birthday balloon! It looks like overtime for me. An overloaded spleen isn't going to break down old and odd-shaped red blood cells as effectively, so their oxygen-carrying ability is also going to be decreased.

The spleen has a lot of blood vessels running into it, which even in the best of times are prone to rupturing in an accident. When your spleen is under back-pressure from your portal vein, it's even more vulnerable to ruptured blood vessels from a sudden jolt.

All the debris of warfare—immune complexes containing dead or dying Boogy Boys or antigens from your food that are impaled with antibodies whose tails are sticking out and "hot"—drift out of the lymph into your bloodstream where they are free to circulate throughout your body until they jam up in some area of poor circulation—like the joints, under the skin, on the membranes, or at the site of a previous injury. When the roving white blood cells spot the hot antibody tails attached to the immune complex log-jams, they zoom in for the kill.

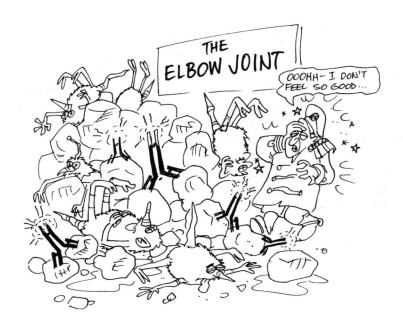

IgM and IgG antibodies especially start the complement cascade and activate neutrophils and macrophages who move in for the finish. Beautiful soldiers with beautiful weapons— built to kill with certainty and effectiveness—that are now about to be used on you, the innocent bystander. You're about to get wounded as the cops and robbers start shooting at each other. Tumour necrosis factor, activated complement enzymes, interleukins, interferons, histamine, serotonin, leukotrienes, major basic protein, membrane attack complex, granzymes, superoxide radicals, hydrogen peroxide, nitric oxide, hydroxyl radicals, hypochlorite, perforins, and lymphotoxins are all from your own immune system.

But, they can make you feel bad—very bad—as they build up in your system. Bacteria dying off release **endotoxin** from their cell walls, and endotoxin can be severely toxic and force **Bloaty** to slam your liver valves tight! Viruses can scuttle out from inside cells destroyed by your immune system and scurry around looking for other places to hide; and yeast die-off can be extremely toxic.

Sometimes, all this is going on quietly in your body without obvious symptoms. Other times, the immune system has the body writhing in pain as you get hit in the shoot-out. There's not much else I can do if **Bloaty** doesn't settle things down at your liver and if she doesn't stop dumping proteins into your lymph. I have to keep your immune system going full-blast. If the thymus gland becomes less active due to stress or low zinc, then allergies can really run amok.

There's only a very fine line between an allergy and an autoimmune disease, but generally, as the spleen gets weaker, the problem gets more serious and mysterious, and peculiar diseases start to appear. Big Momma can lock onto your own IgG in an immune complex—thinking it's a Bad Guy. This is called **rheumatoid factor**.

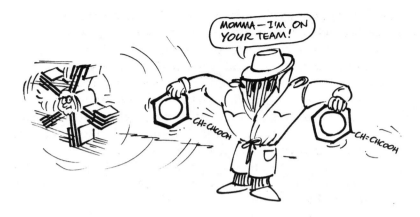

Macrophages that have gobbled up bacteria in the Peyer's patches and then wandered off to other parts of your lymph system might spit the bacteria out instead of digesting them because they are so disoriented from working too hard. This is how the immune system can actually contribute to The Boogy Boys being spread throughout your body.

Yet, there are other potential adversaries with which the immune system has even more trouble than The Boogy Boys. At least The Boogy Boys are easy to identify because they wear cell wall suits that make clear antigens. The others are more elusive. I have a hard time finding them because they change their form so fast. They can hide in the shadows and if you turn up the lights, they quickly change shape and fade away. They can be tiny, like a virus; they can develop into **rods**, like bacteria; they can grow **filaments**, like **mycobacteria**.

They love to reproduce by budding like **yeast**. The official **Liver Dwarves'** name for them is **L-Form**, but I call them **"The Phantom Boogies,"** because as fast as I can pin up a "WANTED" poster of their cell wall in the thymus gland, they've changed their identity by dropping their cell walls and running around half-naked like viruses. What really bugs me to no end is that they enjoy going for joyrides on red blood cells! Then there's **mycoplasma**, which also lacks a cell wall— allowing it to invade your joints so that when your immune system attacks it, you are the one experiencing the pain.

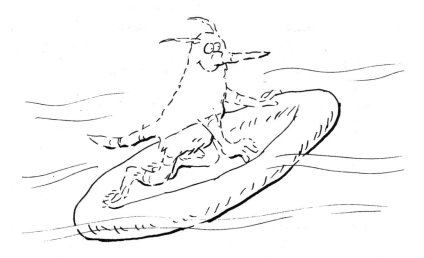

If I could just keep your spleen working well, I could incinerate them when your red blood cells squeeze through your spleen on their regular checkup. But how can I do that if **Bloaty**'s got your liver valves cranked down tight, and your spleen's swollen up like a beach ball? When your spleen's not working right, even "regular" bacteria like Helicobacter can show up inside your body and can be involved in hardening of the arteries.

As if that isn't embarrassing enough, the bacteria **Yersinia** can use toxins to paralyze my macrophages' ability to devour them. Then the whole Yersinia mob climbs aboard the macrophage and goes for a ride around inside you.

Epstein-Barr virus can appear in **lymphoma**, a cancer of the lymph system. Oh, I know that Epstein-Barr's lawyers deny any cause, blame, involvement, association, responsibility, or relationship. They claim circumstantial evidence—pure coincidence that they just happened to be in the vicinity at the time of the crime, minding their own business—but I am highly suspicious.

There's little difference between a persistent nose or skin allergy—where you suffer some discomfort from an enthusiastic but errant immune system—and a full-blown autoimmune disease—where you can suffer serious damage to your body from your own immune system. Any part of your body can be damaged by your immune system. This damage sometimes occurs very quietly, until enough damage is done to create symptoms.

For example, damage to the beta cells of the pancreas by the immune system might take place very slowly and very quietly over a year or two before the symptoms of diabetes would appear. In young children, the antigen triggers could come from cow's milk or other food allergies creating antibodies that cross-react with the beta cells.

When I was a **Liver Dwarf** in New Zealand, I saw that about two years after **influenza B** or **hepatitis B vaccinations** were given, the incidence of diabetes had increased 60 percent. This is because the vaccinations give a sharper rise in the interferon production in the body than a natural infection would. This can cause a slow and destructive autoimmune system reaction in some people, over a long period of time. **Alopecia** (hair loss) can result from high interferon levels triggered by the same vaccinations.

Any part of the body can be damaged by your immune system, but the thyroid is one of the most common. An example of one way that foods can cross-react with parts of the body is the **alpha-gliadin fraction** of **wheat gluten**—it has similar amino acid sequences to thyroglobulin. Thyroid damage can be called **Hashimoto's thyroiditis** or **Graves' disease**, although they actually overlap. Other autoimmune diseases are **lupus**, which attacks the vascular system; **polyarteritis nodosa**, which attacks the arteries; **polymyositis**, the muscles; **scleroderma**, the skin and internal organs; **myasthenia gravis**, the voluntary muscles; **dermatitis herpetiform**, the skin; **Addison's disease**, the adrenal glands; **thrombocytopenia**, the blood platelets; **hemolytic anemia**, the red blood cells; **vitiligo**, the skin; **ankylosing spondylitis** and **rheumatoid arthritis**, the joints—to name a few.

You know by now that all of these problems will have originated back at your liver long before the autoimmune system damage appeared. Toxins from the intestine might have been amplified by the P450 enzymes of the liver faster than your conjugation enzymes could neutralize them, forcing

Bloaty to close down the inlet and/or the outlet liver valves, scattering the toxins into your bile, kidneys, and lymph system.

It pains me immensely to know that my little soldiers—well armed and well intentioned—could, in their haste to clean up your lymph system, further amplify this toxicity and cause damage by creating autoimmune diseases.

There are some things that my little soldiers have been accused of that I think are unjust. **Gastritis** and **duodenal ulcers,** for example, are now being blamed on the immune system. It should be known, however, that I will only send my troops under the membranes of the stomach and duodenum *after* a Boogy Boy—like the sneaky Helicobacter—has already penetrated the membrane. Sure, my troops shooting superoxide radicals may be responsible for most of the damage done, but if your duodenal membrane hadn't been weakened by toxic bile, low zinc, and low bioflavonoids, the Helicobacter never would have gotten under it in the first place.

My dear macrophages have also been accused of causing hardening of your arteries, but this is an accusation very short on evidence. I've questioned many of my leading macrophages and they all have the same story: *NOT GUILTY!* Oh, they were *there* in the coronary arteries and they were *involved*, but they didn't actually *start* it. They say that **low density lipoproteins (LDL)**, which are a type of cholesterol carrier, got into trouble under the membrane of the artery, in the **intima**.

LDL got slightly oxidized by peroxides and they were screaming for help. It's hard to imagine them getting oxidized because I keep them well stocked with membrane protectors like **alpha** and **gamma tocopherol** (vitamin E), **alpha** and **beta carotene**, and **lycopene**. I also keep **high density lipoproteins (HDL)** nearby and they're loaded with the enzymes **paraoxenase** and **platelet-activating factor** to destroy any lipid peroxides on sight.

Anyway, LDL somehow got oxidized, in spite of all my precautions. There was some talk about their defences getting overloaded by a cloud of cigarette smoke and cadmium. Some of my macrophages swore they saw Helicobacter sneaking around in the area but there was a lot of homocysteine obstructing their view. Homocysteine builds up when The

Boogy Boys in the small intestine have stolen the vitamin B_6, vitamin B_{12}, and folic acid that are necessary to convert homocysteine to a less irritating form. Anyway, the alarm bells were ringing so I gave my macrophages permission to go in and try to pull out the LDL—oxidized and in big trouble—deep within the coronary arteries.

Well, okay, okay, so my macrophages *didn't* actually rescue them! As soon as they got in there, they knew by the smell that the LDL were in pretty rough shape and beyond saving. They had to do *something* to clean up the mess so they ate up all the dying LDL. They're not cannibals or anything; they're just very—er—tidy! Very tidy and very efficient.

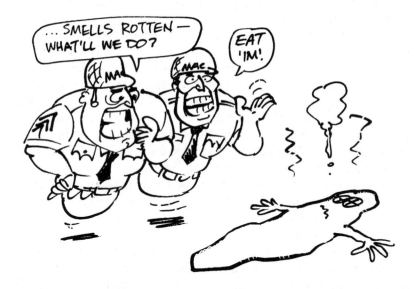

Well, sure, maybe they shot off a few rounds of superoxide and hydrogen peroxide that maybe did a *little* more damage to the arteries, but what do you expect? They're soldiers—trained to kill—not peace negotiators. And many of them gave their lives so that you could live a good life, free of toxic fat. You see, the macrophages who ate a lot of the toxic LDL bloated up so much, they were called **foam cells**—behind their backs, of course. You would never want to call a proud macrophage a foam cell to his face—if you valued your life, that is.

Little did these valiant warriors know that their LDL dinner would cost them their lives. The severe toxicity of the oxidized fats in your LDL killed them! So maybe the macrophages *did* contribute to the fatty plaque plugging up your arteries by dying in your intima from a bellyful of toxic fat. But remember, they *never* started it—and they gave their lives trying desperately to save you.

As the layers of fatty plaque in your arteries pile up, a layer of calcium gets deposited on top, *if* you have low vitamin D activity. Of course, if your vitamin D levels were normal, the calcium would be in your bones where it belongs instead of wandering around in your blood where it could turn your arteries into porcelain. **Itchy** will describe vitamin D next, since that's his department.

You won't know anything about the plaque in your arteries until it's so thick that your coronary arteries are 75 percent blocked. That's when your heart starts to get into serious trouble because of the decreased circulation of oxygen. Of course, the plaque will also be deposited in your other arteries at the same time. If the carotid arteries in your neck were to become substantially blocked, then you would get less circulation to your brain. Plaque in the arteries of the leg can decrease circulation in your legs.

Certainly, if damage is being done to your body by your immune system, then I—as General of your immune army—must be held responsible, but you can rest assured it's not from lack of effort on my part!

Most cancers start in organs that are drained by your portal vein, or cancers may develop because of hormonal imbalances due to problems with the liver enzymes, as **Sluggy** and **Bitchy** will explain later. With all the immune system firepower I have available to give you, you can deal with cancers—if they're caught early when they're small, and if **Bloaty** gives me some room to manoeuvre.

Oh, how I hate pain! I'd do anything to get better! I'll eat anything, drink anything, take any pills! Problem is, I'm allergic to every pill I take, as well as all the foods. Also pollen, dust and dust mites, fur, sun, wind, air. Even hot and cold. I'm sure I'm even allergic to water! In fact, I think I'm allergic to the

whole darn planet! Probably the whole solar system. Hey: I
hear they've found a new planet in a new solar system, only
four light-years away. Maybe I can get a transfer. A fresh start in
a new solar system—sounds pretty good!

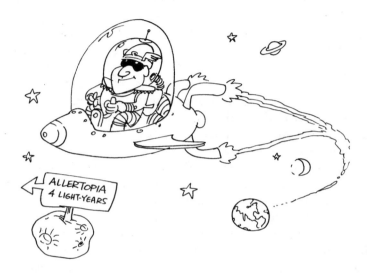

Anything to get rid of all this infernal aching. You can sting
me with bees if you think it would stop this awful pain. I'd
better go check your immune system and see if I can do
anything. I should put every one of those white blood cells up
for a court martial. Attacking their commanding general should
be punishable by death by a firing squad. Actually, a slow,
painful death would be more like what I'm going through now.

Maybe I can find some relief when the new **Liver Dwarf**, the
doctor, gets here. **Itchy** will be along in a minute to give you a
tour of your plumbing. He looks after your kidneys—which
means he's the traitor that let The Boogy Boys into the small
intestine through the ileocecal valve. He ought to be shot!
Never should have let a civilian look after such a strategic point
as the ileocecal valve. Civilians are too soft; should have put
someone tough in charge. Like me! Ouch!!! Did you touch me? I
asked you not to touch me! Don't touch me again—*please*!

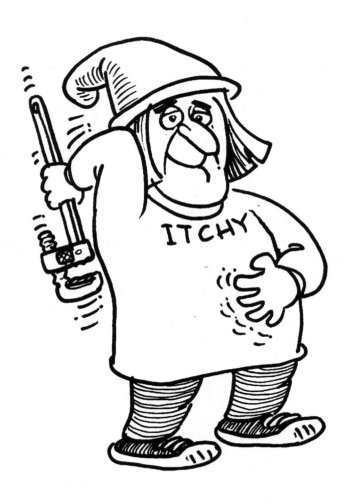

CHAPTER 6

Itchy: Guide to Your Kidneys

Hi: **I'm Itchy, the Kidneys' Liver Dwarf!**

When your **liver's detoxification enzymes** get overloaded, some of the **toxins** spill over into your **blood** and I have to dump them into your **kidneys**, which don't know how to neutralize them. Usually, the kidneys just dump them down your **urinary tract**, irritating the heck out of the whole damn thing, or, if they're in a more rebellious mood, they just dump them out through your **skin**.

Yes, my name's **Itchy**, and boy, am I itching! I just can't stop scratching myself. Would you mind giving me a little scratch between my shoulder blades? I can only reach there with a pipe wrench. Aahhh . . . that feels good. It's been centuries since I've had a good scratch there.

You've probably figured out by now that I'm your **Liver Dwarf** responsible for **skin problems**. Well, I won't beat around the bush. I don't know a darn thing about skin. My job as a **Liver Dwarf** is to keep your kidneys working in harmony with your liver and, since skin problems are usually secondary to liver and kidney problems, then I guess that makes me responsible for your skin, too.

The liver starts the whole process. Normally, your liver detoxification system—the Phase 1 P450 enzymes and the Phase 2 conjugation enzymes—completely deactivates toxins. Then the larger pieces of neutralized debris are removed through the bile by **Burpy**. It's my job to run the smaller pieces out through your kidneys. That's easy for me, unless your Phase 2 conjugation enzymes can't keep up with the Phase 1 P450 enzymes. Remember, the P450s make fatty substances water-soluble by turning them into epoxides. And they spin off a mess of free radicals at the same time—which can generate an ugly mess of fatty peroxides.

The conjugation enzymes need large amounts of specific nutrients to neutralize the toxins and free radicals. If those nutrients aren't readily available, the toxins can't be neutralized so when they leave your liver, the toxins are still "hot." **Burpy** has already told you that all he can do is dump the larger molecules into the bile, resulting in toxic bile and all the digestive problems that it can create. I'm stuck with the same dilemma. If the conjugation enzymes of your liver can't fully neutralize the smaller molecules, then they're passed to me. All I can do is dump them into your kidneys—still hot and still toxic.

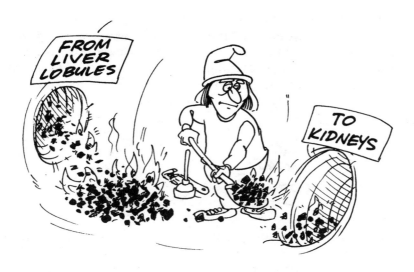

The kidneys are filters, too, but unlike the liver, they're not designed to neutralize these kinds of toxins. All they can do is fire them down the **ureters**, into your **bladder**, and out through your **urethra**. Of course, this can cause a lot of irritation throughout your **urinary system**, especially in your bladder and your urethra.

Irritated membranes become more vulnerable to infections as well, especially if they're low in calcium. Viruses, bacteria, and yeast can then get established there more easily, although the toxins themselves can create a lot of symptoms without an actual infection. If an infection does move up your urinary tract, it can cause serious **kidney problems**.

The kidneys sometimes get a little upset with having to do work that your liver is designed to do so. Sometimes they say, "We're not built for this liver crap; we don't know how to neutralize toxins and we're not going to take it anymore!" and so I have to dump the toxins out through your skin instead—which can weaken it.

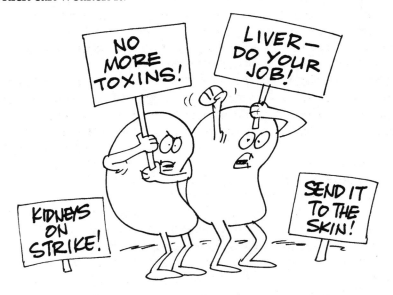

So in a sense, I end up using your skin as an extra kidney. The skin is already covered with bacteria, yeast, and fungus that can now penetrate down into the weakened skin. Oh, you can apply creams and ointments until you're blue in the face, but no topical cream is going to correct your overloaded liver and kidneys.

If **Achy**'s got a lot of antibodies stuck to antigens floating around as immune complexes, many of them attach to the underside of the skin. When the immune system starts shooting away at them, the skin can take a heavy beating that can be manifested on the outside of the skin in the form of rashes, welts, and spots. **Hives** are usually an allergic reaction to **mannan**, which comes from the cell wall of Candida yeast, although hives can also be a reaction to food that's made worse by stress.

With some conditions, like psoriasis, there might even be a little liver damage. Maybe it's passed on genetically through your family tree; maybe it's acquired. As in all chronic disease, you can be sure that there are some allergies present—either obvious or hidden—because you know **Bloaty**'s got the outlet liver valves tightened down and proteins are flooding into the lymph system. Psoriasis usually involves an allergy to the bioflavonoid malvin—'though when you react to one bioflavonoid, you'll usually react to others too, and hundreds of different types of them are found in plants.

There are other ways that your body will use your skin as a kidney. Fluid, in the form of sweat, can be dumped out through your skin. The body would much rather dump out excess through your skin than leave it hanging around internally, where your important organs might get fouled up. So in a sense, your skin is being used as a safety valve to protect your more important internal organs.

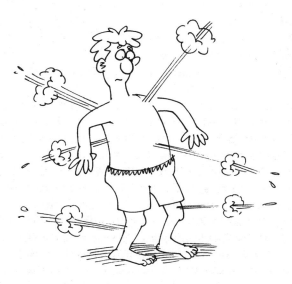

Your skin can also give you some clues as to what's going on inside your body. **Malondialdehyde** is a toxic end-product of lipid peroxidation, made in your body when fats react with free radicals. Malondialdehyde binds with **ethanolamine** to form

lipofuscin. The presence of lipofuscin is seen as brown skin spots; they indicate that peroxides and free radicals have cross-linked fats and proteins together.

These ageing spots are also appropriately called **liver spots**. The *external* spots don't give an accurate picture of the extent of the lipid peroxidation-driven damage *internally*, but you can be sure that what you see—the spots—are just the tip of a fairly large iceberg. Fortunately, it's possible to slow—and perhaps even reverse—a bit of the ageing process, as the doctor, the new **Liver Dwarf**, can hopefully explain . . . if he *ever* shows up!

Your liver can put your kidneys under a great deal of stress in other ways. **Bloaty** may tighten down the inlet valves of your liver to the extent that portal vein back-pressure becomes high enough to open up veins that have been unused since you took your first breath after birth. These dormant veins include the veins that once carried your mother's nutrients from her placenta to you, and that delivered your wastes back to her liver. When back-pressure on your portal vein opens these long-unused veins, they can then dump intestinal toxins directly into your kidneys without any liver detoxification being done first, and that can cause more severe kidney damage.

Another indirect way that your liver puts stress on your kidneys is if **Bloaty** tightens down the valves going out of your liver, so that fluid buildup in your liver causes it to enlarge. As **Bloaty** explained, when the back side or caudate lobe of your liver swells, it can pinch off your inferior vena cava, the vein that drains your kidneys, legs, and pelvic area. Pinching off the inferior vena cava can interfere with drainage from the kidneys, lowering their blood pressure, thus leaving them choking in their own toxins and interfering with their ability to function.

Fortunately, I've found a way to deal with this. You see, I keep some **prorenin** stored away in your kidneys. If **Bloaty** starts swelling the liver up so that it interferes with the inferior vena cava and your kidneys' blood flow is reduced, then I hit the panic button and prorenin turns into the active enzyme **renin**—which activates the release of **angiotensin I**. That tightens up your blood vessels to increase your pressure and get your circulation going.

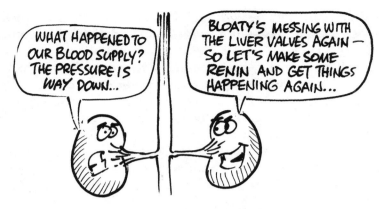

KIDNEY CONVERSATION

If this doesn't work, I run over to your lungs where I borrow an enzyme to convert angiotensin I into **angiotensin II**, a much stronger constrictor of blood vessels, which also causes the kidneys to retain salt and water. This usually gets the job done, and now your blood is flying through the narrowed inferior vena cava. This makes your kidneys happy again. Of course, it also raises the **blood pressure** in the rest of your body above what might be a safe level. But my first responsibility is to look after your kidneys, and I've done my task well. I guess that makes ME a fairly important **Liver Dwarf**!?

If **Bloaty** gets your liver-swelling under control and stops pushing on your inferior vena cava, then I can get your blood pressure back on track in no time. If damage to your liver—like cirrhosis—or damage to the kidneys has been done, I might have to keep your blood pressure high to keep your kidneys working. But if there's no damage and **Bloaty** gives me a chance, I'll get your blood pressure straightened out quickly.

There's another way you can get high blood pressure without the production of renin, yet it still has to do with my work down in your kidneys. If you're low in calcium, your **parathyroid glands**—four pea-sized glands found in your thyroid gland—make **parathyroid hypercytocalcic factor (PHF)**. PHF makes vascular smooth muscle cells in your blood vessels more sensitive to hormones that cause constriction of the blood vessels and, in turn, this constriction causes high blood pressure. People with high PHF are salt-sensitive since salt increases fluid retention, which makes the blood pressure worse.

So you can see that low calcium can cause trouble—which is what makes me your most important **Liver Dwarf**. I'm responsible for your kidneys, which also puts me in charge of your ileocecal valve. Like all the membranes in your body, your ileocecal valve is kept strong by calcium, the "cement" of your body. Calcium keeps things tough. Well, guess who's responsible for getting calcium into your body and keeping it there? Yes, that's right, it's me, **Itchy** the **Plumber—King of your Kidneys**, the key to your health!

You see, calcium is a tough mineral, but it's even tougher to absorb. First, you need **stomach acid** to **chelate** it, which means bind it to a carrier to help it cross through your intestinal membrane. Yet even then, less than one-third of the calcium would be absorbed. The rest goes out with your stool. This is where vitamin D comes in. Vitamin D is made in your skin when it is exposed to the **ultraviolet rays** of the sun. Vitamin D is stored in your liver, but to be stored, it has to be inactive. When it's released from liver storage, your liver converts it from **cholecalciferol (vitamin D_3)** to **25-hydroxycholecalciferol (calcidiol)**, which activates calcium absorption a little.

Let me tell you straight out that this is a pretty weak attempt at improving calcium absorption. It might be good enough for Hawaii, where your skin's making a lot of vitamin D from the sun, but it's never going to get the job done for Eskimos in the winter when there's little or no sunlight.

The real action doesn't start until I activate vitamin D. When I've finished running calcidiol through your kidneys in the presence of **parathyroid hormone**, it has become the strongest form of vitamin D_3; it improves calcium absorption 1,000 times more than that wimpy, weak-kneed stuff made by the liver. Its technical name is **1, 25-dihydroxycholecalciferol** but I call it **calcitriol**, for short. This is *winter-strength* vitamin D. Within two days, my superactivated form of vitamin D stimulates your **intestinal cells** to make a **calcium-binding protein**, which transports calcium from your intestine into your portal vein at a dramatically higher rate.

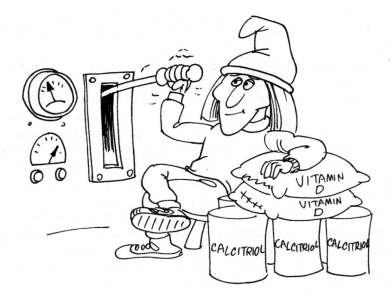

Taking extra calcium in your diet doesn't do you much good if I'm not on the job at your kidneys, activating vitamin D in conjunction with hormones from your parathyroid glands.

Once the calcium has arrived in your blood, I still control the calcium levels because I'm continually running the minerals along the membranes of your kidney plumbing as I maintain the proper fluid and mineral balance levels. **Sodium, potassium, chlorine, calcium, magnesium, urea**, and **phosphate levels** are readily controlled by me. As I'm juggling all these minerals, if one is in excess, it's easy for me to let one drop, and out it goes in your urine!

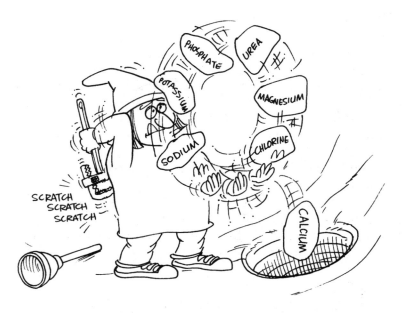

If your insulin levels are high due to high-sugar foods or low levels of **GTF chromium**, then I have to dump a lot of calcium out in the urine, which can lead to the formation of kidney stones. High caffeine intake can make me dump even more calcium out of your kidneys.

The urea that I have to deal with at the kidneys contains **nitrogen** and hydrogen in the form of **ammonia**. Ammonia is released when amino acids are broken down in three places: 1) your liver; 2) your muscles; and 3) your intestines.

The primary place of ammonia production is in your liver when there are too many amino acids to be stored. The surplus amino acids are broken down into sugar to be used for energy or stored as fat. The ammonia leftovers are toxic so, in your liver, I bind two ammonias together with carbon dioxide to create urea, which can be sent safely through the blood to the kidneys where I can eliminate it in your urine.

The second source of ammonia is when amino acids are broken down in your muscles to supply energy when the muscles are working anaerobically. The ammonia is then bound to **alanine** to make it nontoxic for shipping through your blood to your liver for processing.

The third source of ammonia is The Boogy Boys—when they eat amino acids in your intestine. They're not so thoughtful about what they do with their nitrogen wastes. They just dump their toxic ammonia into your intestines where it gets picked up by your portal vein and sent to your liver. The ammonia from both these sources—your muscles and The Boogy Boys—is converted into urea by your liver for shipping to your kidneys. So you can see that creating urea is one way that I eliminate nitrogen safely from your body.

I should tell you that I'm not in a big hurry to eliminate all this nitrogen. As you probably know already, through a genetic mutation that happened a very long time ago, one of your ancestors lost the ability to make **ascorbate** in the body— otherwise known as **ascorbic acid** or **vitamin C**—so now you can only get vitamin C from your diet.

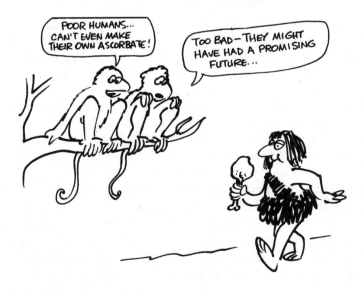

The loss of a steady supply of the antioxidant ascorbic acid could have led to dire consequences for your health and lifespan if I, **Itchy**, the one responsible for your kidney function, hadn't done some quick calculations and adjustments. I figured out that reabsorbing over 90 percent of the **uric acid**—which contains nitrogen—from your kidneys and maintaining a higher uric acid level in the blood might solve some of the problems associated with an unreliable supply of ascorbic acid.

My calculations showed that uric acid could be a good scavenger of free radicals, capable of protecting your DNA and cell membranes from superoxide, peroxides, and even from the deadly hydroxyl radicals just as well as ascorbic acid can. It turns out that my calculations were wrong. Uric acid turned out to be even *better* than ascorbic acid at many of the same jobs of defending you, one of the reasons why you can live to a greater age than animals who can make their own ascorbic acid but who have low levels of uric acid. Of course, uric acid can't replace vitamin C entirely, as there are still some jobs that only ascorbic acid can do.

Your uric acid levels can get too high and form **crystals** of uric acid—often in your big toes—which your immune system then attacks, causing intense inflammation and pain. This is called **gout**. While everyone is quick to give me the blame for this, you should understand that people with gout usually also have blood sugar problems, and high cholesterol due to liver problems. Excess uric acid can also contribute to inflammation of your muscles.

Everybody also tries to blame me for letting The Boogy Boys get through the ileocecal valve into your small intestine. But hey—I'm just doing my job the best I can.

The ileocecal valve problems start when people get me all confused by mixing up their diets and the seasons. You know from **Spacey** that your body adapts to changes of night and day, and to changes in the seasons as measured by the amount of light received by your eyes and their message is forwarded to your pineal gland. The neurotransmitters serotonin and melatonin are adjusted to the *daily* rhythms of sunrise/sunset, and these hormones can have a profound effect on your body and mind. The female hormonal tides are synchronized to the *monthly* cycle of the moon.

I have to adjust vitamin D activity with the seasons, because your skin makes tremendous amounts of vitamin D from the sun in the summer, and often none in the shorter days of winter. Obviously, I've got to activate vitamin D a lot more in winter, and tone it down considerably in the summer. The problem is in determining whether it's swimming weather or skiing weather, and whether to activate vitamin D weakly by the liver, or strongly by the kidneys.

It's completely dark down here in your kidneys, so I can't see whether flowers are blooming or snow is falling. I ordered a periscope from Army and Navy Surplus but it never arrived. I've never even received a complimentary calendar from the local insurance agent. No, I have to guess which season it is, based on the food that's coming in through your diet, and much of my judgment is based on the minerals I detect in those foods.

One of the things I have to do is maintain an equal balance between sodium and potassium. As seasons change, the balance between sodium and potassium in the diet tends to change. This gives me a clue as to what the season is, and allows me to use those fluctuations to warm or cool your body to suit the weather.

You see, when it's been warm for a while in the spring, greens start to come into the body. I can tell it's spring because these foods are fairly high in potassium, which has a cooling effect on your body when I run it through your kidneys.

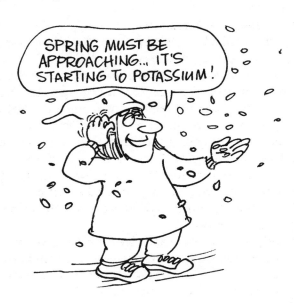

I decrease the activation of vitamin D, knowing you must be out in the sun by now, making vitamin D in your skin from the sun's rays.

After it's been hot for months, berries start to come into the body and they're even higher in potassium, which I use to cool your body down even more; I also reduce the activation of vitamin D more, in expectation of the tremendous hours of sunlight that must be out there to ripen the fruit.

Also, the sugars in these foods give me an important clue that it's been sunny and warm for quite a while because I know it takes months of warm weather to grow sugar. When I see bananas and papayas—and what a whopping dose of potassium and sugars they're carrying!—I cool down your body to the max. I also cut way back on the activation of vitamin D, to allow for the searing levels of tropical ultraviolet rays that you must be exposed to when you're out picking these fruits in the tropical sun.

Of course, things go the other way in the fall and winter. Plants stop growing and so potassium and sugars decrease. This is when foods higher in sodium and fat appear more in the diet.

I can use the higher sodium levels to help warm the body as I run it through the kidneys. I also begin to activate vitamin D more with the shorter days and less sunlight.

What really throws me off, down in your kidneys, is that lately we've been getting fruit and fruit juices year-round— even in cold climates. Watermelon, tropical fruits, and salad in winter. Summer foods in winter. How amazing! How confusing! How do they do that? To make it worse, they're not adding **salt** to anything!

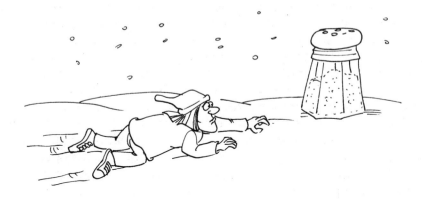

Okay, so too much salt and protein can be bad for you, and drive calcium out of the kidneys, but *no* salt *and* low amounts of animal protein are brutal to me on kidney duty! How can I get enough sodium to keep your kidneys running? One of the things I have to do is always keep an equal balance of sodium and potassium. I use the subtle seasonal shifts in sodium/potassium levels in the diet to aid body temperature regulation, but now here comes a high-potassium, low-sodium diet that I'm supposed to do something with!

I'm a hard worker, I can make it work, for a while—as long as the weather's warm. As soon as the weather cools off, though—BINGO! There go the calcium levels down the tubes, literally, as I struggle to keep your kidneys working. Having to deal with your eating cooling foods in cool weather is too much for me! I get all confused and stop activating vitamin D; within a few days, a lot of your calcium can get dumped because, as you know, less vitamin D means less calcium absorption. Now, this likely won't show on a blood test for calcium levels because I absolutely have to keep your blood calcium levels balanced or you could be dead in minutes. No, I'll have to pull the calcium out of your membranes first, then out of your nerves and your bones.

Now your intestinal membranes, including your ileocecal valve, start to become more sensitive without the toughening effect of calcium. Coarse fibres can really aggravate the valve now. Bran muffins, popcorn, granola, and coarse salads are a few of the things that can aggravate the proper functioning of your now-sensitive ileocecal valve.

To us **Liver Dwarves**, your ileocecal valve is just a trap door through which we toss our table scraps after we've extracted the valuable nutrients out of them. Then we quickly slam the door before any of The Boogy Boys can get into the small intestine. To them, though, your ileocecal valve is like the door to Heaven. They mill around below your valve, waiting for it to open. They jockey like sailboats tacking for position at the start of a race, eager to be first in line when the skies part suddenly and Manna falls from Heaven! They push and shove to get a share of this glorious, divine offering from above.

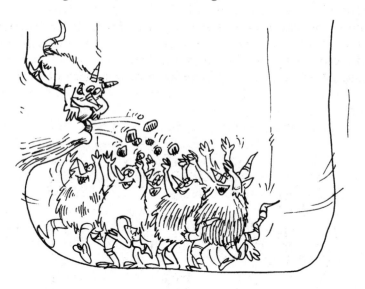

At night, I'm sure they dream of getting through this barrier to the land of "milk and honey." When hungry, they will certainly push and shove en masse against your valve, trying to shoulder their way through. Perhaps their grandmothers sat them on their knees when The Boogy Boys were very young, and told them ancient stories of how this land was once theirs—until they were routed out during troubled times—but that one day, they would be returned to their "promised" land. The Boogy Boys have a legend that their ancestors once controlled the Earth and that magicians among them during their Golden Era solved the riddle of how to capture energy and train IT to work for them. How to make IT remains a secret to them and their descendants.

Yet, IT is in great demand by others. To The Boogy Boys, IT is sacred, and they wouldn't give IT away, never mind sell IT. So those who want IT and ITS powers must take IT from them by force and hang on to IT intently, as they will surely attempt to get IT back. To them, IT is Holy: their Holy Grail. To me, their legends are a crock of hooey. It's just vitamin B_{12} they're talking about, nothing magical about that! They'll never take your B_{12} as long as I can keep them out of your small intestine!

In their brainwashed little minds, they feel they *deserve* to be in your small intestine so they can search for their Grail. What a bunch of stupid bacteria! All this fuss over B_{12}! **I'm** the one that keeps them out by toughening your ileocecal valve with calcium. I told you I was your most important **Liver Dwarf**!

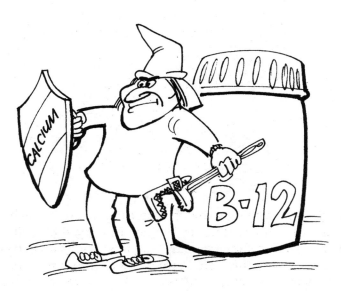

I'd *never* let that rabble into your small intestine if I could run your kidneys according to the seasons, the way I was trained to. How was I to know that you would eat so many summer foods in winter, and then I'd end up being the bad guy by not activating vitamin D and thus end up decreasing your calcium absorption and weakening your ileocecal valve? And even if I did get your calcium absorbed, how was I supposed to know you'd eat so much sugar, coffee, and sodas that you'd flush it right out in your urine?

So one day, The Boogy Boys are milling around your ileocecal valve, jostling for position. They push together against your valve and, because of the low calcium, the walls crumble as if Joshua had blown his trumpet, and the valve pops open when it shouldn't. Then The Boogy Boys—slowly at first—start to crawl out of their dark hole into your small intestine with its booty of bountiful food, its vacuum-cleaner-like absorption, and its complex yet very fragile, velvety walls. Their ugly party has begun. Where will it end? A little bloating and indigestion? Perhaps a little emotional instability or some fatigue? Or maybe it'll go all the way to **MS** or **arthritis** or **cancer** or **mental disease** or the hundreds of variations that your body can come up with as your liver desperately shunts toxins into your bile, kidneys, and lymph.

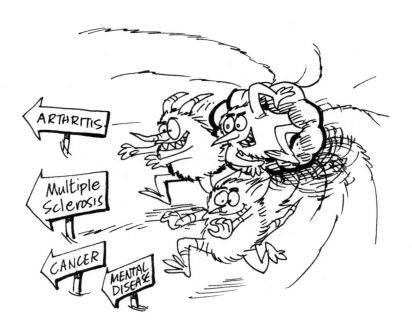

Their party of horror is beginning and suddenly, I'm not feeling very well. I'm itchy. Could you please give me another little scratch between my shoulder blades? Oh, don't stop! It feels so good. **Bitchy** will be along soon to continue your tour. Did I say **Bitchy**? I better get going before *she* shows up. She's scary. I'm outta here!

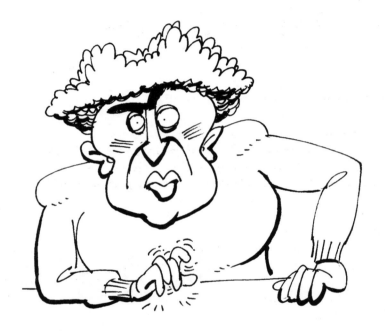

CHAPTER 7

Bitchy: Guide to Hormones

Hey: **I'm Bitchy, the Hormone Liver Dwarf.**
When your **liver enzymes** become **jammed up with toxins,** I can't break down your **hormones** efficiently so I use another **enzyme system** that makes hormones that are MONSTROUS!

What took you so long! I've been waiting two minutes already, you schmuck! I'm **Bitchy**, and I know what you're thinking. You're thinking that I'm a female and my hormones must be out of whack, and that's why I'm Bitchy! Well, you're wrong!

I'm **Bitchy** because those damn doctors and those damn chemical companies they work for have been mucking around with my hormones for too damn long. What am I, anyway? Some kind of guinea pig they get to practise their latest experiments on? I'm going to give you a tour of hormones, but I just might change my mind, so don't ask me any stupid questions!

You should already know that hormones are messengers sent through your blood from one part of your body to other parts, so that the cells work together. For a cell to receive a message from a hormone, it has to have receptors—either on the cell membrane (outside or inside) or deep inside the cell near the DNA—so that a hormone can dock like a boat in a marina.

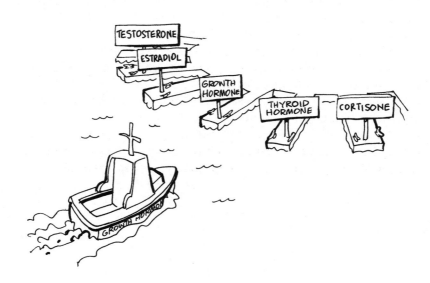

A single cell might have thousands of receptors that can receive messages from a number of different hormones. Without a specific receptor for a specific hormone, a cell can't receive or react to its message. The number of receptors constantly changes, and their sensitivity to hormones can also change!

Almost all cells have receptors for growth hormone from your **anterior pituitary gland** and for thyroid hormone from your thyroid gland because these hormones stimulate growth and increase rates of oxygen use—so important to all cells. Other hormones target more specific cells: for example, the **digestive hormones** primarily affect digestive organs.

The **sex hormones—testosterone, estrogens**, and **progesterone**—are **steroid hormones** that mainly target **sex organs**. All steroids hormones originate from **cholesterol**, which comes from your diet or is made in your body. Much of your steroid-building is done in your **adrenal glands** and involves enzymes—including P450 enzymes—NADPH, and oxygen. The **adrenal cortex** makes small amounts of the sex hormones as well as **adrenocortical hormones**. Cholesterol is turned into **pregnenolone**, which can be turned into progesterone and/or **DHEA**—these can then be converted into adrenocortical hormones, estrogens, and testosterone.

Now, you're probably getting confused. Progesterone is supposed to be a **female hormone** and testosterone is supposed to be a **male hormone**! Looks like you're wrong so far, because both hormones are found in males and females. So your adrenal glands can create many of your steroid hormones. I know a lot of this sounds very complicated, but it's just part of a long list of things that we **Liver Dwarves** have learned to build up from a simple starting compound, **isopentenyl pyrophosphate**.

ALDOSTERONE

ESTRADIOL

CORTISONE

TESTOSTERONE

ESTRONE

CORTICOSTERONE

CORTISOL

ANDROSTENEDIONE

DHEA

PROGESTERONE

PREGNENOLONE

BILE ACIDS

VITAMIN D

CHOLESTEROL

VITAMIN A

RUBBER

VITAMIN E

CHLOROPHYLL

VITAMIN K

CAROTENOIDS

COENZYME Q

Δ^3-ISOPENTENYL PYROPHOSPHATE

At **puberty**, the **testes** and **ovaries** begin to make a lot more of the sex hormones and take the testosterone a step further to make **estradiol**, the strongest of the estrogens. That's what I said—estrogens—plural. There's no such thing as estrogen— there are only estrogens, with an "**s**" on the end. There are over 20 estrogens altogether, but the three most important are **estradiol, estrone,** and **estriol**. You had better remember that because I may give you a quiz later. You better listen more carefully, or I'll leave. Do you think I have time to waste with people who don't listen? So smarten up, or you'll have to stay after class and write lines! And what are you chewing?! Is that gum?! Spit it out right now or I won't continue! And sit up straight!

That's better. Where was I? Oh, yes. Both men and women make progesterone, testosterone, and estrogens. After puberty, women make 6 percent as much testosterone as men do, and men make about 20 percent as many estrogens as women do.

Men make most of their estrogens in their liver, while women make their testosterone in their ovaries. At puberty, increased **luteinizing hormone (LH)** from the **pituitary gland** stimulates the testes in males to secrete more testosterone. The enzyme **5α-reductase** then begins to convert it within the cells to **dihydrotestosterone (DHT)**, which has a much stronger effect for bringing out male characteristics.

LH has a different effect in women. For the first two weeks of a woman's month-long menstrual cycle, her pituitary makes LH as well as **follicle-stimulating hormone (FSH)**; these hormones stimulate a **follicle** in the ovary to make more estrogens. This prepares her body—especially the **uterus**—for **pregnancy**. After about two weeks, an increase in LH and FSH trigger **ovulation**.

The **egg** is released from the follicle and the remaining cells in the follicle become the **corpus luteum**, which secretes large amounts of progesterone and estrogens. If pregnancy doesn't occur, then the production of estrogens and progesterone drops off dramatically, and menstruation soon follows. Progesterone levels stay low until the next **ovum** is released from the opposite ovary about two weeks after menstruation, as the cycle repeats itself.

If the ovum gets fertilized and a **placenta** is formed, the placenta makes large amounts of estriol. At one-eightieth the strength of estradiol, estriol from the placenta is just what the baby ordered for a nice, soothing, nine-month ride. The whole pelvic area thrives on this mild "baby-strength" version of the estrogens—it keeps the membranes moist and strong.

Estradiol is crucial for successful reproduction. Its great strength, however, can overwhelm the tissue it was designed to stimulate. The strong stimulation of estradiol can result in **benign growths**, such as **fibrocystic breast disease**. As a local defence against this overstimulation of the breast, I keep a handy store of **iodine** in the breast to neutralize the stimulation of estrogens. This helps protect the breast from irritants like estradiol, which can result in excess potassium being packaged into **cysts** in the breast tissue.

The other thing I do with these strong hormones—testosterone, estrogens, and progesterone—is that I keep them bound to proteins as long as I can. As long as they're bound, they're out of commission. Also, I break them down into less active hormones as quickly as I can. For example, I only keep estradiol for a very short time; then I convert it into **estrone**, which has only one-twelfth the strength of estradiol. There are two routes for this conversion into estrone—the **C-2 pathway** and the **C-16 pathway**—one of which can lead to cancer, as I'll soon show you.

If necessary, I can also convert estrone back into estradiol. This comes in handy after **menopause** when the ovaries can't make estradiol any more. The adrenals and fat cells can still make estrone, and I can convert it to estradiol, as needed. The important thing is not to have too many fat cells after menopause, or you may end up with an even greater risk of **breast cancer** because of a higher production of estrogens.

Today, there is a steady increase in breast cancer in many countries, and where breast cancer goes up, **prostate cancer** goes up, as well. This tendency runs in families also. In fact, my mother and aunts all died of breast cancer. My father and his brother died of prostate cancer. My brother has already died of it, too. I know I'm going to get cancer. I'm doomed! (*Sob!*)

I shouldn't have taken those **birth control pills** all those years. Those **synthetic estrogens** and **progestins** probably pushed me over the edge! There are probably little tumors growing in my breast right now. I should go for a mammogram! No, the x-rays will probably make it grow faster.

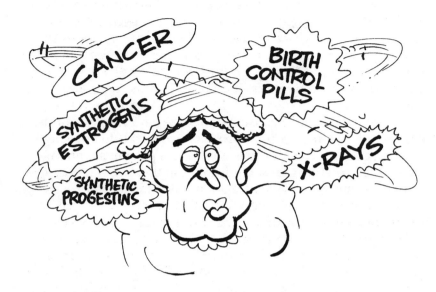

What can I do? I wish the doctor, the new **Liver Dwarf**, would hurry up and get here. Maybe he can help me! I must go on; after all, I'm a **Liver Dwarf** and **Liver Dwarves** never give up!

The important thing to do is run the hormones through the liver as quickly as possible, so it can turn them into much milder forms. But there are problems sometimes. Broken down by the liver and **conjugated**, most of the estradiol and estrone is then quickly secreted out through the kidneys. Twenty percent, however, passes into the bile, which is then secreted into the intestine by **Burpy**, especially when fat is eaten.

If the bowels are working well and the intestinal flora is normal, the fibre in the stool will pull out most of these hormones. But sluggish bowels, high-fat, low-fibre diets and Boogy Boys partying can not only lead to reabsorption of these hormones, but The Boogy Boys can also convert them back into . . . the (*screech!*) the . . . dreaded **16α-hydroxyestrone**. How I *hate* 16α-hydroxyestrone! It's the Monster of the estrogens. I know The Boogy Boys are out to kill me with 16α-hydroxyestrone. I need help! Oh, when is the doctor going to come and save me?

I must go on. I have to be strong (*sniff*). I must learn to stand up and face the dangers of 16α-estrogens, especially 16α-hydroxyestrone. You see, there's more than one method of breaking down estradiol into estrone. There are two different ways to run estradiol through the liver enzymes, and each produces different results. The C-2 pathway creates **2-hydroxyestrone**, which is fine by me—it's mild and I call it my angelic estrogen because it's so sweet and lovable—but the C-16α pathway makes 16α-hydroxyestrone, a B-I-G problem. That nasty stuff doesn't want to bind to a protein so it hangs around the receptors longer, stimulating them way too long— and that can spell trouble with a capital C for cancer.

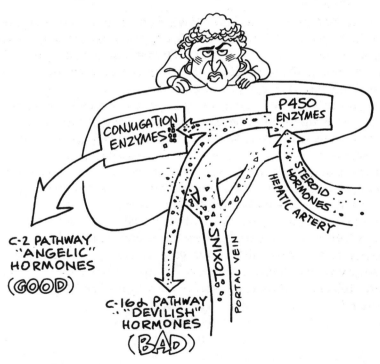

I call 16α-hydroxyestrone the devilish estrogen because it gets this devilish glint in its eye as it struts over to the *susceptible* organs—you know: the breast, uterus, and ovaries—and then proceeds to kick the crap out of them, at the same time spearing them with its sharp three-pointed spear, the trident.

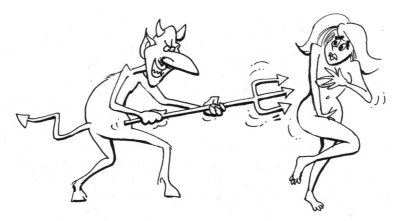

I try to be a good little **Liver Dwarf** and run all the hormones from the hepatic artery through the C-2 liver pathway as I was taught so many years ago at **Liver Dwarf College**. But the C-2 pathway needs the same P450 and conjugation enzymes as the toxins entering the liver via the portal vein.

The success of the C-2 pathway in producing mild, angelic hormones lies in quick, effective access to these enzymes. So what the heck do you think I can do if the damn C-2 pathway's all jammed up with all that #&!*$% **chemical crap from plastics**, like **bisphenol-A**, which lines the inside of tin cans and gets into the food. Or **phthalates** found in plastic wrappings that can also get into food. Or **red dye number 3**, which is deliberately put into food like hot dogs. And **pesticides**, like **endosulphan, alachor, chlordane, dieldrin, heptachlor, atrazine**, and **mirex**—all of which can screw up your ability to break down your steroid hormones. And what about **formaldehyde** in the glues used in carpets and pressed-wood products!

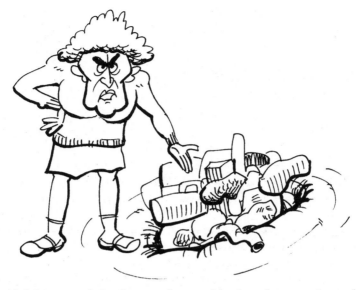

As if this weren't bad enough, you're already carrying a load of **PCBs**, **DDT**, **dioxins**, and **metals** that I wasn't able to deal with years ago when you were first exposed to them so I just stored them in your fat cells. Dioxins and PCBs in meat and dairy products, along with bleached products, like tampons, can also cause **endometriosis**. These chemicals have spread to the far corners of the world, so even moving to the country won't get you away from their dastardly influence on C-2 hormone breakdown.

And then there are chemicals like **nonylphenol ethoxylates** in **laundry detergents** and **household cleaners**, **toluene** in **makeup**, and **isopropyl alcohol**, **ethylene oxide**, and **dioxane** in **shampoo**—to name a few. **Cocamide DEA**, which is also found in shampoo, can form cancer-causing **nitrosamines** if it combines with **nitrites** or formaldehyde.

Benzene is a solvent found in **lubricants** intended for sexual purposes, and also in **disinfectants**; benzene suppresses your immune system by destroying your bone marrow. Solvents like benzene, **acetone**, and toluene are used to process and extract fat from some foods, such as **"diet," "fat-free," "salt-free," "decaffeinated," "lite,"** and **"imitation"** foods. **Benzoic acid**—also known as **methylparaben** or **propylparaben**—is a version of benzene that's used as a **food preservative**. These chemicals may cause health problems for some people.

There are 71,000 more chemicals. They're everywhere and they're profitable, so they're not likely to go away. They're in the food, the water, and the air. What am I supposed to do when all these chemicals have overloaded your liver? And what am I supposed to do when you use drugs that really muck up the C-2 pathway? And what can I do with all that fried food and sugar crap you've been shovelling down all these years, and that have been jamming up your liver even more?

Hey—look at me when I'm speaking to you! I'm asking you a question and I demand an answer! What am I supposed to do with those damn estrogens if the C-2 pathway is all plugged up?! And just because you may be a man doesn't mean this won't apply to you! Men make estradiol, too, and if you want to keep your precious manhood working right, you'd better pay closer attention. These same hormone-mimicking chemicals can give you testicular cancer, lower sperm counts, and smaller penises. These chemicals have already made you half the man your grandfather was, and I'm not just talking about the amount of hair on your head, big boy!

Do you see what you've done to me? Do you see that you've given me no choice? I must run your steroid hormones through the C-16α pathway. What else can I do? So I run estradiol through the C-16α pathway and you get 16α-hydroxyestrone, the MONSTER hormone! I hope you survive it. I hope I can survive you!

Estradiol isn't the only hormone I run through the C-16α pathway, and 16α-hydroxyestrone isn't the only hormone made on this pathway. But 16α-hydroxyestrone is the scariest, because it can *kill*. Oh sure, the C-16α pathway hormones can create all kinds of menstrual problems, like irregular periods, cramping, fluid retention, and even infertility. Some of the other **Liver Dwarves** even think that these 16α-hormones can make you moody and irritable, but look at ME! I'm normal! And I'd kill the little bastards if they'd ever said that to my face!

Things like dioxins and cigarette smoking stimulate the C-2 pathway, but why prevent breast cancer with **lung cancer**? Maybe the doctor can give us more insights when he shows up.

Melatonin can help inhibit breast cancer, but the pineal gland's ability to create melatonin decreases with age, and can also be interfered with by bright lights at night and overexposure to electromagnetic waves from computers and other electrical gadgets. Shift work and its constant changes can also throw the pineal gland's production of melatonin off, because it takes about six days for it to adjust to a bedtime change.

What I'd like to talk about next are thyroid hormones because they also burn me up. The thyroid gland in the neck selects **iodine** and the amino acid tyrosine from the blood and builds them together into large units called **thyroglobulin**. For iodine to be bound to tyrosine, the peroxidase enzyme and hydrogen peroxide are needed. Thyroglobulin can store two to three months' supply of the thyroid hormones **triiodothyronine** (T_3) and **thyroxine** (T_4). When thyroid hormones are needed, the body splits them from thyroglobulin, and releases them into the blood, mainly as T_4—which contains two tyrosines and four iodines.

T_4 is relatively inactive, and only the brain prefers to use it. Other tissues would rather use T_3, which has one less iodine than T_4 and a much stronger effect. One of my jobs is to split off one of the iodines from T_4—mainly at the liver—to make the more active T_3.

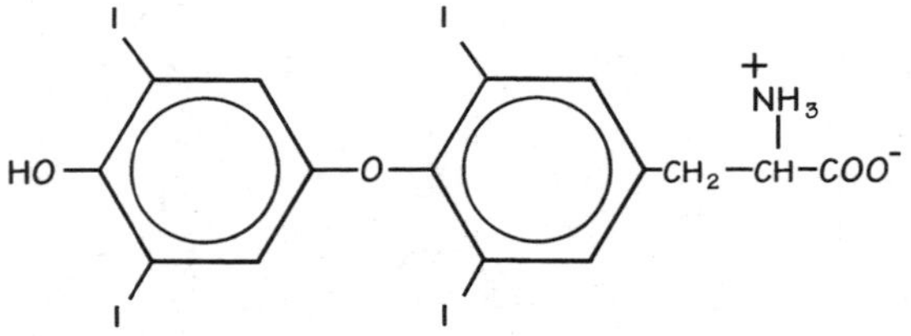

THYROXINE (T_4)

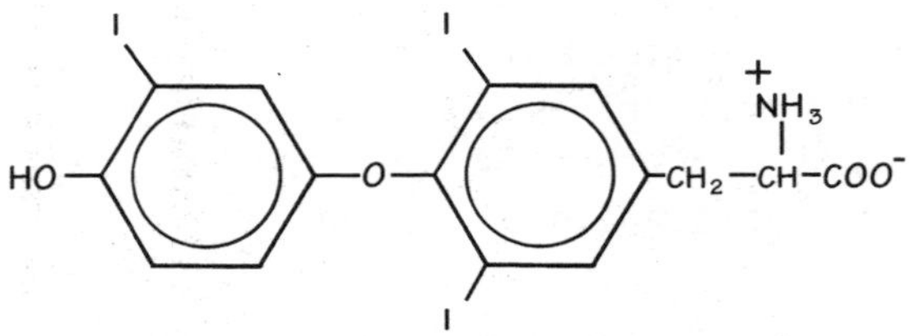

TRIIODOTHYRONINE (T_3)

The receptors for the thyroid hormones are found deep within the cells, close to their DNA. When thyroid hormones, especially T_3, bind to their receptors, these cells quickly get to work and increase their enzyme production up to six-fold, which can dramatically increase their use of fuel and oxygen and, of course, this process gives off heat.

In blood tests, large numbers of people are found to have abnormal thyroid function and are put on thyroid hormone—usually synthetic—with little consideration given as to why their thyroid is malfunctioning. Even if the use of thyroid hormone corrects the blood test, and some of their worst symptoms are improved, many of the other nagging complaints may refuse to go away entirely. This is because the blood tests are *missing the underlying problems*.

Thyroid hormone doesn't work in the blood, *it works inside every cell* of the body, particularly in those that must be the most active. If T_3 isn't available at the cellular level, then those cells can't function properly. The one universal characteristic of low thyroid activity is low body temperature. Since a side effect of work is heat, then low body temperature indicates low work levels in the body as a whole, especially in cells that have a lot of work to do.

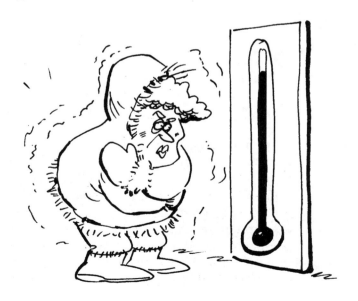

For example, the liver needs a lot of T_3 to handle fats in the blood properly. Maybe even more important, the stomach needs T_3 to make **hydrochloric acid (HCl)** because that is hard work: it takes more than 1,500 calories to make one litre of gastric juice—which is mainly HCl, as **Bloaty** probably told you.

Low hydrochloric acid production can allow The Boogy Boys to creep further up the small intestine after they've gotten through your ileocecal valve. Taking HCl capsules can alleviate many of the digestive symptoms that accompany low HCl production but this doesn't solve the mystery as to why your stomach wasn't making acid in the first place. What has been overlooked is that even if you have the correct amount of T_4 in your blood, it's not fully active until broken down into T_3. And even if you have the right amount of T_3, it's going to have no effect on the cellular DNA until it binds to the T_3 receptors.

The common missing link in all of these biochemical reactions is **zinc**.

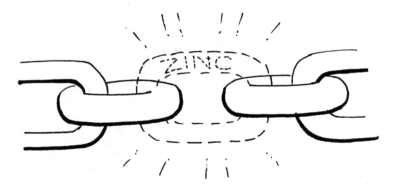

Zinc is necessary in over 200 enzyme systems in the body, including the enzymes that convert T_4 to T_3. Zinc is also the key ingredient in many of the cell receptors, as well as being the hub of the **templates for DNA transcriptions**. Zinc forms very distinctive structures called **zinc fingers**.

If T_3 is in low supply in the stomach due to low zinc, the stomach may be unable to make enough hydrochloric acid. And as Burpy probably told you, HCl is needed so that minerals—such as zinc—can be chelated and absorbed. So zinc is necessary for the production of HCl, and HCl is necessary for the absorption of zinc.

Using **acid blockers** like **cimetidine** or **ranitidine** can further depress zinc absorption. And I'm sure that **Burpy** has already told you that he makes picolinic acid from tryptophan to absorb zinc—so tryptophan is important for zinc absorption. Toxic metals such as copper or cadmium can also interfere with your absorption of zinc.

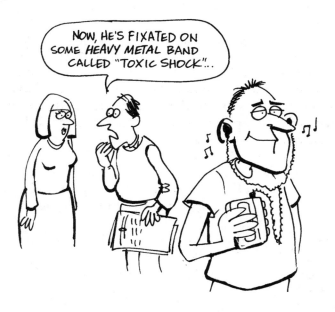

The thing that most depletes your body's zinc supply is elevated adrenal gland activity. Fear, worry, emotional stress, illness, excessive fasting and cleansing diets, and toxic stress can all put your body under great strain. As the adrenal glands' activity goes up, your body's zinc levels go down, quickly—as does the function of your thymus gland. Thymus and zinc are two things that are crucial for stimulating your T cells into regulating your immune system.

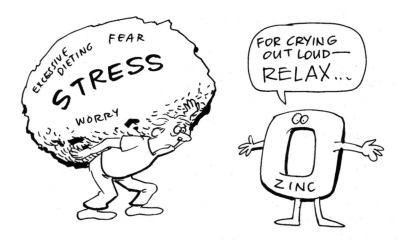

I have a trick to help deal with the high demands for zinc when there's a low supply. When T_4 is converted to T_3, I make an equal amount of **reverse T_3 (r-T_3)**. While r-T_3 can dock in the thyroid receptors, it can't activate the cells' DNA. So it blocks the activity of T_3 and thus slows down the body's use of fuel and oxygen. If things improve quickly, the r-T_3 is broken down, and T_3 begins to again activate the DNA to get the cells back to work.

If the stress drags on for extended periods of time, large quantities of zinc may be lost by the ongoing **adrenal overfunction,** which can result in the underfunctioning of dozens of **zinc-dependent enzymes.** And if the stomach is no longer making acid due to low T_3, you now may be unable to absorb enough zinc to get things back to work.

How are you going to break this cycle? In younger people, this is greatly counteracted by the large nightly production of melatonin that shuts down the adrenal glands overnight, allowing the body a reprieve during which it can restore zinc levels. As the pineal gland ages, it's less capable of shutting down the adrenals with its now-reduced melatonin production, and zinc levels gradually decrease.

Reduced zinc levels can lead to the following:
- Decreased production of hydrochloric acid by the stomach and sluggish fat metabolism by the liver
- Decreased function of the brain
- Decreased immune-regulating activity of the thymus hormones
- Decreased detoxification ability of the liver

I don't see how giving a synthetic hormone to correct a short-sighted blood test is going to correct all of this. To fix the thyroid, you've got to fix the minerals of the body—iodine, zinc/copper, calcium/magnesium, sodium/potassium. **Itchy** has already told you that most of these minerals are controlled by your kidneys—also called **the renals**—and by their little buddies who sit on top of them—your adrenals.

The other key organ is the liver. If your liver is producing peroxides that aren't being neutralized by your conjugation enzymes, then they can directly affect peroxidase function in your thyroid. Or even worse, your immune system can create even greater peroxide activity that can cause autoimmune thyroid problems. Either way, know that thyroid problems are secondary problems, preceded by problems with your diet, kidneys, liver, and/or stress.

So I'm **Bitchy**, and now you know why!

Your next **Liver Dwarf** guide is **Sluggy**. He was once a powerful magician who could virtually pull energy out of the air, but now he seems to have lost his spark. He still tries hard to do his chores; he's not old but he's tired. His wand has lost its power and doesn't create miracles anymore.

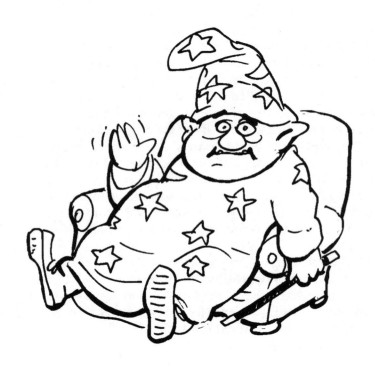

CHAPTER 8

Sluggy: Guide to Energy

Um: **I'm Sluggy, the Mitochondrial Liver Dwarf for Energy**.
Your **energy** comes from **food** and must be made useable by
your digestive system. The last stage of **digestion** takes place
in your **mitochondria**. If the mitochondria are not working
well, you can feel **tired**, really tired. Like me!

I'm your guide to Energy. I hope you don't mind if I sit; I'm just too tired to get up. Too pooped, no pep, petered out. To think that I was once thought to be a great magician because of the endless energy I could pull out of thin air. I could go, go, go—day and night. I hardly needed to sleep and could go all day without eating. Yes, those were the days (*sigh*). I truly was a great magician. I'm not now, though, since my mitochondria got barbecued. Let me tell you how it happened.

Mitochondria—I used to call them my Mighty Chondria because they made so much energy—are where the last stage in the digestive process takes place: that is, the process of turning crude food into useable energy. All the work that **Burpy** does with your stomach and pancreas and bile and intestine is to get the food small enough to travel through the bloodstream to each of your cells.

Your mitochondria are found inside each of your cells. The number of mitochondria in each cell can vary from fewer than a hundred to several thousand; the harder-working a cell is, the more mitochondria it has. Heart, nerve, liver, muscle, and immune cells have the most mitochondria because of the strenuous jobs they have.

It's your mitochondria's job to convert your food into a "super-high-octane" fuel called adenosine triphosphate or ATP. ATP contains **triphosphate,** which is three molecules of phosphate—that contain **phosphorus**—lined up in a row, with one end bound to adenosine and the other end sticking out, and very unstable. Its phosphorus in a match head that explodes into flame when a little friction is applied. Removing one phosphorus from ATP unleashes this power for you to use and leaves adenosine diphosphate or ADP, which I can "recycle" with a third phosphorus when it returns to your mitochondrial workbench. ATP is the explosive powder that your cells use for energy and heat, and most of it's made by your mitochondrial power plants, with the help of oxygen.

You probably already know from **Spacey** about ATP being your main source of energy, and she probably told you how she can make quick energy without oxygen, in an emergency. And she really can do all that. This is, however, a messy and inefficient use of glucose. The lactic acid given off by anaerobic metabolism can make you tired, and two ATP per glucose is the same as what the primitive Boogy Boys get when they ferment sugar. I, **Sluggy**, the **Liver Dwarf** in charge of your latest high-tech mitochondrial machinery, can get you a far better deal—with the help of oxygen. And I'm not totally dependent on glucose; I can use fats for fuel as well.

It might take me a couple of minutes to get things started, but once I kick in your magic mitochondrial machinery, you're going to get your "second wind" and you'll have the stamina to go for hours and hours. From each molecule of glucose, **Spacey** can get you only two ATP and two pyruvic acids, which is only 3 percent of the energy available in glucose. I'm better than **Spacey** because after I split the glucose to get the two ATP and two pyruvic acids, I run the two pyruvic acids through my **citric acid cycle** inside your mitochondria. This gives me a couple more ATP, some carbon dioxide—which **Gaspy** sends out through the lungs—and most important: a whole bunch of hydrogens.

Yessir, I'm a hydrogen hog. I combine these hydrogens with NAD (which, of course, is made from tryptophan) to form NADH. Once I'm finished with these hydrogens, you'll have extracted 66 percent of the energy in glucose, which shows that I'm a far more important **Liver Dwarf** than **Spacey**, with her measly 3 percent effectiveness. Why, I can even take her lactic acid waste products and reconvert them into pyruvic acid and glucose for use as needed. Let's take a closer look at your Mmmmarvelous Mitochondria.

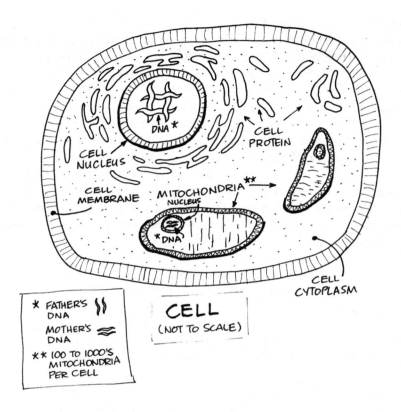

CELL
(NOT TO SCALE)

* FATHER'S
   DNA
   MOTHER'S
   DNA
** 100 TO 1000'S
   MITOCHONDRIA
   PER CELL

A cell has a **nucleus** containing **DNA**, yet every mitochondrion within the cell has its own nucleus, also with DNA, but from a different source. The DNA in your cell nuclei came equally from your father and mother, but the DNA in your mitochondria came entirely from your mother. The inner membrane of each mitochondrion is its workbench for the phenomenal energy transactions that take place here, and it's folded back upon itself many times to provide more room to do its valuable work.

Along the inner membrane are complex structures containing enzymes that carry out the last step of turning food into energy for your heat, action, or thought. Together, these membrane structures are called the **electron transport chain** because they transport **electrons** and **protons**, which do the actual work.

Glucose and fatty acids are the main sources of fuel (ATP) in your body. When they are broken down within your cells, they release hydrogen atoms. These hydrogen atoms are then transported by carrier molecules—such as NAD—to the electron transport chain.

Glucose products are transported from the cell into the mitochondria where they are further broken down to release hydrogen. The breakdown of fatty acids takes place within the mitochondria. The long-chain fatty acids that are to be sacrificed in your honour are transported into the mitochondria by **carnitine**, which then carries out the shorter fatty acid residues of the previous "offering." Inside the mitochondria, the long chains of fatty acids get pieces chopped off to provide fuel for the electron transport chain machinery.

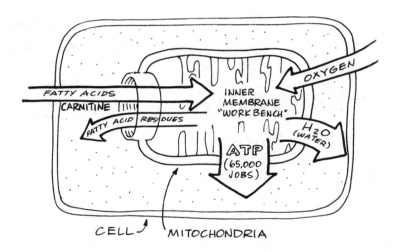

NADH brings a hydrogen atom—from the breakdown of glucose or fatty acids—to **Complex I** of the electron transport chain. Complex I passes the proton (H+) *through* the membrane and the electron (E-) *into* the membrane. **Complex II** receives electrons from propionate via succinate and also passes them into the mitochondrial membrane.

NAD is the water-soluble electron carrier within your cell fluids, and it can't function in the fat of your cell membrane. It takes a special fat-soluble substance called **coenzyme Q_{10}** (**CoQ_{10}** or **ubiquinone**) to receive the two electrons from Complexes I and II, and hand them off down the membrane to **Complex III**. Then Complex III passes them to a single electron carrier called **Cytochrome C**, which passes them to **Complex IV**—where I bind them to hydrogen and oxygen to make water. This is where a cell's tremendous need for oxygen is finally fulfilled.

INSIDE MITOCHONDRIA

GLUCOSE AND LONG CHAIN FATTY ACIDS NADH

PROPIONATE

COENZYME Q10 (UBIQUINONE)

SUCCINATE

ATP SYNTHETASE

HYDROGEN & OXYGEN

ATP

COMPLEX I

COMPLEX II

COMPLEX III

COMPLEX IV

INTERMEMBRANE SPACE

THE BODY'S "INTERNAL COMBUSTION ENGINE"

All this need for oxygen just to make water!? Well, there's a little more to it. As you know, opposite charges attract and like charges repel. Electrons and protons have opposite charges and are strongly attracted to each other. By running the flow of electrons through the mitochondrial membrane, I create an attractive energy current that lures protons through Complex I, III, and IV into the **intermembrane space**. Thus, with a little cunning, I've tricked the protons into the intermembrane space by baiting them with the sexy electrons.

When I turn the electrons into water in Complex IV, that ends the negative charge of the electrons and leaves the large buildup of protons trapped in the intermembrane space.

When they realize they've been tricked into the presence of a horde of other ugly protons, they desperately need to move away from each other and, in a mad panic, they hurl themselves away from the other protons. But the only way they can get out of the intermembrane space is to shoot through an opening in **ATP synthetase**, which uses the fleeing proton—like a turbine would use falling water—to generate **ATP** by adding a phosphorus to ADP.

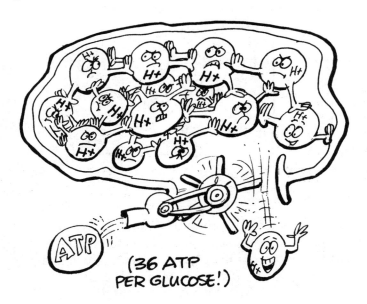

(36 ATP PER GLUCOSE!)

We **Liver Dwarves** find ATP as useful to run your body as you would find batteries to power your flashlight. In fact, we **Liver Dwarves** use ATP to power 65,000 different jobs we carry out in the body.

I know this probably looks like a lot of very complicated mumbo jumbo—with all these protons whizzing around just to make ATP—but **Liver Dwarves** learned long ago that it's well worth it!

If a Boogy Boy were to ferment one glucose molecule, the best he could do is create 2 ATP (never mind the stinking mess he might make doing it). I, however, using oxygen and my mitochondrial electron chain helpers, can trick **38 ATP** out of one molecule of glucose. That's what I call magic, and that's why *I'm* your most important **Liver Dwarf**!

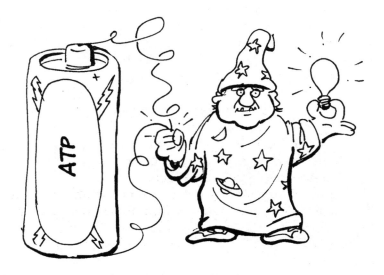

Of course, all of this mitochondrial magic fails if there's not enough oxygen. Athletes have some debts to pay off after vigorous exercise. One is the **glycogen debt**, which is the glycogen that's used up during anaerobic exercise, and the other is the **oxygen debt**, which comes from the depletion of oxygen stores. The oxygen stores allow your body to switch from anaerobic metabolism to aerobic metabolism for a minute or so without your having to breathe deeper—by letting you use some of the two litres of oxygen stored in your lungs, red blood cells, and fluids.

After you finish strenuous exercise, you need to keep breathing heavily for a while to replace the two litres of oxygen borrowed from storage. Plus, I need another nine-and-a-half litres of oxygen to regenerate the creatine phosphate levels within minutes and, over the next hour, to reconvert lactic acid to pyruvic acid and glucose. If the muscle glycogen levels have been greatly depleted due to major anaerobic exercise, it can take two to six days to recover those glycogen stores.

Here are a few ways you can have low oxygen.

- If your spleen isn't breaking down old red blood cells— so the old geezers get so stiff, they can't squeeze through the capillaries to pick up or drop off oxygen.
- If you have iron or zinc deficiencies or not enough vitamin B_{12} to make fresh, new red blood cells.
- If you have lung or heart damage from smoking.
- If you have congestion or allergies (from an overloaded lymph system) that interferes with sinus-made nitric oxide so the blood vessels of your heart and lungs are less dilated, which gives you less circulation of blood and therefore less precious oxygen.
- If you have magnesium, thiamin, riboflavin and vitamin B_6 deficiencies from bad diet or from Boogy Boys eating these nutrients up in the small intestine.
- Or, if you're just plain out of shape from sitting on your butt too much!

And, of course, where there's demand for oxygen, there's need for active thyroid hormone, too.

And if oxygen does get furnished, there can be a tremendous benefit in energy, but with it comes an equally great danger. You get all those electrons flying around, with all that oxygen, and it's like playing with matches at a gas station. Big danger!

If an oxygen gets loose with only one electron, it will desperately try to find another electron in order to feel stable, even if it has to rip it out of one of your membranes. In other words, it becomes a deadly free radical.

In the mitochondria, the most frequent place for free radical production is at coenzyme Q_{10} (CoQ_{10}) because it's such a show-off that it tries to pass two electrons at once.

Even at the best of times, CoQ_{10} tends to fumble a few hundred electrons a day, which become superoxide radicals and then hydrogen peroxide. I keep a good supply of water-soluble vitamin C in the cell fluids—to protect the cell proteins—and fat-soluble vitamin E on guard in the fatty membranes. I also keep Super OD and Gladiator Glutathione enzymes nearby, to protect you against damage from these errant sparks.

Obviously, the harder you push CoQ_{10}, the more likely it is to fumble electrons and generate free radicals. Since the whole purpose of the electron transport chain in the mitochondria is to turn food into energy, overloading this system with an excess of foods can dramatically push this system—especially its weakest link, CoQ_{10}—into a big increase in wild energy, in the form of free radicals. So the price of overeating is overproduction of free radicals in your mitochondria.

Another thing that can cause free radical trouble in your mitochondria is your immune system. When your cells are attacked by invaders, especially viruses, they make interferon to warn neighbouring cells to make antiviral proteins. Large quantities of interferon, over extended periods of time, can affect your nervous system. The sensitivity of the receptors in your nervous system is controlled by **NMDA (N-methyl D-aspartate)**, which makes nerve receptors—and therefore nerves—*more excitable*, and by **GABA (gamma-aminobutyric acid)**, which inhibits nerve receptors and therefore makes nerves *less excitable*.

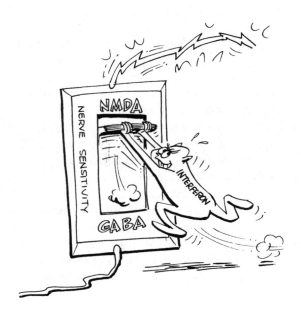

Interferon can leave your nerve receptors dominated by NMDA, which results in small pain stimuli being perceived as large pain. The pain feels real enough to the person experiencing it, but can be puzzling to an observer because the person's reactions seem so exaggerated.

But the most important thing to me as the energy **Liver Dwarf** is that the production of interferon requires tremendous quantities of ATP from your mitochondria. This is why sick people often lose so much weight very quickly if they're unable to eat. To make the pounds of ATP necessary to make large amounts of interferon, I will even break up your own body in order to aid the immune system. So, while excess eating can *push* CoQ$_{10}$ into making more free radicals, the demand of your immune system for more ATP can *pull* more electrons into CoQ$_{10}$ and also generate more free radicals.

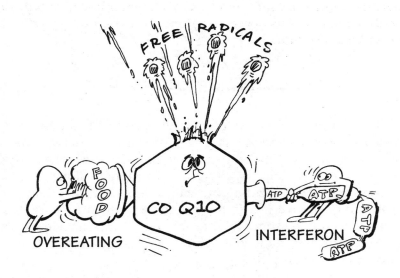

If you run low on fat-soluble antioxidants like vitamin E, these free radicals can do damage to cell membranes. And being low on water-soluble antioxidants like vitamin C can lead to damage of cell proteins.

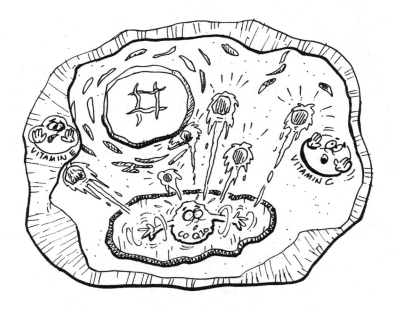

Of course, if damage is done to the DNA inside the cell nucleus, it could become a runaway cancer cell. That's why I keep a full crew of DNA repair specialists at work, constantly splicing and repairing any damage that might be done.

They are very meticulous at making sure they have everything repaired just right—no matter how much energy it takes. And so they should, because your DNA is priceless! In an average workday, they will repair a thousand pieces of damage to your DNA in *each* cell.

Let's take a look at your DNA. Most cells in your body have a large nucleus that contains the genetic blueprint that you inherited from your parents and their ancestors. This blueprint is called DNA and it's stored in coded form on two strands that are bonded together and twisted into a helix shape.

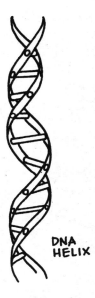

DNA
HELIX

Since the DNA stored in each of your cells is two metres long, I have to "supercoil" it by further twisting it so it gets very kinky, the way your telephone cord kinks up if you don't untwist it once in a while.

The backbone of each DNA strand consists of alternating sugars and phosphates. Your genetic code consists of a sequence of bases on one strand that are bonded to different bases on the other strand. There are four bases that are always paired the same way. **Thymine** is always linked to **adenine** with a double bond, while **guanine** is always bonded to **cytosine** with a triple bond.

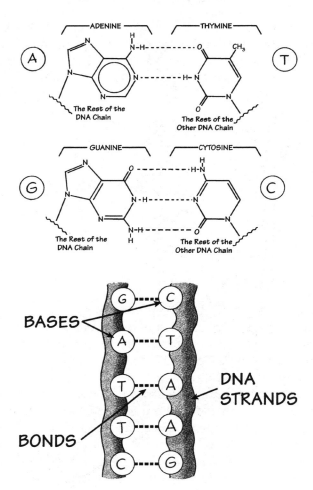

If the sequence of bases on one DNA strand is guanine, cytosine, thymine, and adenine, the sequence on the other DNA strand *must* be cytosine, guanine, adenine, and thymine—since the pairs never change. When a cell is actively working, the DNA is unwound and becomes the *blueprint* that the **RNA** construction crew *reads* to know how to *assemble* more of *you*. RNA does this by building proteins.

Every three bases that the RNA reads on a DNA stand tell RNA to add one specific amino acid to a protein that it's constructing. This is called **triplet code**. For example, if RNA reads thymine, guanine, guanine, sequenced on a DNA strand, it knows to add a tryptophan to the chain of amino acids that it has already assembled. If the next three DNA bases are adenine, thymine, guanine, then RNA knows to add a methionine amino acid to the chain.

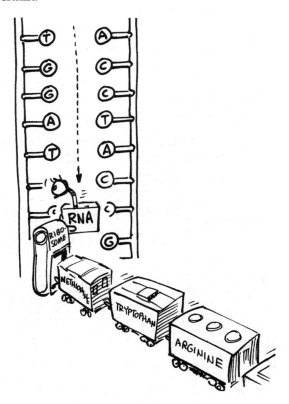

Since only four bases are used, and they are used in triplet code—that is, three bases equal one amino acid—there are 64 possible combinations of triplet code. Since there are only 20 amino acids to be coded, most amino acids have more than one triplet code to represent them. For example, if the DNA blueprint says thymine, thymine, thymine, or thymine, thymine, cytosine, either of these two triplet codes will tell RNA to add a **phenylalanine** to the protein that it's assembling. Sixty-one of the triplet codes are used up by specific amino acids, while the other three—thymine, adenine, adenine;

thymine, adenine, guanine; and thymine, guanine, adenine—
are stop signals that shut off the RNA production machinery.

It's your DNA triplet code sequences that guide your RNA
construction crew as it builds the proteins that take you from a
tiny egg fertilized by the head of an even tinier sperm, into the
full-grown marvel you are today!

Since it has taken thousands of years of triumph over famine,
drought, pestilence, and war for your ancestors to have given
you the right batch of "success" genes stored away in your
DNA, I have to guard them vigilantly against damage. I'll give
you these secret triplet codes as long as you promise not to
show them to anyone else.

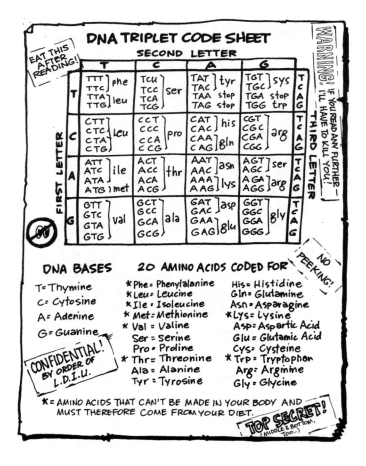

If damaged genes were to be read by your RNA, it might end up adding the wrong amino acids when building your proteins. For example, hemoglobin is a protein containing 150 amino acids. Since each amino acid is coded by three bases, 450 DNA bases must be in the correct sequence to make perfect hemoglobin. The triplet **guanine, adenine, guanine** is the code for **glutamic acid**, one of the amino acids in hemoglobin. Yet some people's DNA have the adenine replaced with thymine, so it reads **guanine, thymine, guanine**, which tells RNA to build in the amino acid **valine** instead of glutamic acid. That small variation of one amino acid in hemoglobin is what creates **sickle cell anemia**. Even the **malaria parasite** has difficulty living on such fragile, flawed hemoglobin. Most mutations are detrimental to the individual and some can lead to cancer development.

Your liver's P450 enzymes can make a number of different types of expoxides. Some epoxides can be harmless; some can be toxic, which means that they can bind to your DNA; some can be **mutagenic**, which means they can damage your genetic code stored in your DNA. Some can even be **carcinogenic,** which means that the genetic damage they cause can lead to the formation of **cancer**. This wide range of epoxide trouble is especially prevalent when the epoxides originate from **polycyclic aromatic hydrocarbons**.

Now don't be afraid of this word because **Achy**'s already explained what it is. **Hydrocarbon** means it contains only hydrogen and carbon. **Cyclic** means circle-like, and **aromatic** means that it shares internal electrons in the form of an aromatic cloud. In other words: **benzene**. And **poly** means many. So polycyclic aromatic hydrocarbons are simply many benzenes joined together.

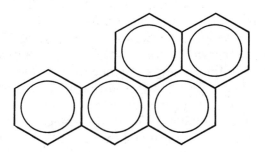

Benzo[a]pyrene (BP)
(A polycyclic aromatic hydrocarbon
consisting of five benzenes)

It's the P450 enzymes' job to add oxygen to the polycyclic hydrocarbon to make it water-soluble. And it's this oxygen that can take an innocent thing like **benzo[a]pyrene** (**BP**)—a polycyclic aromatic hydrocarbon—and turn it into a monster that can damage your genes and send them toward a wild journey of self-destruction called cancer.

Benzo[a]pyrene might enter your body when you eat smoked or charbroiled food, or when you inhale smoke from cigarettes, cigars, smelters, or power plants. Here's an example of two forms of **benzo[a]pyrene dihydrodiol** that are created in your body from benzo[a]pyrene. Notice that the left cyclic ring has had two oxygens added to it already, which resulted in its loss of the aromatic cloud.

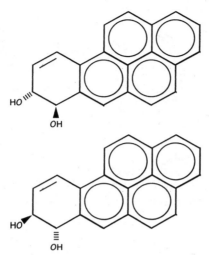

Benzo[a]pyrene dihydrodiols

There are two versions drawn here to show you that the two oxygens were added to benzo[a]pyrene in two different ways. When oxygen is added to benzo[a]pyrene, it must attach at an angle. The dash lines in the diagram mean the oxygen is angled away from you. The other oxygen will attach angled toward you, and this is represented by the darker shape that looks like a little triangle.

As *each* benzo[a]pyrene dihydrodiol goes through the P450 liver enzyme system, another oxygen molecule (O_2) is split; one oxygen is added to the benzo[a]pyrene dihydrodiol and the other becomes a free radical. The free radicals that are formed are turned into peroxides by Super OD and the peroxides must be quickly neutralized by your conjugation enzymes.

The new oxygen that's added has no hydrogen to hang onto, so it hangs on with both hands to two carbons. Since the new oxygen will also be added at an angle—on one side or the other of the benzo[a]pyrene dihydrodiol—each of the two benzo[a]pyrene dihydrodiols can end up with two versions. So altogether, you can end up with four versions, all called **epoxides**. They are **(-)-BP-diol-epoxide 1**, **(-)-BP-diol-epoxide 2**, **(+)-BP-diol-epoxide 1**, and **(+)-BP-diol-epoxide 2**.

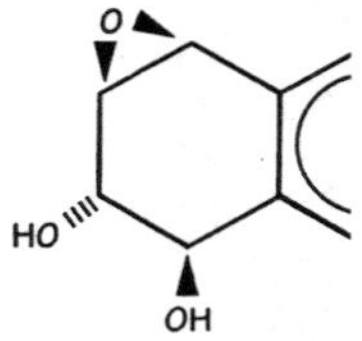

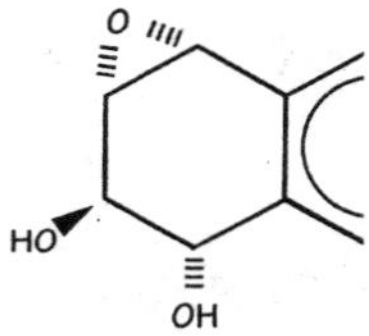

(-)-BP-diol-epoxide 1

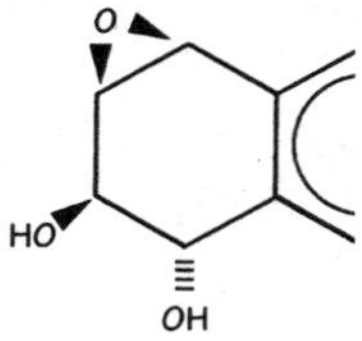

(-)-BP-diol-epoxide 2

(+)-BP-diol-epoxide 1

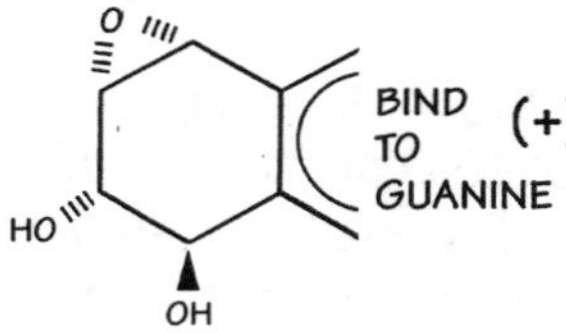

BIND TO GUANINE   (+)-BP-diol-epoxide 2

Of these four epoxides, at least one of them will be more able to bind to your DNA because of the favourable angle of its oxygen. It's their ability to bind to your DNA that makes them *toxic* epoxides.

When toxic epoxides come into contact with guanine in your DNA, the last oxygen that was added makes a swap with a nitrogen of the guanine base in your DNA. Oxygen gives up one of its benzo[a]pyrene carbon handholds for a hydrogen that was bound to the nitrogen on the guanine, and the nitrogen then latches onto the carbon of the epoxide released by the oxygen. A quick little two-step dance and now your precious DNA has a polycyclic aromatic hydrocarbon stuck onto it. This is called an **adduct**.

(+)-BP-diol-epoxide 2 →

GUANINE ADDUCT

DNA ADDUCT

Do not panic! This is not a big problem. Within a day or two, your detoxification processes will have cleaned up this hydrocarbon mess stuck to your DNA. Of course, if new toxic epoxides are constantly being added by your P450 enzymes faster than your detoxification system can remove them, damage to your DNA could occur. The damage, however, is not likely to occur to guanine. Guanine is pretty tough and not easy to damage.

Adenine is another of the four bases that make up your genetic code recorded in your cells' DNA. Polycyclic aromatic hydrocarbons only bind to adenine one-tenth as much as they do to guanine, but adenine is much more vulnerable to being damaged. This is because adenine is the only DNA base that has an aromatic structure—and within a day of having a polycyclic aromatic hydrocarbon toxic epoxide bound to it, adenine can become deformed by the greater energy currents of this bulky, stronger aromatic intruder.

Of course, my DNA repair crew will quickly splice in new adenines to replace any that are damaged, and life will go on smoothly.

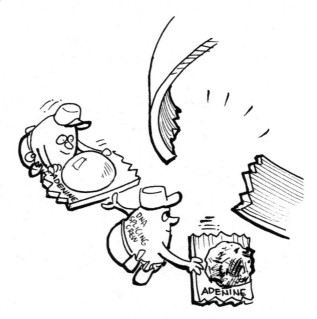

ADENINE REPAIR

If your liver's P450 enzymes continually bombard your DNA with greater quantities of the damaging toxic epoxides than my repair crews can keep up with, then things can get more serious. Yet this is still not permanent. Damage to your genes only becomes permanent if your DNA were to replicate—that is, make an exact copy of itself—before my repair crews have fully repaired it.

When DNA replicates, the copy becomes "carved in stone" as the new blueprint for the real you. If this new DNA has errors in it, it's called a **mutation** and the thing that caused the mutation is **mutagenic**.

Toxic epoxides are only mutagenic if the damage is done to your genes faster than repairs are made *and only if* this damage is recorded permanently *after* the replication of your DNA. Replication must take place if a cell is to reproduce.

Carcinogenicity is the ability of the mutation (gene damage) to lead to the development of cancer.

If the oxygen that binds to DNA is next to a part of the polycyclic aromatic hydrocarbon that has a bay-shaped indent, then it's more likely to generate cancer. The example we used—a version of benzo[a]pyrene—has a bay region that amplifies the effects on the DNA, and therefore makes it more likely to cause cancer.

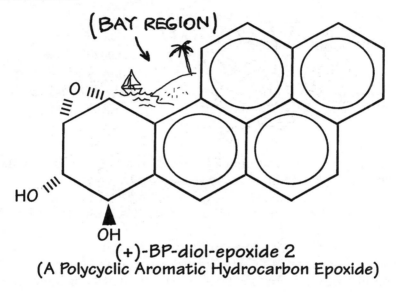

(+)-BP-diol-epoxide 2
(A Polycyclic Aromatic Hydrocarbon Epoxide)

Of course, cancer can't occur if the damage is repaired before replication records the mutation permanently. Since the tightly twisted DNA has to unravel before it can replicate, I keep my most competent supervisor—**p53 protein**—locked onto the DNA strands to make sure replication can't be completed until DNA repair is finished. After the DNA strands have duplicated, p53 protein makes them pause for a spell-check; that is, it makes sure that all DNA bases have been repaired correctly.

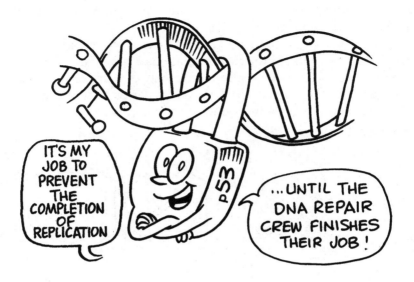

The p53 has an additional job as well, that's somewhat hush-hush. If p53 should in any way sense the DNA trying to replicate with damage still unrepaired, and if p53 had the slightest doubts about its ability to block this replication, then p53 is under direct orders—not from me: from higher up . . . **General Achy**—to commit the entire cell, including its DNA, to apoptosis. As you will have heard from the great General himself, *no cell shall fall into enemy hands.* It is better to have a cell blow itself up than to have its DNA become a slave to viruses or cancers.

Speaking of **General Achy,** I've been meaning to talk to him about the behaviour of some if his troops—but I've been too tired to make it over to his barracks. Every time toxic epoxides pass by in the blood, his neutrophils start sucking up oxygen, and about 40 seconds later, they blow a burst of superoxide radicals and hydrogen peroxide all over the place!

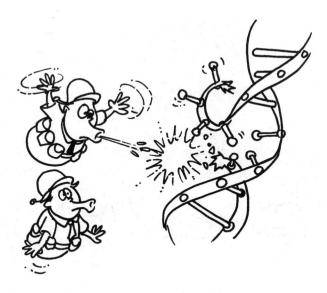

My DNA repair crew has reported numerous breaks in the DNA strands from this peculiar behaviour. My repair crew can fix the damage, but this takes a lot longer than simply splicing in a new adenine base—and the margin for error is much greater.

You see, when adenine is damaged beyond recognition, they still know it's adenine because the strand across from it has thymine—which can only bind to adenine. But when a strand of the DNA gets broken, the whole DNA spiral twist can pull out of shape, making it harder to know which bases were originally lined up with each other. Still, given time, my repair gang will usually get it done right. The important thing is for the repair to be done before the cell completes replication and imprints the damage in new DNA. That's why I've got p53 supervising every strand of DNA.

The shape of p53 is what suppresses DNA replication, and it's zinc that keeps p53's shape taut and true.

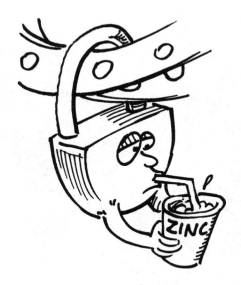

You know by now the story of low zinc levels; surely you recall that The Boogy Boys in the small intestine can steal tryptophan so your pancreas doesn't have enough picolinic acid to absorb zinc. Or even if the zinc is absorbed, a lot of adrenal stress can flush it right out of you. And you know that free radicals can come from your liver's P450 enzymes along with peroxides and toxic epoxides, and that every cell's mitochondrial CoQ_{10} can also generate free radicals. These free radicals can generate fatty peroxides anywhere in your body. And now you know that your own white blood cells can drastically amplify the damage and destruction with the same peroxides and hydroxyl radicals.

If a continual bombardment of free radicals and peroxides eventually distorts your zinc-depleted p53 protein so that it can't suppress your damaged DNA's replication, your one hope left is that it will at least blow the whole cell up by stimulating apoptosis.

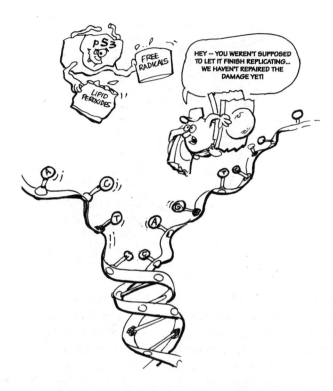

If p53 is too bent out of shape to do that, and your DNA completes replication—with damaged DNA now recorded forever as "your genes"—then there is *still* little possibility of your getting cancer.

One mutation does not necessarily a cancer make. It takes at least two or even six mutations in a cell's DNA before it can run amok—out of control—as cancer. I had a bad dream the other night that p53 protein was so deformed that it became a **growth stimulator**, and whipped your mutant DNA into reproducing faster and faster.

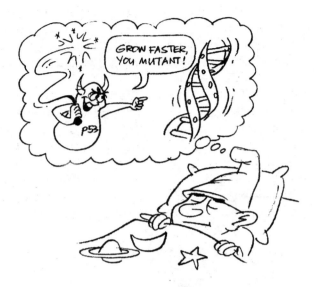

There are some enzymes that may play a role in stimulating cancer development. Recurrent exposure of the skin to carcinogenic hydrocarbons can increase the activity of the enzymes **ornithine decarboxylase** and **methionine decarboxylase**. These enzymes convert the amino acids **ornithine** and **methionine** into **putrescine, spermadine**, and **spermine**, which create an increased rate of growth—which can gradually create **benign tumours**. Greater activity of the decarboxylase enzymes could eventually result in **malignant tumours**. Of course, bacteria and yeast also have decarboxylase enzymes that can turn your amino acids into toxins in your small intestine—should they manage to get in there.

You know that your liver's P450 enzymes are the source of the toxic epoxides, and many of the free radicals. Your mitochondria also make free radicals, and their greatest free radical production occurs when I run low on CoQ_{10}, especially if your mitochondria are being pushed or pulled by overeating and/or viral infections. With low CoQ_{10} levels, your mitochondria spin off thousands of free radicals per day, and even large amounts of vitamins C and E and other antioxidants may not be enough to prevent damage to the mitochondria or to the rest of the cell.

I try to keep your CoQ_{10} levels up, but it's hard to do that if your liver's jammed up by **Bloaty** closing down your outlet liver valves, because it's your liver that has to assemble CoQ_{10} from food. All living things use coenzyme Q but with many variations off a similar stem.

The **basic stem** is the same in all life forms, but the number of **isoprene side chains** vary from CoQ_1 in some microorganisms, to CoQ_6 in some plants, and CoQ_9 and CoQ_{10} in most animals. Your liver's job is to strip the **isoprenes** from the CoQ stem and then reassemble them on the stem so that it has a total of 10 isoprene side-chain units—CoQ_{10}—another proud **Liver Dwarf** product! Your liver can also make CoQ_{10} directly from tyrosine but it needs vitamin B_6 to complete one step in the process.

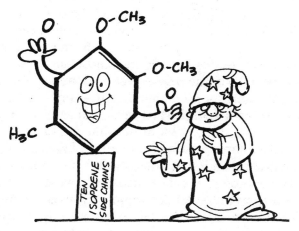

COENZYME Q_{10} — "ANOTHER PROUD LIVER DWARF PRODUCT"!

The problem is that CoQ_{10} can't be made if your liver isn't working well, which is particularly apparent with ageing. Low CoQ_{10} levels may not be obvious right away, but eventually the burden of excess free radicals will make itself known, especially if overeating, infections, antioxidant deficiencies, and/or ageing are involved.

What happened to me was that I got a sore throat and slightly swollen glands, which then developed into a flu, and then the lymph glands under my chin got larger and sorer. I had a fever. I took antibiotics, and after a few days, I seemed to get better for a while, but then gradually I got weaker and weaker.

How could this happen to me? I'd been eating so much better. I had been a strict vegetarian for a year, and I'd been feeling so good! No animal products, low fat, no salt, five servings a day of fresh fruits and vegetables, whole grains—just like all the researchers have been saying. Maybe I had been under a little stress; I had been trying to get a lot done. I had a vaccination to which I had a reaction for a few days and since then, whenever I tried to do anything strenuous or got under stress, I'd just fall apart.

Now, I'm always tired. My lymph glands have slowly gotten better, but now my digestion is really bad. I never had any problems like that before. Now I get gas and bloating after eating *anything*. I react to any chemicals—from food additives to perfume—yet skin testing for allergies didn't show anything. Even water seems to bother my digestion. My bowels are undecided: first constipation, then diarrhea. I'm tired physically and mentally and my muscles are weak and achy. I'd rather sit down than stand, and lie down rather than sit. I haven't been able to work for a long time, but sometimes I get feeling a little better, and then I go and do a little research. Gradually, I've been able to piece together what happened to me.

I found out from **Itchy** that by cooling down my kidneys too much with foods out of season, I stopped activating vitamin D and got low in calcium—which weakened my ileocecal valve, thus allowing The Boogy Boys into the small intestine. The antibiotics I took killed the intestinal yeast's natural enemies, thus enabling the yeast to run rampant. The strong absorption from the small intestine resulted in their toxins flooding into the portal vein and the liver's P450 enzymes amplified their toxicity up to 60 times more. The low-protein, high-carbohydrate diet I was on interfered with the conjugation enzymes' ability to keep up. **Bloaty** told me she had to shut down the outlet liver valves, which began to dump toxins, fluid, and proteins into the lymph system.

   My white blood cells attacked the proteins as invaders and a fibrin net was thrown around their victims so they couldn't escape. That created congestion in the lymph, which laid the foundation for a viral picnic. Oh, this wasn't a viral infection in the commonly used sense of the word. The virus was already in me, but dormant.

   There's a whole family of viruses that—once in your body— don't go away. Normally, your immune system gets onto them, and they go dormant. They're different from most viruses in that their genetic code is in DNA, like yours, rather than the RNA that most viruses have; so they're a little larger than most viruses but also less dependent on needing your cells' DNA to reproduce. That allows them to sit dormant in your body for years, catching up on their reading or shooting a little pool, waiting for your immune system—either **locally** or **systemically**—to relax its guard. Then they reproduce quickly, causing a number of diseases, depending on the type of virus they are. This is the **herpes simplex virus (HSV)** family that I'm talking about.

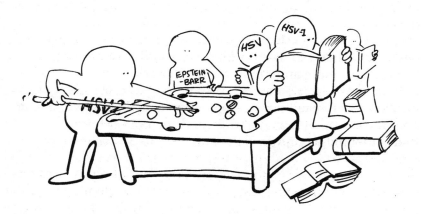

   HSV-1 usually causes painful blistering of your lips and can be triggered by damage to your lips from the sun, wind, and cold temperatures. These elements weaken your local lip area, which can allow the HSV-1 to activate. **HSV-2** is usually found in your **genital area**, although some sexual practices can reverse the location of these two viruses.

Varicella-zoster virus causes **chicken pox** in children, and painful **herpes zoster** or "**shingles**" in the nerves of adults, when their immune systems are down.

Cytomegalovirus is found in most adults, but like other HSV, rarely causes symptoms in adults whose immune systems are working well. Once your immune system is weakened, however, cytomegalovirus can be involved in everything from hardening of the arteries to colitis to cancer. **HSV-6** is another virus that is common and normally dormant in most adults, but in a body with a weakened immune system, it can pop up and contribute to serious problems.

Epstein-Barr virus is usually associated with **mononucleosis**, 'though many people who are exposed to it don't manifest the full symptoms of swollen lymph glands, fatigue, weakness, muscle aches, etc. What I had was Epstein-Barr virus taking advantage of my clogged-up lymph system. I immediately started making interferon to warn all the other cells of this viral threat. The demand for ATP literally drained the energy out of me and burned up some body weight because I was too sick to eat.

My liver was too sluggish to make enough CoQ_{10} to keep up with the demand for ATP and my mitochondria started spinning off more and more free radicals. My mitochondria took the brunt of the free radicals and their membranes got all swollen and twisted out of shape. Now they look like cars that got hit head-on by a freight train and then caught fire. Barbecued mitochondria is the only way to describe them.

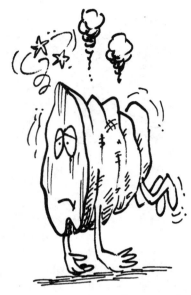

MITOCHONDRIA —
"HEAD-ON CRASH & BURN"...

Achy eventually got the immune system somewhat under control and he thinks the virus is dormant now. The problem is, I'm left with the residue of the battle: swollen and distorted mitochondria. They can still make ATP but not nearly as much as before. A healthy, active person might turn a few pounds of food into a few pounds of ATP each day, to power all the ambitious projects he or she has to do in a day. I can't make much ATP so I don't get much done. I'm always tired.

Bitchy recently told you a bit about certain hormones that are made in specific glands or organs, and that are often sent on long journeys to distant cells where their messages are read after being docked on specific receptors. This is the "long-distance call" in the world of **hormonal communications**. Cells can also communicate over shorter distances in a way that can be even more powerful. Cells talk to their immediate neighbours through their membranes, the way you might talk to your neighbour over your backyard fence.

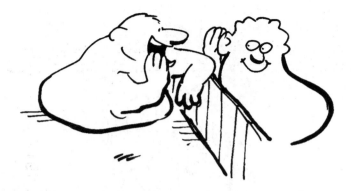

The membranes of every cell (except red blood cells) make and release a large variety of very short-lived, short-range, hormone-like messengers called **eicosanoids**. The three types of eicosanoids—**prostaglandins, thromboxanes**, and **leukotrienes**—can be made in a staggering variety of forms that can have a dramatic influence on neighbouring cells. Their actions on membranes can affect both the release of other hormones and the sensitivity of the hormone receptors.

The profound effect of these short-range hormones depends on the enzymes that make them and, more important, on the type of fat that they're made from. In each cell membrane, there are numerous enzymes, including **delta 6 desaturase** and **delta 5 desaturase**. These two enzymes are capable of turning two types of fats—**omega 6** or **omega 3**—into fatty acids, which can then be transformed into eicosanoids by **cyclooxygenase (COX) enzymes** or by **lipoxygenase (LOX) enzymes**.

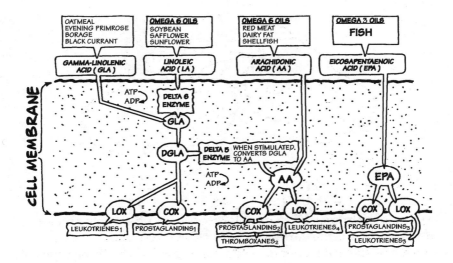

For the delta 6 and delta 5 enzymes to work properly, they need ATP, and spare ATP I don't have right now, so I don't make eicosanoids properly. That can create a wide range of problems, from physical to mental and emotional. In fact, I have all the symptoms of allergies, yet none were found on testing. **General Achy** said it had something to do with eicosanoids, but I've been too tired to talk to him for quite a while.

There is hope, though. We're supposed to be getting a doctor from the **Liver Dwarf Agency**. I think I'll stick around with you and see if he can help me straighten out this mess I'm in.

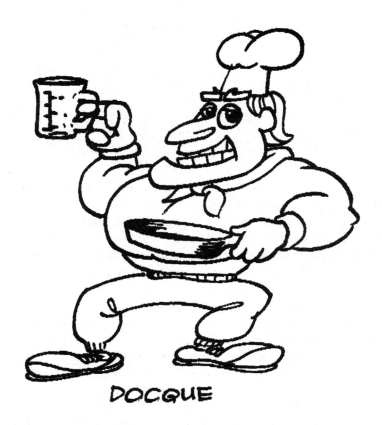

DOCQUE

CHAPTER 9

Docque: Guide to Food

Hi! I'm the new **Liver Dwarf** you've been expecting. I was sent by the **Liver Dwarf Agency**.

Sluggy: Oh, you must be the doctor. Boy, are we ever glad to see you! We've been taking quite a beating. We've all been working overtime big-time, trying to win the Liver Wars. We've got eight casualties, most of whom are barely able to get by.

- **Burpy**'s got indigestion.
- **Bloaty**'s swollen up like a balloon.
- **Gaspy**, I'm not sure if she's still alive.
- **Spacey**'s not even on this planet.
- **Achy**—wow, is he in pain!
- **Itchy**: well, he's preoccupied with scratching.
- **Bitchy**'s about ready to blow a gasket.
- And I'm **Sluggy**. I'm too tired to even shake your hand.

So, welcome, doctor; we sure do need your expert medical opinion!

Docque: Medical opinion?! There must be a misunderstanding. My name is spelled "D-o-c-q-u-e," not "D-o-c." I'm not a doctor—I'm a cook!

Sluggy: Oh, oh! It looks like the Agency goofed up big-time. I'd better call the rest of the **Liver Dwarves** over the PA system.

"Calling all **Liver Dwarves**, calling all **Liver Dwarves**. Code Blue! I repeat, Code Blue! Proceed immediately, I repeat—

immediately—to **Liver Dwarf Headquarters**." They should be here soon and are *they* going to be disappointed! I don't think they'll be able to go on without immediate medical care.

Burpy: (*Burp*) This better be important 'cause I've got toxins running into the bile, and we're heading for a big case of indigestion if I don't do something soon.

Bloaty: And I've got all the liver valves tightened down to Warp 3. If I don't watch her closely, she could blow!

Gaspy: I'm just going to lie down here on the floor. Tell me if I die. By the way, could you give me a light for my very last cigarette?

Spacey: What's "Code Blue"? Is it my birthday already? It can't be, I just had it last year.

Achy: Ouch! What's all this Code Blue stuff? I hurt every joint in my body hurrying to get here!

Itchy: For a minute there, I stopped scratching, but now it's back with a vengeance.

Bitchy: Who signalled Code Blue?! Don't you know that's only to be used for emergencies? I've got important work to do, regulating hormones. I've got no time for false alarms!

Sluggy: I've got bad news for you all. There is no doctor. This is the new **Liver Dwarf** and his name is **Docque**—spelled D-o-c-q-u-e—and he's a cook.

Gaspy: A cook? I'm nearly dead and they send me a cook? I'm finished—it's over. Don't send flowers to my funeral; instead send a cheque to the **Liver Dwarves' Broken Heart Fund**. I know my heart is finished.

Achy: (*Sob*) I can't go on with all this pain. Somebody put me out of my misery!

Spacey: Where'd you get a name like **Docque**?

Docque: Docque is actually my nickname. You see, I've been a ship's cook for centuries. The place where I'd first meet people was at the *dock* when the ship came in, so for some strange reason, people started calling me "Dock." Because I'm French, I spell it D-o-c-q-u-e instead of D-o-c-k. As a ship's cook, I've cooked on galleys and galleons, steamships and cruiseships, fishboats, and even a pirate ship. I've seen every corner of the globe, and learned much from the many cultures I've encountered.

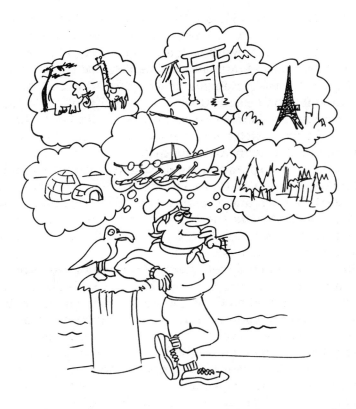

I'm very sorry you're so disappointed with my arrival; I'd return to the Agency immediately and find you someone better suited—except there *is* no one else. **The Liver Dwarf Agency** is bare; there's no one there. There's such a demand for **Liver Dwarves** these days that they pulled me out of retirement— they said you were desperate. I'm sorry, but I'm all you're going to get!

Gaspy: I'm finished!

Bitchy: Wait a minute, **Gaspy**. Let's give him a chance. You say you can cook?

Docque: Absolutely. I have experience with food from all around the world.

Burpy: Does it taste okay?

Docque: I've cooked for every culture, in every corner of the world. I've cooked every kind of food, with many different herbs, so that every palate might be appeased. I should also say that many of the cooks I've met believe that their work is at the root of healing—of the stomach, the mind, and the spirit.

Itchy: Are you saying you could make us better?

Docque: (*Laughing*) Remember, I'm not a "doc." All I can do is find out what you need to change, and then you're in charge from there on. So I'll talk to each of you and find out what problems you're having, and then work up some diets for you. How about I start with you, **Sluggy**?

Sluggy: My mitochondria got damaged when my immune system was fighting a virus, so they make less ATP and more free radicals, which makes me really tired. And now my cell membranes don't make the proper eicosanoids. I sure don't feel well.

Docque: Next . . .

Bitchy: I've got crazy estrogens because my liver's not breaking them down properly, and my thyroid is going a little berserk. I'm sure I'm going to get breast cancer; it's probably started growing already, or maybe it's in my uterus or ovaries. I'm sure it's in the ovaries.

Itchy: Oh, I'm just downright itchy because my kidneys are trying to do some of the liver's detoxification work. They're so upset about this—doing something they're not designed for—that they're dumping toxins out through my skin.

Achy: I'm achy because my lymph system is jammed up with phenols, epoxides, and proteins. My immune system is in overdrive trying to clean up all this junk in the lymph, and I'm the innocent bystander getting hit by all the flying bullets.

Spacey: My brain doesn't work so well when my blood sugar is up and down like a yo-yo. Drives me to eat more sweets, which is making me fat, even though I'm on a low-fat diet and I exercise regularly.

Gaspy: My heart acts up because it doesn't get enough oxygen, because **Bloaty**'s got the blood backed up below the liver. It's got nothing to do with my smoking, so don't start on that!

Bloaty: I get bloated when toxins overwhelm the liver's detoxification enzymes, and I have to close the liver valves to prevent the toxins from getting past the liver.

Burpy: I get indigestion when the liver's detoxification enzymes get overloaded with toxins, and I dump them into the bile.

Docque: (*Laughing*) Well, you certainly have a wide variety of complaints. But there are even more similarities than there are differences. Let me see if I can sum up most of your problems in a simple way.

Eating refined carbohydrates leads to loss of chromium—and other nutrients. And loss of chromium leads to a decrease in glucose tolerance factor (GTF). Less GTF means that insulin is less effective and more abundant in your blood. High insulin causes your brain to crave more sugar, your body to store excess sugar as fat, and your kidneys to dump out calcium; it also activates your delta 5 desaturase enzyme, which may increase pain and inflammation. Low calcium causes narrowing of the jaw, weak bones and teeth, and leaves the membranes of the sinuses, nose, throat, bladder, nerves, and intestine more sensitive. In addition, low calcium will make your ileocecal valve sensitive to coarse fibres, causing it to open when it shouldn't. This, in turn, will allow bacteria from the large intestine into your small intestine where they can steal nutrients like vitamin B_{12} and tryptophan, disrupt absorption of other nutrients, and dump toxins into the portal vein, which delivers these toxins to the liver.

As long as your liver can filter out portal vein toxins, there are no problems. Even after your liver's detoxification enzymes become overwhelmed, there still may be no apparent symptoms immediately because there are very few nerve endings in your liver. Symptoms may not appear until the toxins have been scattered into your bile, lymph, or kidneys so that you get problems that are seemingly far removed from your liver.

Itchy: I've been talking this problem over with a **Dwarf** brother from the electrical union; we could easily wire up a detection system that would activate as soon as the liver's detoxification enzymes started to run out of sync with each other. We could install flashing red lights in the eyes and sirens in the ears so that people would know *immediately* when their diet was throwing off their liver enzymes.

Bitchy: You missed the most important element in your

alarm system—a trap door in the mouth that slams shut when you're eating the wrong stuff.

Docque: These are all good ideas and I'll send them in to **Liver Dwarf Headquarters** for consideration. In the meantime, we're stuck with a whole mess of trouble from the inadequate system that now exists. Though altogether, it sounds like an average job for a **Liver Dwarf** cook. I'll see if I can work out a generalized program that might cover all of your main problems. Of course, you'll need some individualized attention to get started.

Let's start with **Sluggy**. The enzymes that you were talking about are **delta 6 desaturase**, **delta 5 desaturase**, **COX**, and **LOX**. These enzymes can make you feel good, bad, or great—depending on how well you keep them running. They're involved in the conversion of **fatty acids**—located in your cell membranes—into **eicosanoids**. Eicosanoids are very powerful, short-lived, short-range hormones that control the membranes and therefore, the receptors; eicosanoids can thereby override other hormones—even the long-range hormones. There are three types of eicosanoids—**prostaglandins, leukotrienes**, and **thromboxanes**—and they belong to three major families.

Sluggy: How did you know that?

Docque: I was a **Liver Dwarf** for many centuries before you were born, and I've learned much. The first enzyme in a cell membrane is delta 6 desaturase. **Chronic viral infections** can dramatically weaken this enzyme—as can **ageing**, especially around menopause in women. **Caffeine** in coffee, colas, and chocolate can interfere with it, too. **Stress** can throw it off and, since all enzymes need specific vitamins and minerals, deficiencies in these can also interfere with the optimal function of delta 6 enzyme. **Hydrogenated oils** can gradually gum it up. **Alcohol** in very small amounts can stimulate it, but excess alcohol can dramatically interfere with it. I'll draw you a picture as we go, so you can follow along.

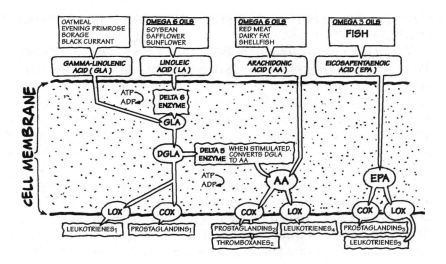

Delta 6 enzyme converts **linoleic acid (LA)** to **gamma-linolenic acid (GLA)**. Linoleic acid is an essential fatty acid—meaning that it must come from fat in your diet. It's found to some extent in almost all foods and it's particularly high in oils such as safflower, sunflower, and soybean. GLA, on the other hand, is found in only a few foods—in very small amounts in **oatmeal**, more abundantly in **black currant seed oil** and **evening primrose seed oil**, and most copiously in **borage seed oil**. Since these oils already contain GLA, the delta 6 enzyme isn't needed to convert them to GLA.

GLA easily becomes **dihomogamma-linolenic acid (DGLA)** and from here, it should be an easy downhill slide to become eicosanoids of the **1 Family**—the "**feel great**" family. The 1 Family eicosanoids all originate from DGLA, as opposed to the **2 Family** eicosanoids—the "**feel bad**" family—which are all made from **arachidonic acid (AA)**, and the **3 Family** eicosanoids—the "**feel good**" family—which are made from **eicosapentaenoic acid (EPA)**.

There are two enzyme pathways that convert DGLA, AA, and EPA into eicosanoids. **Cyclooxygenase (COX) enzymes** make prostaglandins and thromboxanes, while **lipoxygenase (LOX) enzymes** make leukotrienes. Even though all of these eicosanoids are short-lived, short-range hormones, they can have a profound effect on your physical, mental, and emotional health.

Prostaglandins—especially **PGE₁**—and other eicosanoids of the 1 Family decrease inflammation, improve immune function including suppression of cancer development, improve fat metabolism, and inspire the sense of well-being and confidence that comes with serotonin and growth hormone. All in all, the 1 Family keeps you feeling like Numero Uno, the centre of the universe—fit, strong, and stable.

Spacey: Why don't I feel that way then, because I take evening primrose seed oil supplements? They're already high in GLA and therefore must make lots of DGLA.

Docque: The one little obstacle in the way of this perfect ending for your DGLA is that even though it doesn't need the delta 6 enzyme, it still has delta 5 to deal with. Delta 5 enzyme will sit on the sidelines cheering DGLA on as it scores in the 1 Family end zone—*unless* you have high insulin from eating too much sugar. High insulin will kick-start delta 5 into grabbing DGLA and will drag it, kicking and screaming, over to the 2 Family side, where it will be turned into arachidonic acid and the "feel bad" family of eicosanoids.

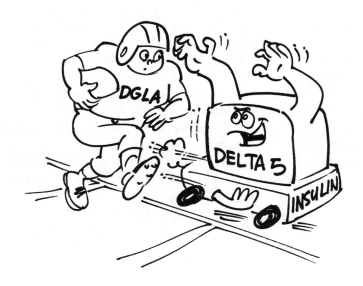

So, foods that are high in sugar can activate insulin to make your precious DGLA into arachidonic acid, especially if you have low glucose tolerance factor (GTF).

Excess eicosanoids from arachidonic acid can cause a wide range of symptoms. Every symptom that all eight of you **Liver Dwarves** have—in fact, virtually every disease, from asthma and arthritis to heart problems and cancer and all the rest—can be traced back to an excess of eicosanoids made from arachidonic acid.

For example: **prostaglandin E$_2$ (PGE$_2$)** is what causes much of the pain of inflammation such as in arthritis. It's also involved in migraines, dermatitis, insomnia, diarrhea, irritable bowel, and schizophrenia. **PGD$_2$** can cause flushing, sneezing, sleepiness, and skin reactions. **PGF$_2\alpha$** can create high blood sugar, depression, diarrhea from the small intestine, and chemical sensitivities.

Thromboxanes (TX)—such as **TXA$_2$** and **TXB$_2$**—can cause edema in the lungs and clotting, as in heart attacks. They can also cause the kidneys to leak protein and are involved in fetal alcohol syndrome. These are just a few of the conditions to which thromboxanes can contribute when they're present in excess.

The LOX enzymes make **leukotrienes (LT)** of the **4 Family**, which, for convenience, we'll include in the 2 Family, since they're also made from arachidonic acid. **Leukotriene B$_4$ (LTB$_4$)** is involved in dermatitis, rheumatoid arthritis, and colitis. **LTC$_4$** can cause sneezing, hypertension, angina, asthma, and anaphylaxis. Anaphylaxis can be fatal.

Dozens of different variations of these eicosanoids can be made and they can be found together in many combinations. For example, high levels of PGE$_2$, PGF$_2\alpha$, TXB$_2$, and LTB$_4$ can be found in irritable bowel syndrome.

So you can see that most physical and emotional—and even some mental—problems come from an excess of arachidonic acid eicosanoids.

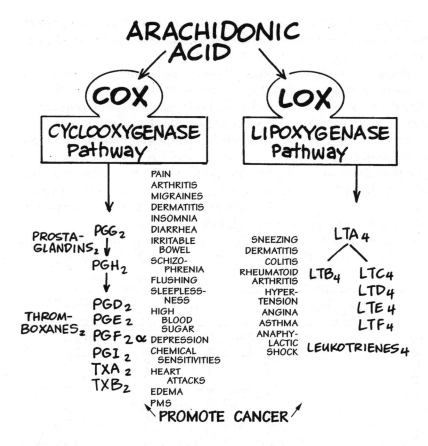

Bitchy: Omigawd, **Docque**. How do we get rid of arachidonic acid? It sounds so *bad*!

Docque: Arachidonic acid isn't bad; it's just a fatty acid that's built into your membranes and it's totally harmless. In fact, it's also very beneficial as a source of many eicosanoids that are crucial for cell membrane conversations. The eicosanoids from arachidonic acid only become "bad" when they're made in excess over long periods of time, and *then* they're the root of all lingering, chronic diseases.

Gaspy: I still don't like the sounds of arachidonic acid. Where does it come from?

Docque: Arachidonic acid comes directly into your diet from red meat and, to a lesser extent, from dairy fat and shellfish.

Sluggy: But **Docque**, I'm a vegetarian; I don't eat *any* animal fat and haven't for years, and just look at the terrible shape *I'm* in!

Docque: Arachidonic acid plays a major role in your first line of defence when your cell membranes are threatened with direct attack by "aliens," so your body must be able to make arachidonic acid from other fatty acids, under certain conditions. As I said earlier, insulin can activate delta 5 enzyme to convert DGLA into arachidonic acid; this would mainly apply to **Spacey**, since she's the one with high insulin. The rest of you are making arachidonic acid from a different pathway. You have an enzyme called **phospholipase A₂** that's converting **phosphatidyl choline** into arachidonic acid.

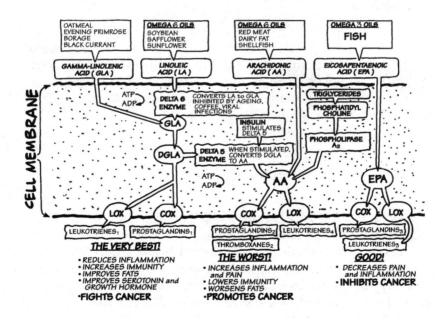

Gaspy: And to think I was taking phosphatidyl choline to lower my blood pressure.

Burpy: And I was taking it to thin down my bile to help my fat digestion.

Docque: Taking phosphatidyl choline isn't necessarily a problem because large amounts of phosphatidyl choline can be made from triglycerides anyway, and triglycerides can be made from carbohydrates. The amount of phosphatidyl choline isn't that important. Most crucial is the activity of phospholipase A_2 enzyme that converts phosphatidyl choline into arachidonic acid and makes it readily available for the COX and LOX enzymes to make eicosanoids. So even a diet low in arachidonic acid can result in an excess of eicosanoids made from arachidonic acid *if* phospholipase A_2 is activated. This is the way that the rest of you are getting excess arachidonic acid eicosanoids.

Sluggy: So what activates phospholipase A_2?

Docque: Mainly your immune system—such as when it attacks aliens trying to break through your cell membranes.

Achy: All right, blame it on my little soldiers. Everybody else is blaming their problems on those hardworking guys. You might as well just dump another load of guilt on them!

Docque: Of course, the immune system is just doing its job of responding to a cry for help from the cells. The cells shriek out in horror whenever an alien docks in their receptors, and the distress signals they send are the eicosanoids made by the COX and LOX enzymes from arachidonic acid.

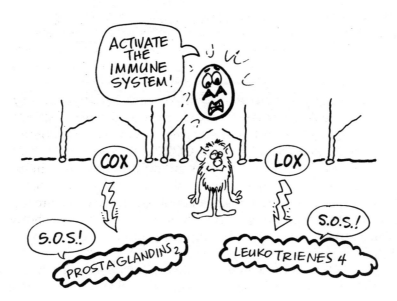

When the nearby macrophages hear these distress signals, they rush to the rescue, followed shortly thereafter by their neutrophil assistants. If they see any aliens nearby, they open fire with superoxide radicals as you have trained them to do, **General Achy**. The superoxides will create hydrogen peroxide and hydroxyl radicals that will rip the would-be invaders' membranes to shreds. Of course, your own membranes will take a severe beating as well. If that membrane is in your nose, you might get rhinitis; if it's in your lungs, you might get asthma; if it's in your joints, you might get arthritis—and so on throughout your body, from your bowels to your brain.

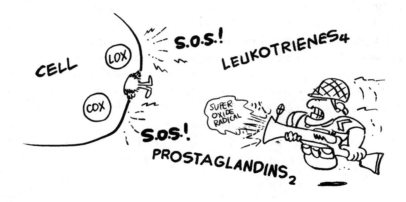

The resulting peroxides and hydroxyl radicals also activate phospholipase A_2 enzyme to make more arachidonic acid available to the COX and LOX enzymes—which also become more reactive. So you can see that COX, LOX, and phospholipase A_2 work together as an important team to help save your membranes when they're in danger. Together these three enzymes call in the troops when suspicious aliens are spotted, and they continue shrieking for help if the alien should survive the first assault by your immune system.

Achy: Those Boogy Boys would *never* live through a barrage of my soldiers. I keep them armed with the latest and best weaponry. Did you know that I personally designed IgA so that it could withstand the heat of battle? That's a fact! The Boogy Boys wouldn't stand a chance.

Docque: That's true, General. The problem comes when the aliens *aren't* Boogy Boys. If chemicals such as epoxides made by your liver, or phenols and proteins from food get into your lymph via your liver or a "leaky gut," then they're just as foreign and unwelcome as a Boogy Boy, and they're attacked just as vigorously.

Of course, if **Bloaty**'s continually dumping more phenols from plants and chemicals into your lymph and blood systems, your cell membranes will keep screaming for help in dealing with aliens. And as your immune system attacks over and over again, the hydroxyl radicals generated by your immune system against the aliens will also create tremendous stress on your own membranes. This irritation can be found anywhere from your nose or sinuses to your intestine, skin, or joints. And the same phenols might be present in pollens and perfumes so that you start cross-reacting with a wide range of external substances.

If your membranes rupture from this assault, or from apoptosis, and leak out metals and proteins, your immune system can mistakenly identify and attack bits of *you* as the enemy. So, from simple allergies, complex autoimmune disease can grow.

Sluggy: But I don't have any allergies! I had skin testing done and only dust mites showed up. And feathers.

Docque: An allergy is an oversensitivity to something because the immune system is reacting to it. Skin testing is only looking for immediate reactions involving IgE. There are many other ways that your immune system can cause strong reactions that may not show on skin testing. In fact, skin testing for food reactions might reveal only 10 percent of the problems with foods.

When IgE causes the release of histamine, the skin can develop symptoms within an hour—but soon after, the histamine is decreasing, and **prostaglandin D_2 (PGD_2)** from arachidonic acid is increasing. PGD_2 is what sustains the skin symptoms five or six hours later. So while histamine from IgE may initiate an allergic reaction rapidly, it's prostaglandins from arachidonic acid that maintain it over a much longer period of time. Other parts of your immune system may stimulate the same prostaglandins, without any IgE being involved.

Children who eat a high-sugar breakfast—like highly processed cereal—can get a surge of serotonin building up in their platelets, due to high insulin levels increasing the absorption of tryptophan. Then, exposure to a food that has triggered an immune reaction—such as IgG—could cause a sudden release of the serotonin from the platelets. This release of serotonin stimulates the production of arachidonic acid eicosanoids, which can cause a wide range of physical, mental, and/or emotional symptoms. By definition, these reactions should be called an allergy because the immune system plays a key role. Skin testing for allergies, however, could show IgE levels that are normal or even low—so a person with very strong immune reactions to a food could be told that he or she doesn't have allergies.

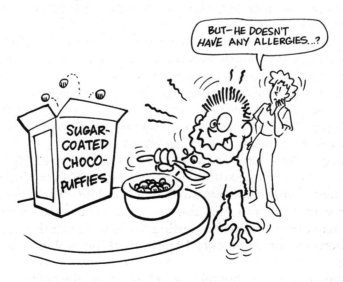

Platelet serotonin release contributes to the joint inflammation of rheumatoid arthritis in a similar way. Of course, chemical intolerances to food additive phenols—such as **salicyclates** like **tartrazine** (yellow dye #5) or the preservative **benzoic acid**—could also result in the release of serotonin and the subsequent cascade of arachidonic acid eicosanoids. In people sensitized to acetaldehyde, even a whiff of phenols in perfume or petroleum products can be enough to cause a dramatic release of arachidonic acid eicosanoids. These eicosanoid cries-for-help quickly attract the soldiers of the immune system and they attack immediately, 'though IgE or other antibodies need not be involved.

Sluggy: Is that right, **Achy**?

Achy: Basically correct. My solders will always respond to a cry for help. If there's danger, they attack; that's what I trained them to do.

Bitchy: It seems to me they're too well armed and not very bright. They're shooting up the whole body just to knock out a few little pieces of food that happened to get into a person's body.

Achy: They've been trained that the only good alien is a dead alien. They spot alien material but they can't tell that a phenol from food is less dangerous than a **typhoid bacteria**. That's not for them to decide. Their job is to *kill everything* that isn't you. It's up to you to keep bits of food and chemicals out of your lymph so that my soldiers don't waste a lot of your precious ATP energy attacking nonhazardous targets.

Sluggy: By the way, **General Achy**, I've been meaning to tell you that lately my DNA repair crew has seen your neutrophils damaging the DNA strands with their peroxides whenever chemicals have been passing by.

Achy: Has it gone that far that they're even damaging the precious DNA? I'm so humiliated, I should rip the stars off my epaulettes. Yes, I must resign, turn in my stars, and then take the honourable way out of this embarrassment by committing apoptosis.

Docque: Not so fast, General. You're right that your white blood cells are only doing their job by reacting to things they perceive as dangers, even if they're only bits of food, pollen, or chemicals. It's your liver's detoxification enzymes that are really to blame for this whole mess.

If your liver's P450 enzymes turn simple chemicals into epoxides that your conjugation enzymes don't fully neutralize, then these toxic epoxides may end up binding to and damaging your DNA bases; if this happens, it's not the fault of your immune system. If the same chemicals stimulate your neutrophils to blow apart your DNA strands, and then this DNA damage leads to cancer, I would say that your liver was at fault, not your immune system.

Also, if the peroxides made by your liver's P450 enzymes aren't neutralized by your liver's conjugation enzymes and Bloaty is forced to shut your outlet liver valves, then proteins and phenols would be spilled into your lymph system, thus forcing your white blood cells to clean it up. If *this* resulted in allergies, sensitivities and intolerances to foods, chemicals, and pollens—and eventually in autoimmune diseases, including cancer—then I would *still* say that your liver was the cause of the problem, not your immune system. Your white blood cells are just good little guys doing their best to help. It's poor liver function that forces them into this difficult situation.

Achy: Did you just say that cancer is an autoimmune disease!?

Sluggy: I think he's referring to your neutrophils damaging the DNA strands.

Achy: Oh, I see.

Docque: It's true that your immune system can accentuate the negative effects of eicosanoids made from arachidonic acid, and it can even promote the growth of cancer. The good news is that this can be greatly affected by diet. Let me explain a little more about how phospholipase A$_2$ works, and then I'll show you how diet can improve your liver enzymes so that you don't get into this jam again.

Sluggy probably already told you that there are things that make your nerve cell receptors more sensitive or less sensitive. NMDA receptors release calcium, which is what stimulates phospholipase A$_2$ to produce arachidonic acid. Interferon from your immune system makes NMDA receptors even *more* sensitive, which releases calcium more readily and activates more arachidonic acid production from phospholipase A$_2$.

For example, if you have sensitive NMDA receptors because your immune system is making interferon, then if you eat glutamate—such as **monosodium glutamate** (**MSG**)—which also stimulates NMDA receptors, you could get such a flood of arachidonic acid eicosanoids in your system that you could feel quite ill. Such a strong reaction may not show on an IgE allergy test, but you can be sure that your immune system was indirectly contributing to your reaction to MSG; therefore this should be called an allergy, although some might call it an intolerance or a sensitivity to MSG.

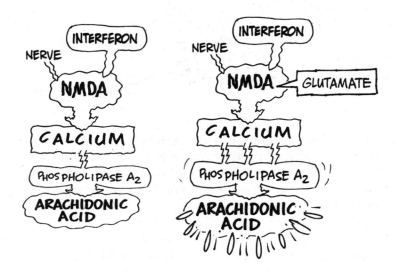

Bee stings and wasp stings contain phospholipase A_2 right in the venom, which immediately begins the arachidonic acid cascade into leukotrienes. If the person's NMDA receptors have already been made very sensitive by his or her immune system, a bee or wasp sting can lead to anaphylactic shock and even death.

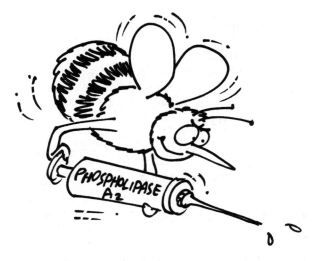

Achy: I've had *my* near-death experiences with leukotriene C_4 and wouldn't want that again. There I was, swimming in a sea of interleukin-4 that was stimulating IgE that was stimulating histamine and leukotriene C_4, and all of a sudden, I wasn't swimming anymore, I was *drowning*—my past lives flashing before my . . .

Bitchy, Bloaty, Burpy, Gaspy, Itchy, Sluggy, Spacey: Enough, already! We've heard it many times before!

Achy: Is there anything that can be done?

Docque: **Magnesium**.

Bitchy: So what are you going to do now—show us how to make a magnesium parfait?

Docque: (*Laughs*) No, but magnesium might keep you alive long enough to enjoy my cooking. A doctor might give you cortisone to inhibit COX, LOX, and phospholipase A_2 enzymes, but what I use in an emergency is magnesium. It's not as strong as cortisone but it reduces your NMDA receptors' stimulation of phospholipase A_2 by blocking calcium release, thus reducing arachidonic acid production. It could also greatly reduce an anaphylactic reaction. Of course, in the long run, getting your liver working well enough so that it stops dumping proteins, phenols, and epoxides into your lymph system will cure autoimmune diseases and allergies, and reduce reactions to insect stings.

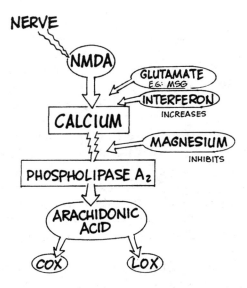

Achy: In the meantime, I'm staying away from bees as much as I can because I know my immune system is *way* overactive.

Docque: And yet bee sting venom, used in small doses, could relieve your symptoms since something that's poisonous at one dose could be an antidote at a smaller dose. This is the essence of **homeopathy**.

Achy: Thanks **Docque**, but I think I'll pass on the bee buffet.

Docque: Once your immune system has activated phospholipase A_2, the casein found in milk will stimulate it further. Human milk protein has less than 25 percent casein, while cow's milk has over 80 percent. This may be no problem for a truly healthy person, but someone with a tendency to arachidonic acid eicosanoid problems—which is virtually everyone with a chronic health problem—will likely be made worse since casein is a stimulator of phospholipase A_2 as well as LOX enzymes.

A calf's stomach protects itself from casein by making **rennet**, which contains a milk-coagulating enzyme called **rennin**. Rennin turns the casein into curd; the curd then slowly releases casein into the calf's small intestine. Since *your* stomach can't make rennet, the casein in cow's milk is released directly into your small intestine at a rate that could overwhelm you.

Casein, however, is not the only protein in milk. After the casein has been turned into curds, whey proteins remain in the milk. Whey consists of **beta-lactoglobulin**, **alpha-lactalbumin**, immunoglobulins, **peptones**, and **serum albumins**—all of which are much less allergy-causing than casein.

In addition, whey is high in **cystine**, which consists of two cysteine amino acids joined together. As **Burpy** may have told you, cysteine is one of the three amino acids that make up glutathione, which is crucial for detoxification and immune system function. So whey is a good way to increase your glutathione levels. In serious diseases, a stronger way to increase glutathione levels is by taking **N-acetylcysteine** (NAC); it's a variation of cysteine, the sulphur-carrying amino acid in glutathione, and it's absorbed from your intestine much better than glutathione.

Breast milk, with its low casein and high whey content, is the best milk for babies. **Goat's milk** is much closer in protein content to human milk than is cow's milk.

For those who have trouble digesting lactose sugar in milk, letting The Boogy Boys ferment the sugar in the production of yogurt may help. Yogurt also inhibits your adrenal glands from making cholesterol. When I was working in Lebanon—where people treasure the yogurt they make every night for the next day's use—I saw that the first thing people do when they get rich enough is trade in the cow for a goat.

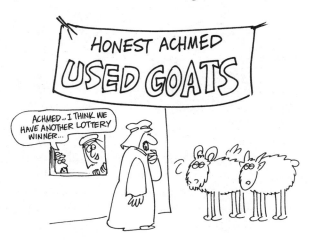

Burpy: So maybe *that's* why Dad always referred to his mother-in-law as "the old goat." It must be a term of endearment!

Docque: Another thing that makes phospholipase A_2 more active is cold, damp weather. Both arthritis and asthma are a result of excess eicosanoids from arachidonic acid, and both can be worse in cold, damp weather because of the increased activity of phospholipase A_2 enzyme. This is one reason why saunas, steam rooms, and sweat lodges are found so universally in the colder climates and why active exercise that heats you up can be so important in the winter.

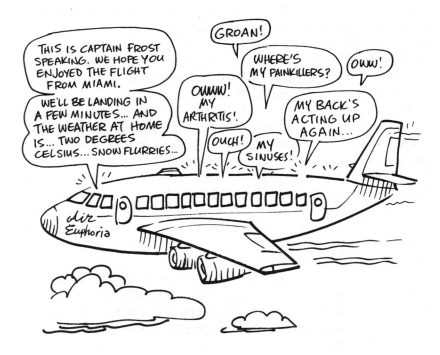

Of course, allowing your body to get cold can also stimulate the production of arachidonic acid eicosanoids due to phospholipase A_2, and the congestion they produce can contribute to more colds, flus, and infections. It's important to keep warm in the winter—it's especially important to keep the kidneys warm. Dressing warmly is one way to do this; eating warming foods is another.

Itchy: I knew that. I told you it's important. They're all eating too much sugar and potassium. All that fruit and salad in winter makes for low calcium and a sensitive ileocecal valve, as well as driving me crazy!

Docque: That's right, **Itchy**. To keep your bowels working, you may need *some* fruit in winter. It's better to use the more northerly fruits, like berries. Eskimos—or Inuit, as they prefer to be called—dry cranberries to use over the winter. In Scandinavia, they dry lingonberries, which are similar.

If **constipation** is a problem, then raisins or even prunes are dried fruits that can loosen you up a little more when they're soaked thoroughly or stewed. Raisins and their cousins, currants, are high in **tartaric acid**, which can reduce your bowel transit time by half. This might help until you get The Boogy Boys out of your small intestine where the indoles they're making from tryptophan are the likely cause of really stubborn constipation.

If extra fibre is needed, try taking **psyllium**, the seeds of the **plantain plant**. This forms a soft bulk in your intestine and usually won't irritate a sensitive ileocecal valve, unlike many of the coarser fibres from grains. Taking a teaspoon to a tablespoon of psyllium, mixed thoroughly in water before breakfast and dinner, can help get those bowels working better.

Sluggy: My bowels work great, Docque, but what about those bad eicosanoids from arachidonic acid that you say we're all making too many of?

Docque: There are herbs that slow down COX, LOX, and phospholipase A_2. **Ginger** is one that is very warming, and it also inhibits arachidonic acid production. **Turmeric** and its most active portion **curcumin** are the parts of curry that give it a distinctive yellow colour. Turmeric and curcumin are very good at slowing down arachidonic acid eicosanoid production. A more obvious way is to eat less arachidonic acid—less red meat, dairy, and shellfish—and eat more fish.

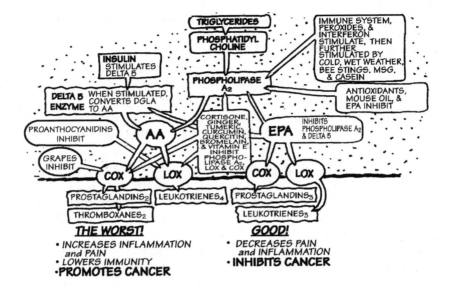

Fish is high in two oils: EPA and **docosahexaenoic acid
(DHA)**. DHA is used widely in the nervous system as a
building block—for brain cells, for example. In other words, it
helps make you smarter. DHA can also be converted into EPA.
EPA inhibits delta 5 enzyme from converting DGLA into
arachidonic acid. EPA also inhibits phospholipase A_2 enzyme,
and competes for COX and LOX enzymes, resulting in the less
war-like 3 Family eicosanoids. So you can see that EPA is one of
the best things for reducing eicosanoids from arachidonic acid.
Fish that is high in EPA oil is also high in CoQ_{10}—so important
to help make ATP for energy.

Fish is also high in vitamin B_6—necessary for your liver to
make CoQ_{10}—as well as chromium, which helps stabilize your
insulin levels. Virtually any fish has some EPA, so it's easy
enough to find some that suit your taste. The oilier ones have
the most EPA. If someone is already quite healthy, all he or she
has to do to maintain that health is eat less sugar and red meat,
and increase the intake of fish. That won't be enough for most
of you **Liver Dwarves** because your immune systems will
continue to activate phospholipase A_2 enzyme into making
arachidonic acid, until we can get it calmed down. That will

take some time because of the **memory cells** that your immune system makes when it attacks an "enemy." In the meantime, more fish!

Sluggy: That's fine by me, Docque, because I like fish and I hope to soon have enough energy to go fishing.

Bitchy: I thought you were a vegetarian.

Sluggy: I *was* a vegetarian for health, not spiritual, reasons. Obviously what I was doing before wasn't working too well. If **Docque** says EPA will help me out, then I should eat some fish!

Docque: EPA comes from fish directly, but can also be made from **alpha linolenic acid (ALA)**, which is found in some plants, particularly **flax seeds**.

Sluggy: Is there anything I can do to repair my damaged liver?

Docque: I'm going to make up some **liver juice**. Liver *juice,* because eating regular liver would give you too much arachidonic acid. The water-soluble liver extract has properties that stimulate your liver cells and your mitochondria to regenerate.

Sluggy: Boy, could I use some new mitochondria! Mine look like they've already been through the wrecking yard.

Docque: Actually, all of you could get some improvement from liver juice.

Spacey: Even me?

Docque: Yes, **Spacey**. Liver juice can also help you because it's high in cysteine, which binds to lactic acid to form **pyruvate**—also known as **pyruvic acid**. Pyruvic acid raises thyroid activity and decreases insulin levels. This will result in fewer fat deposits and more burning up of stored fat. In other words, YOU LOSE FAT.

Spacey: You have my full attention, **Docque**.

Gaspy: It's probably the first time in years that anybody's had your *full* attention.

Docque: In addition, liver juice can dramatically increase stamina. Liver juice is high in vitamin B_{12}, folic acid, and **heme iron**. Heme iron is up to 35 percent absorbable as opposed to nonheme iron (found in iron salts), which is—at the most—3 percent absorbable. Heme iron doesn't create the tremendous free radical activity that nonheme iron does; this free radical activity can lead to digestive upset, constipation, and cancer, especially of the colon.

Sluggy: Now you have *my* full attention, **Docque**!

Docque: **Malic acid**—from apples—and magnesium help to strengthen your mitochondrial membranes, **Sluggy**. And we'll use a little of the amino acid **methionine** because it aids in liver detoxification and also helps the liver to repair.

Burpy: Well, **Docque**, I just want to warn you that when methionine comes into the digestive system, my helpers convert it to **homocysteine** for shipment to the liver. And as you may know, homocysteine can be an irritant to membranes.

Achy: Ahhhhh, so *that's* the source of the homocysteine that my macrophages have reported hanging around the scene of the crime in "The Case of the Hardening of the Arteries."

Docque: That's true, **Burpy**, but homocysteine is converted back into methionine in the liver. The most active form of methionine is **S-adenosylmethionine (SAM)**, which is made from homocysteine by your liver. Folic acid and vitamin B_{12} are necessary for this conversion—and you know what happens to vitamin B_{12} when The Boogy Boys get into your small intestine. Homocysteine can also be converted to **cystathionine**—which is then converted to cysteine—but vitamin B_6 and/or the amino acid **serine** are required for this to happen. Serine combines with homocysteine to produce cystathionine. High levels of homocysteine can contribute to hardening of the arteries as well as age-related decreased mental function, such as Alzheimer's disease. Homocysteine levels can be reduced within two weeks of increasing your intake of folic acid, vitamin B_6, and B_{12}.

In addition, SAM may play a role in the pineal production of melatonin—by regulating the activity of one of the enzymes—and it may also be involved in the synthesis of myelin. Your levels of SAM can be increased with the use of **betaine**, which is found in beets. Betaine enhances the activity of **betaine homocysteine methyltransferase (BHMT)**, an enzyme that converts homocysteine to methionine.

Every aspect of your health depends on your two liver detoxification enzyme systems working <u>together</u>. Your P450 enzymes can take pesticides, herbicides, drugs, **aflatoxins**, and smoked foods and turn them into deadly DNA-damaging toxic epoxides or membrane-destroying peroxides. It's up to your conjugation enzymes to intercept all of these—as well as deactivate any metals—and neutralize them before they can force **Bloaty** to dump them into your lymph system—where they can go on to create coronary heart disease, cancer, or the hundreds of other diseases from "A" for allergies to "Z" for, um, Zzz . . . Zzz . . . er, Zzzzz . . .

Spacey: Zebras?

Docque: Thanks, **Spacey**. I got stuck trying to think of a disease that started with "Z."

Spacey: I didn't know that zebras were a disease.

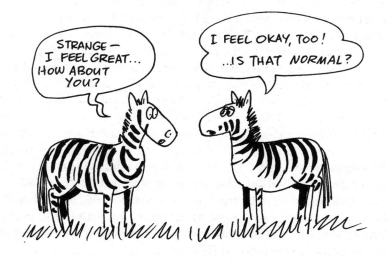

Docque: Anyway, most people with diseases have their P450 enzymes making epoxides and peroxides faster than their conjugation enzymes can neutralize them. Of course, they weren't designed to work this way; the P450 and conjugation enzymes were designed to run at the same speed. It's the little day-to-day bad habits that throw the liver's detoxification enzymes out of harmony with each other.

Alcohol and tobacco speed up the P450 enzymes, and high carbohydrate diets—sugar, in other words—dramatically slow down the conjugation enzymes. Coffee, even decaffeinated coffee, can throw off liver function in general and can create a myriad of mental symptoms. Coffee is a nerve stimulant and, like all stimulants, it'll eventually weaken the organ that it stimulates; this is particularly true of the liver.

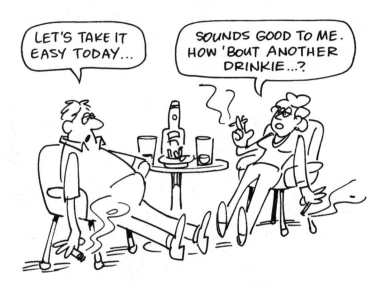

Bloaty: Did you say sugar slows down conjugation enzymes? Could that be what makes my magnificent Super Hero conjugation enzymes fall asleep after eating? Then the free radicals, peroxides, and epoxides force me to slam the liver valves shut—and spread the toxins into the bile, lymph, and kidneys.

Docque: Sugar shuts down the conjugation enzymes quickly and the more processed the sugar is, the faster it shuts them down. The conjugation enzymes need protein. Of course, if your P450 enzymes are making more carcinogens by the stimulation of alcohol and tobacco—while at the same time, your conjugation enzymes are being "knocked out" with sugar—then you're heading for big health problems.

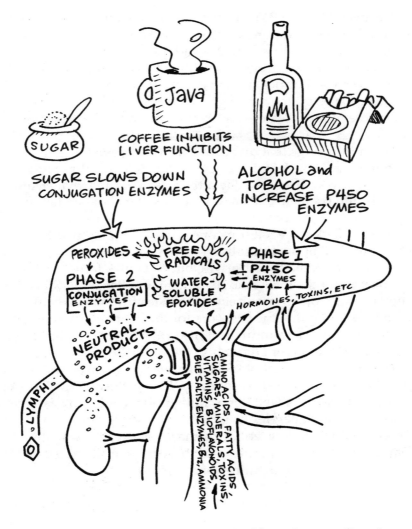

Alcohol, tobacco, and sugar can quickly twist your liver's detoxification enzyme function so that instead of protecting you from dietary and intestinal toxins, the detoxification enzymes can make these toxins up to 60 times worse and can even make them cancer-causing. Coffee can throw your liver off even further.

Gaspy: Seems to me that a little coffee, sugar, and alcohol never hurt anybody in the old days.

Docque: Well, the P450 enzymes were designed to make our steroid hormones water-soluble and in the Olden Days, that's about all they were used for. Nowadays, with thousands of petrochemicals and drugs—which your P450s can convert into carcinogens—it's much more crucial that you have your conjugation enzymes running at least as fast as your P450s, so that these modern water-soluble epoxides don't damage your DNA.

All of the things that disrupt your liver's detoxification enzymes are habit-forming or even addictive. It's those little things that you do wrong day after day, over time, that create most health problems. It's best that you get rid of bad habits <u>before</u> they get rid of you.

Spacey: Didn't we tell someone once about the **Liver Dwarf** code: survival of the fittest liver?

Achy: I think that was Darwin, but ol' Chuck forgot to add the part about the liver. And then there was Benjamin Rush. We showed him how every disease originates from the liver. But then he decided that the best cure for the liver was mercury; he even taught that to hundreds of medical students . . . that was a heavy period in **Liver Dwarf** history.

Docque: A great deal of social pressure is put on people to see who has the fittest liver—especially during "festive" events. As you **Liver Dwarves** well know, indigestion, colds, flus, fatigue, depression, and allergies usually flare up shortly after Thanksgiving, Halloween, Christmas, New Year's, Valentine's Day, Easter, birthday parties, and the other socially accepted liver-enzyme-damaging times of the year.

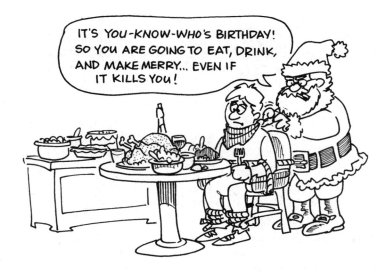

Spacey: When I was stationed in Iceland, I noticed that babies born in October had a high incidence of diabetes, especially if they were boys. Their average date of conception was January 17. You know what conception means, right? You know—when the Boy thing goes into the Girl thing, and the little Spermy thing swims into the big Egg thing, and a Baby starts.

Burpy: So *that's* how it works; I always wondered!

Spacey: So anyway, I did a little digging around and found out that during the two weeks of Christmas celebrations, the Icelanders eat a lot of smoked mutton that has been preserved with **nitrates**. Something in this food seems to cause the high incidence of juvenile diabetes seen in children born in October.

Docque: The Boogy Boys could easily turn nitrates into nitrites—which can bind to other nitrogen compounds to form nitrosamines, which can cause genetic damage. And, the polycyclic aromatic hydrocarbons from the smoked mutton could be turned into toxic epoxides by the liver's P450 enzymes, to further compound the risk of DNA damage and cancer development.

Of course, a developing fetus will be much more likely to be damaged than a full-grown adult. And speaking of nitrates, kids who eat a lot of **hot dogs** containing nitrates are more prone to **leukemia**.

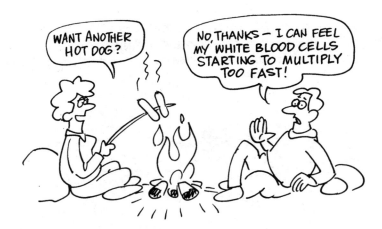

There's a price to be paid for partying, not only by the partiers, but also by the children that these adults conceive. Right, **Sluggy**?

Sluggy: Not me, **Docque**. I'm too wrecked to party. Isn't there anything I can do to get my enzymes working better?

Docque: There *are* things that can slow down your liver's P450 enzymes. **Grapefruit** has a bioflavonoid called **naringen**, which can slow the P450s down quite dramatically. If you're taking prescription drugs, you might have to reduce the dosage you're taking because when your P450 enzymes slow down, the drugs will stay in your blood longer. **Sprouted wheat** or foods high in **ellagic acid**, such as raspberries, grapes, strawberries, walnuts, or pomegranates all have anticancer properties because of their ability to slow down your P450 enzymes.

What I personally prefer, however, is **green tea**. It gently dampens down the P450 enzymes and also stimulates the conjugation enzymes at the same time, which gives your liver a *big* break. Green tea is 25 percent bioflavonoids—such as **quercetin**, **myricetin**, and **rutin**—which stimulate glutathione peroxidase, catalase, and **quinone reductase** in your liver, small intestine, and lungs, and glutathione transferase in your small intestine and liver. Now those attributes alone will give you a degree of anticancer protection, but there's even more good news. If any toxic epoxides get past the conjugation enzymes, **catechins** from green tea can bind to them and neutralize them before they can bind to your DNA. In addition, green tea is great at nabbing those lipid peroxides before they can go bowling in your membranes and it also blocks the formation of toxic nitrosamine compounds. Other antioxidants, including vitamin C, work similarly.

Gaspy: I prefer **black tea**; it's got more of a kick!

Docque: It does have more caffeine and greater aroma and flavour, but it doesn't have the medicinal properties of green tea. When I was working in Southeast Asia—okay, three or four thousand years ago—the leaf of the plant **Camellia sinensis** was already recognized as having healing properties when sipped as a tea. It was also known that those healing benefits were lost shortly after picking.

Being a curious **Liver Dwarf**, I studied it carefully and found that on picking the leaf, an enzyme in the leaf—**polyphenol oxidase**—began to oxidize the bioflavonoids, greatly lessening their activity. So I worked out a way to heat the leaves quickly after picking—to neutralize the enzyme and yet retain the medicinal qualities.

Years later, I heard that foreigners went to Asia and decided that the green tea didn't have enough flavour. They found that chopping up the Camellia sinensis leaf activated the polyphenol oxidase enzyme to rapidly oxidize the bioflavonoids and, in the process, release more aroma and flavour. This is how black tea came to be—by oxidizing green tea.

Spacey: You mean that black tea is just rusted green tea?

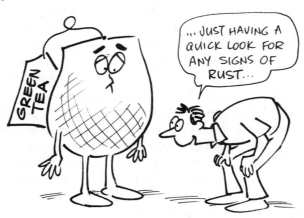

Docque: I guess you could say it that way, **Spacey**. The difference is that green tea has six times more medicinal properties than black tea, although less flavour.

Bitchy: I find it too acidic, so I put milk in it.

Docque: Unfortunately, adding milk to either black or green tea completely blocks their medicinal activity. The Japanese added a little more flavour by adding roasted rice to their **sencha**—which is what they call green tea. Sencha is made by steaming the leaf for less than a minute, just enough to neutralize the polyphenol oxidase enzyme. The roasted rice makes the tea less acidic, and adds a little flavour. **Oolong tea** is partially oxidized, and so it sits between green and black tea in benefits.

Spacey: What about me? I can't take any caffeine because it makes me too nervous. Isn't there anything I can take to help my liver's conjugation enzymes?

Itchy: What about those chocolate bars I always see you gnawing on? Those have caffeine in them. And those sodas you're always sucking on? They're full of caffeine! And the sugar in both those things is going to dump your calcium out of your kidneys.

Spacey: Well, I need them to keep my brain clear and bright, **Scratchy**, so lay off me, will ya?!

Docque: When you get a slump in blood sugar—especially around 3 P.M., when your adrenal glands begin to fade out—the obvious thing to do is force the blood sugar back up quickly with more sugar or stimulants like coffee or chocolate. This can work fast but sugar—in its many forms—or stimulants will soon throw your liver's detoxification enzymes off and create a whole range of digestive and immune system problems.

Ginseng and **licorice** are stimulants that can get you through the afternoon slump without throwing your liver enzymes off. In fact, both are also immune system boosters. Licorice can raise the adrenals' cortisone production enough that some people are able to reduce their use of **synthetic cortisone**. The **glycyrrizinate** in licorice can also raise the blood pressure in some individuals, so it's best for them to use **deglycyrrizinated** licorice—licorice from which the glycyrrizinate has been removed.

As people get older, their adrenal glands tend to dominate the hormones in the body and as adrenal activity increases, thymus gland and nervous system activity tend to decrease. This can be antidoted somewhat by large doses of **ginkgo biloba**. Ginkgo biloba is an antioxidant that works in the brain, the eyes, and also the cardiovascular system, where it helps improve circulation. Dating back to the days of the dinosaur, ginkgo biloba is the oldest living tree species in the world.

Green tea has only 3 percent caffeine; the other compounds in green tea seem to antidote the negative side effects of that small amount of caffeine. But for those who can't take caffeine at all, there is another **flavonoid** that can stimulate glutathione activity throughout your intestine and in your liver. It is **silymarin**, which comes from the seeds of the herb **Silybum marianum**, otherwise known as **milk thistle**.

Spacey: Well, my bum might look silly *now*, but wait till I go on a diet! But I can't take any milk, **Docque**—I'm highly allergic to it. Or sensitive, or intolerant, or something. Anyway, I get a stomach ache.

Docque: *(Laughs)* Don't worry, **Spacey**, there's no milk in milk thistle. The green leaf has streaks of white in it that give it a milky appearance. The double benefit of milk thistle is that it not only stimulates your Gladiator Glutathione enzyme, it also stimulates your other Superhero, Super OD, to break down superoxide radicals. Most of silymarin is conjugated by your liver and dumped through the bile into your intestine where The Boogy Boys reactivate it so that it gets recycled, and it stimulates the intestine and liver all over again. You're protected for most of a day from just one dose.

In fact, if you have a continuous circulation of silymarin in your intestine and liver, the enhanced glutathione activity can protect you from a wide range of toxins. Taking it after an acute poisoning has occurred isn't much good since it takes a few days to get your glutathione enzyme levels up. This wonderful benefit of silymarin stimulating your Gladiator Glutathione will be lost if you're eating a lot of sugar because sugar can knock glutathione down faster than silymarin can pull it up.

Another benefit of silymarin is that it makes the membranes of your red blood cells and mast cells stronger, which means more oxygen and less histamine, and therefore fewer allergic reactions.

Achy: I'll vote for less histamine. Did I ever tell you about the time I was drowning in histamine and my past lives were flashing before my . . .

Bitchy, Bloaty, Burpy, Gaspy, Itchy, Sluggy, Spacey: YES!!!

Docque: **Boswellia serrata** also has antiinflammatory and liver-protecting properties; it was once known as **frankincense**.

Spacey: Hey, I knew Frank. Wasn't he one of the Three Wise Guys? Or was it the Three Stooges?

Bitchy: What about me? Should I slow down *my* P450 enzymes?

Docque: No, it's very important for you to keep them breaking down your hormones as fast as possible. In fact, ideally, everyone should keep his or her P450 enzymes running as fast as the conjugation enzymes can keep up.

Estradiol, estrone and dihydroxytestosterone (DHT) are strong hormones designed to be active for only a short period of time—the shorter the better—because they can overstimulate cells. The breakdown of these strong hormones requires liver enzymes. Since these hormones are all steroids—that is, they're all made from cholesterol—the P450 enzymes have to make them water-soluble before the conjugation enzymes can work on them. So the quicker the P450 enzymes begin the breakdown of your steroid hormones, the better for your long-term health.

There are things that you can include in your diet that will both help and hinder this process. Mother Nature was thinking of you when she designed the **Cruciferae** family of plants, otherwise known as the **cruciferous vegetables**. They include cabbage, cauliflower, broccoli, kale, kohlrabi, brussels sprouts, collards, rutabaga, turnips, and mustard (including radish). These vegetables contain a wide range of **glucosinolates** that, when activated by your digestion, become **isothiocyanates**. These isothiocyanates stimulate the P450 enzymes that begin the breakdown of your steroid hormones, *as well as* stimulate the conjugation enzymes, which finish the job.

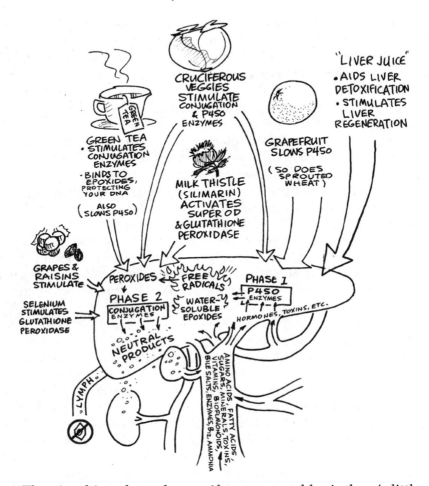

The nice thing about the cruciferous vegetables is there's little direct toxicity from these natural compounds—unlike **dioxins**, which also stimulate the P450 enzymes. The two most active cruciferous ingredients are **indole-3-carbinol** and **sulforaphane**. Both are found in high amounts in broccoli, cabbage, and brussels sprouts.

Indole-3-carbinol quite dramatically stimulates the P450 enzymes to begin the conversion of estradiol to milder forms, such as estrone.

Bitchy: It's not going to stimulate that damn C-16α pathway that's trying to give me breast cancer or endometriosis, is it?

Docque: As you obviously know, there are several enzyme pathways by which steroid hormones can be broken down, and the breakdown of estradiol into 16α-hydroxyestrone is bad news. It's hard to change this pathway directly, but indirectly, it can be affected by stimulating the competing pathway—the C-2 pathway—to create 2-hydroxyestrone.

The good news is that indole-3-carbinol, from eating lots of cruciferous vegetables, stimulates the breakdown of estrogens through the C-2 pathway and thereby reduces the estrogens going into the C-16α pathway. It's probably even smarter to use **organic vegetables** and herbs when possible, since sprayed vegetables may contain chemicals that could be turned into toxic epoxides. Pesticides are some of the many things that can interfere with the C-2 pathway.

Bitchy: It's those damn chemical companies again. First they try to knock me down with all those pesticides, and then they try to finish me off with synthetic hormones. I knew they were out to kill me!

Docque: I'm not so sure that it's you personally that they're after, **Bitchy**, but women have definitely been guinea pigs for chemical engineers. Men are having their own problems as well, though, with lower sperm counts and higher testicular cancer rates. When I first started as a **Liver Dwarf**, men had twice as much sperm as they do now. Higher levels of DHT— the active form of testosterone—can lead to prostate enlargement and subsequent urination difficulties, and can also choke off the hair follicles, leading to baldness. The production of DHT from testosterone by 5α-reductase can be strongly inhibited by the herbs **saw palmetto** and **pygeum africanum bark**.

Your liver's detoxification enzymes break down DHT. Certainly many of the problems associated with higher levels of DHT are the result of man-made chemicals—whether from food or drugs or even shampoos or cosmetics—affecting the liver enzymes.

Using indole-3-carbinol from the cruciferous family is a cheap and effective way to fight back. It helps in two ways: it assists your liver enzymes to throw chemicals out of your body *and* it helps you quickly break down your strong hormones into more gentle ones. Indole-3-carbinol helps to get the hormones into a water-soluble form that the conjugation enzymes can then neutralize.

I'll even come up with a few easy recipes for you that will help the C-2 pathway break down estradiol, shed pesticides at the same time, and probably even burn off a few of those unwanted pounds.

Bitchy: Thanks, **Docque**, that would be helpful.

Docque: Of the more than 100 P450 enzymes, each one has a special substance or two that it works on. **P450 1A1** works on steroid hormones, aflatoxins, and polycyclic aromatic hydrocarbons, from smoke and smoked or charred foods. P450 1A1 turns polycyclic aromatic hydrocarbons into epoxides, some of which can be very toxic. Since indole-3-carbinol stimulates P450 1A1 to break down steroid hormones faster, it— at the same time—may increasingly turn any polycyclic aromatic hydrocarbons into toxic epoxides that can be cancer-causing.

It's not a bad idea to minimize the intake of smoked or barbecued foods to lessen the risk of epoxide formation. Wrapping food in aluminum foil when barbecuing prevents the direct contact between the food and the hydrocarbons from the flame, and thus reduces this potential side effect. Barbecues can also be constructed more like convection ovens to reduce the direct contact between the food and the hydrocarbons.

Aflatoxins are made by the fungus **Aspergillus niger**, when grains and nuts are dried too slowly, and can cause similar problems when processed by your liver. Epoxides made by P450 enzymes from polycyclic aromatic hydrocarbons and aflatoxins can be deadly toxic if they're not deactivated before they bind to your DNA. Of course, now you know that green tea and milk thistle bioflavonoids can block many of these side effects by activating glutathione and other conjugation enzymes in your intestine and liver.

While indole-3-carbinol primarily helps prevent hormonal-type cancers—such as breast and prostate—sulforaphane helps fight a wider range of cancers by directly stimulating the immune system and enhancing Phase 2 conjugation enzymes. Sulforaphane is found in many cruciferous plants, especially broccoli. **Broccoli sprouts** can provide even more cancer protection; broccoli seeds that have been sprouted for three days have up to 50 times more anticancer properties than full-grown broccoli. One pound of broccoli seeds can produce over 10 pounds of sprouts with the anticancer properties of about 1,000 pounds of mature broccoli.

The cruciferous family has a lot of other compounds that stimulate the conjugation enzymes and that stimulate glutathione, which helps the conjugation enzymes eliminate mild hormones into the bile or kidneys.

Bitchy: What the heck's the point of dumping mild hormones into the bile? The Boogy Boys in the intestine just make them into strong forms, like 16α-hydroxyestrone, by which they'll surely kill me with cancer one day. In fact, it may already be too late!

Docque: There are ways to prevent The Boogy Boys from doing that, and there are also ways to encourage them to help you in your fight against getting cancer. All it takes is to eat the right foods. You see, all plants are under constant attack by bacteria, viruses, and fungi so they've developed dozens of different chemicals, called **phytoalexins**, to protect themselves. Plants themselves make natural pesticides that can be toxic. Diseased **celery**, for example, can make enough **psorolens**—a natural pesticide made by the plant to defend itself—that people who handle the celery can get a nasty rash. **Potatoes** that are diseased or even exposed to light can have high levels of the **glycoalkaloids solanine** and **choconine**—which when eaten, can be fatal.

A seed must sit in warm, moist soil full of microorganisms before germinating, so it must be especially high in protective phytoalexins. The outer fibrous coating of the seed, grain, berry, or nut is the physical line of defence against microorganisms. Just underneath, but bound to it, is the **aleuron** layer, the chemical line of defence.

Achy: I'm sure that in one of my past lives, I must have set up those defensive lines.

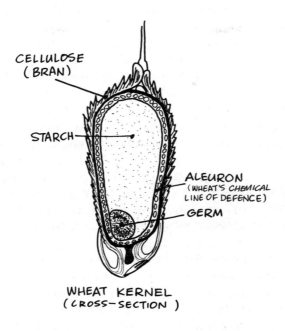

CELLULOSE
(BRAN)

STARCH

ALEURON
(WHEAT'S CHEMICAL
LINE OF DEFENCE)

GERM

WHEAT KERNEL
(CROSS-SECTION)

Docque: In the aleuron layer are the phytoalexins, such as **lignans**. In the intestine, the lignans are eaten by The Boogy Boys, who convert them into **enterolactone** and **enterodiol**; these are plant estrogens, or **phytoestrogens**, that look and act like very mild estrogens.

One thing that enterolactone and enterodiol do is trick the body into making more **SHBG** (**sex hormone binding globulin**), which helps to bind up estradiol and testosterone, therefore lowering their availability and their activity. The next thing that these phytoestrogens do is park themselves in the hormone receptors, thus blocking the much stronger estradiol and estrone from docking in the same space—therefore reducing your risk of cancer.

Bitchy: I love lignans. Where do I get them?

Docque: Seeds have them—especially berries like lingonberries and cranberries—and so do currants and sesame, but most people get them from grains. Because the lignans are bound tightly to the outer fibre or bran, the process of milling and separating the flour from the fibre will remove the lignans.

In other words, pastries, cookies, croissants, and white bread will have no lignans.

By using the whole grain, your body benefits in the following ways.

1) The fibre of the grain pulls the hormones released in the bile out with the stool before The Boogy Boys can convert them into strong hormones again.

2) You feed The Boogy Boys lots of lignans from which they can make enterlactone and enterodiol to keep you protected from cancer.

3) The germ of the seed is loaded with vitamins—especially the vitamin E family—and minerals that your body needs to create stamina and endurance. Of course, after milling, these vitamins will be exposed to oxygen from the air, which can soon make them rancid. The removal of these nutrients thus increases the shelf life of the food product. In fact, the processing and preservation—freezing and canning—of other foods, in addition to grains, can result in decreased levels of vitamins B_6, B_{12}, E, and folic acid, as well as chromium.

Until recently, unprocessed wheat flour was bleached using a chemical called **nitrogen trichloride**. This created a toxic byproduct called **methionine sulfoximine**. Although this process is now banned, it was used for about 50 years. The past use of this toxic flour may be linked to an increase in neurological diseases such as Parkinson's and **amyotrophic lateral sclerosis**.

Bitchy: I bet those food processing companies are owned by the chemical companies that are out to get me. Before you know it, those companies and their flunkies will be controlling the hospitals so they can kill me off slowly with drugs, killer bugs, *and* bad food.

Gaspy: **Bitchy**, you're so paranoid. You should learn to trust them like I have.

Docque: I learned long ago, while cooking in Finland, that rye is the grain highest in lignans. The dark rye bread I used to bake kept the hormones under control. It was only after the city people switched from my pleasant-peasant rye bread to Danish pastries and French croissants that they started getting so much breast and prostate cancer.

Bitchy: What about the Asians? They don't eat many whole grains but they don't get a lot of breast or prostate cancer.

Docque: Actually they do get less breast and prostate cancer. Also, when they *do* develop these cancers, the cancer doesn't grow much because their diet keeps it under control. Their lignans are fairly low—'though they do get a bit in green tea—but their diet is high in an even stronger phytoalexin group called **isoflavonoids**, found mainly in legumes and especially in soy products. These isoflavonoids are also converted into phytoestrogens by The Boogy Boys.

Bitchy: I'm starting to like The Boogy Boys.

Docque: Oh, yes! They can be your very best friends because you certainly won't get as many phytoestrogens if The Boogy Boys have been killed off by antibiotics. Soy has isoflavonoids that can be turned into phytoestrogens, which increase SHBG and block the hormone receptors, reducing estrogens' irritation on the breast, uterus, and ovaries; similar protection applies to the prostate in men. Soy also has one even bigger trick up its sleeve. It contains **genistein**, which can also inhibit the development of cancers by inhibiting the **tyrosine kinase enzyme**—which is a stimulator of cancer growth. Therefore, genistein can inhibit many tumours from growing. Just 50 mg of genistein per day can sometimes inhibit cancer growth, which would come from about 50 g of soy protein per day.

In addition, genistein inhibits 5α-reductase enzyme. Genistein also increases the transcription of the **p21WAF1 gene**, which helps to get cancer cells to commit apoptosis.

Achy: Yay! Finally a *bad* guy committing suicide!

Docque: There's another advantage to genistein. While all the lignans and isoflavonoids are antioxidants, genistein is the strongest antioxidant, which helps protect against coronary heart disease.

Bitchy: I think **Gaspy** could use it more than me.

Docque: You're right about that, because smokers are much more prone to hardening of the arteries. Even teenage smokers around the world have been shown to have the beginning stages of hardening of the arteries.

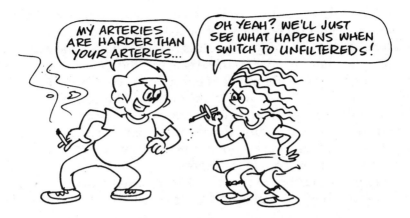

In your case, **Bitchy**, I think you should try using soy milk instead of cow's milk because recently the estrogen levels in cow's milk have increased dramatically. In the old days, a cow would only deliver milk after it gave birth to its calf. The estrogen content in this milk was reasonably low. Now, the farmers can inject a cow to stimulate the animal to produce milk even while it's still pregnant, drastically increasing the amount of estrogen in the milk. Your sensitivity to strong estrogens indicates that soy milk would be a wiser choice.

Also, when I worked in Asia, I noticed that few older women got **hot flushes** during menopause. I found it was because of the mild estrogen-like effect of the lignans and especially the isoflavonoids in **tofu**.

Spacey: Toad food! Who wants to eat toad food! Sorry, **Docque**, but this is where I get off the bus. No toad food for me! I don't want to get warts!

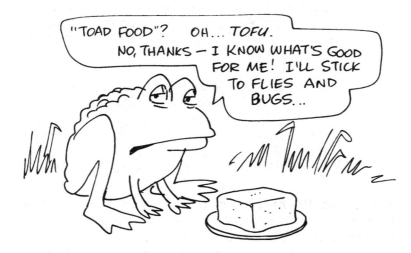

Docque: I didn't say toad food, I said "tofu," also called **bean curd**. Tofu is made from soybeans. There isn't much taste to it, which is an advantage, since it allows the cook to develop flavour using his or her skill with other ingredients. **Miso** and **tempeh** are other soy products, but they're fermented. The advantage of eating fermented foods is that it lets The Boogy Boys perform the early stages of digestion for you, before you even eat the food. The Boogy Boys love to come to the fermenting party when miso, tempeh, **sauerkraut**, and yogurt, are being made. For instance, in the making of miso, letting The Boogy Boys ferment the soy before you eat it, gives your digestive system a bit of a break from having to work on the complex molecules that legumes have.

With the cruciferous family, The Boogy Boys ferment cabbage into sauerkraut, which aids in digesting its coarse fibres and enhances the anticancer properties of indole-3-carbinol. In the making of yogurt, The Boogy Boys break down lactose in the milk, and at the same time, they fortify it with vitamins. Soy can be made into a form of yogurt by fermentation by The Boogy Boys.

It's not a good idea to use *unfermented* soy products—such as tofu, soy milk, etc.—as your <u>main</u> source of dietary protein since they can inhibit trypsin and other enzymes that are required for protein digestion. *Fermented* soy products, such as tempeh, soy yogurt, and miso, don't block the action of these enzymes—the fermentation process destroys the inhibitors.

Achy: Some of us are a little nervous about that "f" word, **Docque**. We've been having some trouble with fermentation in the small intestine lately.

Docque: You've got to learn to use The Boogy Boys' many talents to your advantage. They can make your life much easier by fermenting your food, but *do* confine them to doing their fermenting in your large intestine or the kitchen—not in your small intestine!

Bitchy: And if soy's plant estrogens aren't strong enough to help in menopause?

Docque: Well, when I worked in Mexico, I discovered that Mexican yam was even more beneficial.

Bitchy: Oh, good! I love baked yam.

Docque: No, not that yam. **Wild Mexican yam** is quite different and tastes awful. You take one to four capsules of it per day as your ovaries weaken with age. It doesn't contain hormones, but it contains precursors that the adrenals can use to make some hormones—just like they did before the ovaries kicked in at puberty. Or an even better idea is that I could do a little **Liver Dwarf** trick of treating the wild yam with hydrochloric acid to convert it directly into progesterone—then you'd just have to rub a half-teaspoon of it into your skin every day.

If the **vagina** is too dry, this shows that it could use more estriol—the mildest of the estrogens—in which case a little **estriol cream** could help. Or you can add **black cohosh** herb into the diet, which has an effect like estriol: it's particularly good for the pelvic area but also can help settle down moods.

Your pituitary gland hormones tell your ovaries to make estrogens, and if your ovaries aren't making enough estrogens, your pituitary hormones start yelling and screaming at the ovaries to get to work. All this pituitary ranting and raving can cause hot flushes and sweats. Black—or even blue—cohosh or the Chinese herb *dong quai* have enough estrogen-like activity to quiet down the pituitary gland and make it think that the ovaries are finally listening to it.

Bitchy: Thanks for the tip; I'll try it when I get older.

Docque: I've got one more thing for you, **Bitchy**. I know how sensitive you are about breast cancer and all, so I wanted to tell you that your breasts use iodine to inhibit the estrogens from overstimulating them. Iodine deficiency can therefore allow estrogens to aggravate the breasts to create breast cysts and breast cancer.

Bitchy: Why, I knew that, **Docque**. That's why I always make sure I use iodized salt.

Docque: Iodine salts can be used by the thyroid gland because it can convert the salt into a more useable form of iodine, but the breasts don't have the same bag of tricks. They can't convert salts into a useable form nearly as well as the thyroid. They need more simple iodine such as that found in seafood. Since sea fish also have anticancer properties because of their effects on eicosanoids—and are loaded with iodine—I would highly recommend eating them.

If you can't eat fish, you should at least eat some **sea plants**—they're rich in vitamins and minerals like iodine and selenium. **Brown algae** (such as the **seaweeds wakame, kombu, hijiki,** and **arame**) contain **alginic acid**, which binds to radioactive substances and heavy metals (such as lead, mercury, and cadmium) and removes them from the body. Algae also inhibit phospholipase A_2, which gives them antiinflammatory properties.

Eating sea plants or sea fish—which are high in iodine—can also protect you from iodine loss. Iodine loss can occur when you eat large amounts of cruciferous vegetables because they tend to block the absorption of iodine. Also, everything I tell **Spacey** applies to you as well because abnormal insulin levels can also stimulate cancer. The more stable your liver and pancreas are, the better your health will be.

Bitchy: Thanks, **Docque**. I think I'm beginning to like you.

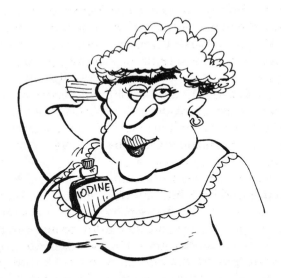

Docque: I take that as a real compliment.

Bitchy: What will help against **osteoporosis**?

Docque: **Osteoblasts** are cells that build up bone and **osteoclasts** break bone down. Progesterone stimulates osteoblasts to make more bone. **Chaste tree bark** is one herb that will stimulate the ovaries to make more progesterone, as long as they're still working. Once the ovaries are too old to make progesterone, then progesterone creams can be used. Estrogens stimulate osteoclasts to commit apoptosis—so the estrogens *slow down* bone loss, but they don't actually renew bone, like progesterone does. The phytoestrogens—plant estrogens—can slow bone loss by stimulating osteoclast suicide.

Also remember that PGE_1 plays a big role in healthy hormones because it affects hormone receptors on cell membranes. Using borage seed oil or evening primrose seed oil will help bypass the delta 6 enzyme, which especially weakens as a woman nears menopause.

The other thing that has such a profound effect on delta 6 enzyme is a viral infection—while coffee and hydrogenated oils can also weaken it. A viral infection can knock out your delta 6 enzyme, decreasing your flow of "feel great" eicosanoids, which can lead to low serotonin and its associated depression and/or anxiety. Since your weakened immune system is now unable to toss the virus out, it makes interferon as a warning to the other cells that a virus is snooping around. Of course, interferon is a tremendous drain on your energy and can lead to severe fatigue.

The interferon also activates phospholipase A_2, which can dramatically increase pain and inflammation, such as in **fibromyalgia**. Once phospholipase A_2 is activated by your immune system, it can be further stimulated by MSG, insect stings, casein from dairy products, and cold, wet weather. So a virus can weaken your immune system and affect your serotonin and mood by inhibiting delta 6 enzyme—and by creating interferon, it can make you feel tired and sore.

Itchy: I just want to stop scratching; I'll do anything!

Docque: As you probably know, **Itchy**, your skin problems come from your liver's conjugation enzymes not being able to keep up to the P450 enzymes, so the toxins are being dumped into the kidneys; they in turn dump the toxins out through the skin. This is compounded by the immune system attacking any of the phenols in the blood. Histamine and acetylcholine— which functions somewhat like histamine—can increase the itching considerably.

The first thing to start taking would be milk thistle to aid your liver's conjugation enzymes. The next thing would be **burdock root**. It helps the kidneys and lymph system work better, thereby taking a big load off the skin.

Itchy: Should I take some nice chilled grapefruit juice to slow down the P450 enzymes as well?

Docque: It's not for *you*, **Itchy**. Grapefruit is a tropical fruit, and your kidneys are already too cool; they aren't activating the vitamin D properly, so you're losing calcium. Low calcium has weakened your ileocecal valve, allowing The Boogy Boys into the small intestine.

Itchy: Well, how come **Sluggy** can have it, then?

Docque: Because he lives on the sunny side of the liver, his skin can make vitamin D directly from sunlight, and living in a warm place like that, his kidneys could use a little cooling. On your side of the liver, things are dark and cool, and you'd really confuse your kidneys if you started drinking a lot of fruit juice.

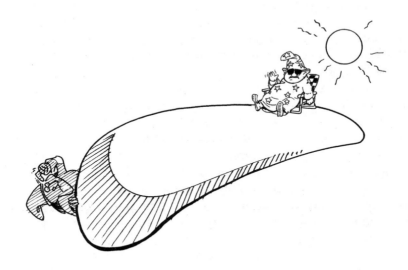

You might be better off if you use **ginger tea**, which has a strong warming effect. Green tea might be an even wiser choice for you, however, because it also slows down the P450 enzymes.

Itchy: I'm moving to Hawaii so I can eat bananas and papaya and hang-10 on my surfboard.

Docque: (*Laughing*) That's fine, but until you do, we have to work on a warming diet so you can *hang onto your calcium*. In the north, during the months with an "r" in their name, your body usually needs to get extra vitamin D from supplements. Take a little **halibut or cod liver oil** to get vitamin D in the winter: one capsule of 400 IU per day. In the months of May through August, you will generally get enough vitamin D from the great outdoors, unless you live in a cloudy area or the Southern Hemisphere or you don't get outside much. Dark-skinned people are going to have less activation of vitamin D, which can be detrimental in the darker days of winter. Also, as you age, your vitamin D is activated less effectively. A 70-year-old might activate only one-third of the amount of vitamin D activated by a 20-year-old. As you get older, supplementing with 800 IU of vitamin D per day might be more appropriate.

If you eat warming foods in the cold weather, your kidneys will quickly realize you're not living in a hot, sunny climate and will activate your vitamin D 1,000 times stronger than the liver could do. Within nine days, you'll have lots of calcium absorption.

Until we get your kidneys activating vitamin D, you can take some spring-picked **horsetail** herb. The silica in it will trick the kidneys into hanging onto your calcium longer.

Bitchy: Because I live on the sunny side of the liver, does that mean I should only eat fruits and vegetables?

Docque: You can eat a small amount of fruit and raw vegetables because you live in a hot, sunny place, but there are limits. Some people thrive on a high fruit and salad diet; others fade away very quickly without lots of animal protein. People with **blood type O** tend to need more animal protein; **AB blood types** can often lean more toward vegetarianism. The other blood types—**type A** and **type B**—tend to need a diet that's somewhere in the middle of these two.

A person who's working hard physically, especially in a cold climate, may need more animal protein than a sedentary person in a hot climate. In other words, have you ever seen a vegetarian Eskimo?

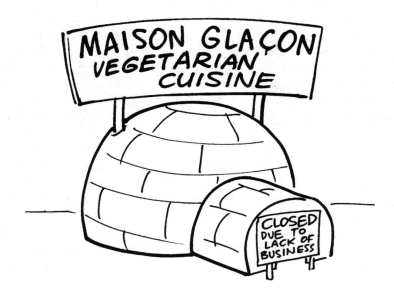

Bitchy: Inuit, **Docque**, Inuit!

Docque: Sorry. No matter whether you're an omnivore or vegetarian, it's important to get the appropriate amount of salt, because the kidneys need equal amounts of sodium and potassium. In fact, we have highly evolved salt and thirst mechanisms that will tell us exactly when to take salt, and when to drink. Our mind can be fooled, however, into ignoring the body's pleas for salt by the belief that salt is bad for us. This need for salt may manifest as cravings for potato chips or other salty foods.

All animals know what they need, and will go to great efforts to get it. For example, a deer—a vegetarian—living on a high potassium diet has a very strong desire for salt and will go for miles to get it. A cougar, however, couldn't care less for salt, as he gets his from eating the deer. In other words, animal products have the perfect mineral balance that our body needs; vegetable products are imbalanced and need extra sodium to antidote their high potassium levels. Products from the sea, whether animal or vegetable, have the further advantage of containing a myriad of trace minerals that have been lost from the soil due to leaching or intensive farming.

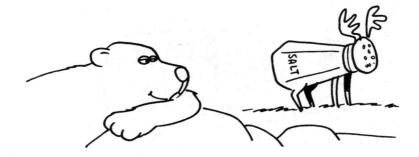

Animals know what they need because they listen to their true brain: **the Gut!** It tells them when to drink water and how much. It tells them when salt is necessary and how much. It tells them how much protein, fat, and carbohydrate are needed. If they eat the wrong things, their bodies will make them sick to let them know that something is wrong. The gut will even tell an animal which herbs to eat to cure an illness, like when a carnivore such as a cat or dog suddenly knows it's time to eat grass to make itself regurgitate.

The brain in your head and the brain in your gut both developed from the **neural crest** when you were an **embryo**. They use the same hormone-like substances such as serotonin, melatonin, dopamine, glutamate, and norepinephrine and they can give feedback to each other through cholecystokinin, gastrin, insulin, enkephalins, and benzodiazepines. Your head-brain and your gut-brain are also directly linked by the vagus nerve.

The brain in your head is just a big filing cabinet that can get information and misinformation mixed up. It's your "gut feelings" that keep you in harmony with the world around you. If your guts aren't right, you're doing something wrong, like listening to more misinformation from your head-brain. Of course, if your guts aren't right, that can also mess up your head-brain and create anxiety, depression, confusion, aggression, moodiness, insomnia, memory problems, and even suicidal desires as well as psychiatric disorders. So if your gut says it needs salt, then give it salt, even if your misinformed head-brain tries to tell you that salt is bad.

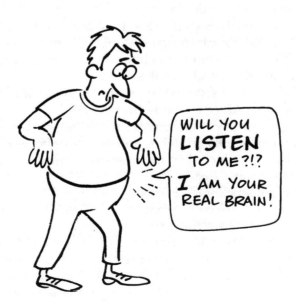

Gaspy: But won't salt give me high blood pressure?

Docque: Low calcium and liver and kidney problems create high blood pressure. Salt may aggravate some people's high blood pressure, but it's not the cause. The word "salary" is closely related to the word "salt" because, to ancient farming communities, salt was more valuable than gold. Hunting communities, however, had little use for salt other than as a food preservative. The original salt was crude and coarse and often straight from the sea. It contained a myriad of the trace minerals that are found in the ocean. Modern salt is industrial-grade pure **sodium chloride**, stripped of its valuable trace minerals, and it's especially low in magnesium. **Processed sea salt** is the same. Unprocessed sea salt retains the important trace nutrients.

Achy: Will that help my sore joints?

Docque: **Salt packs** can help bring down swollen joints, **Achy**, but to actually cure your joints, it'll take work from the inside. Remember, I told **Sluggy** that EPA from fish is better for you than arachidonic acid from animal fat—the eicosanoids of the 3 Family made from EPA don't shout as loudly for help as do the eicosanoids from arachidonic acid, so the immune system is less likely to do damage to your membranes. You should eat more fish as well—to at least provide some relief until you can get your immune system back under control. To help your immune system, you have to get your digestion, intestinal flora, liver, and lymph system fixed up.

Your allergies and sensitivities are not only causing high levels of eicosanoids to be made from arachidonic acid, they're also making your liver valves more sensitive—which increases the amount of phenols, proteins, and epoxides being dumped into your lymph, which then increases your immune system's attacks against these toxins.

Achy: So I'm stuck in a vicious cycle?

Docque: Right. But eating more fish will at least slow down the cycle a bit, until we can break it.

Achy: I can tell you right now that I'm allergic to fish.

Docque: It's the protein in the fish that you're reacting to, and cooking the protein is usually what makes it more allergenic. Raw fish—like sushi—may not be such a problem, but be careful: allergic responses to fish can cause anaphylactic reactions.

Achy: Raw fish! They're full of worms! You're going to give me worms!?

Docque: Freezing fish thoroughly for three days before it's to be eaten raw should kill any parasites in the flesh. When I was stationed in Japan, I also learned that a skilled sushi chef can spot parasites in unfrozen fish, and can easily remove them. I never saw a major parasite problem when I was in Japan.

For some people, food processing increases the **antigenicity** of some foods. For example, the more that milk is heated—such as during pasteurization—and the longer the lapse time till the milk is used, the more the milk casein and lactose will react with each other to create "browning reactions." Browning reactions are most obvious when you slice an apple with a knife and the apple soon starts to "brown" as oxygen comes in contact with the sugars. The browning effect greatly increases the antigenicity of milk, which makes it more likely that your immune system will attack it. Milk fresh from a cow, without any processing, may not cause any allergic reaction at all in a person who reacts to processed milk.

Achy: I hope you're not going to try to kill me with raw milk as well—because I know that's *full* of dangerous bacteria!

Docque: Even pasteurized milk still has lots of bacteria in it, although the more dangerous ones would have been killed by the pasteurizing process. Also, there are filters that can be used to remove some of the bacteria.

Dangerous bacteria don't originate in the milk. They come from the cow, and most cows don't have dangerous bacteria. Safe raw milk can be provided by a responsible farmer if regular testing of the cows is done to make sure they don't have harmful bacteria. I saw the testing done when I was stationed in California. Even with large-scale production, some of the dairies in that state have provided the public with raw dairy products for many years. Of course, making yogurt from it gives additional nutrition, and yogurt is *full* of millions of bacteria—bacteria that are good for you. Cheese is also full of bacteria, and many of the finest European cheeses are still made from **unpasteurized** milk.

The sugars present in overripe tomatoes also create browning reactions when they react with other parts of the tomato and that increases allergic reactions for some people. Canned tomato sauces and pastes are more likely to be made from overripe tomatoes and might cause allergic reactions in individuals who have no problem with fresh-picked tomatoes. **Sulphites** are used in salad bars to block browning reactions, but many people—especially asthmatics—can be made much worse by sulphites because they interfere with glutathione.

Achy: It sounds like I'm going to have to grow my own food. From General to Farmer. Turn swords into plowshares. It has a familiar ring to it. I wonder if I didn't write that in one of my previous lives . . .

Bitchy, Bloaty, Burpy, Gaspy, Itchy, Sluggy, Spacey: *STOP!*

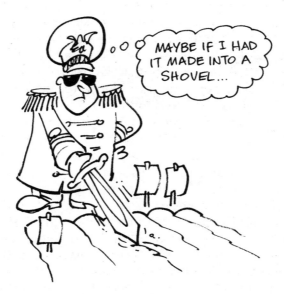

Docque: Doing your own gardening could be a wise step toward better health—both for yourself and the soil. Or find farmers or markets that put food quality and the best interests of your health—and the health of the soil—on the same level.

The real key to reducing your allergies is to fix your intestinal flora, particularly the fermenters. Yeast are especially troublesome because they can make steroid hormones,

cinnamic acid, gallic acid, and acetaldehyde; these can make
you allergic to just about anything and everything. Let's get
your intestinal floral straightened out, your liver working better
and, to help your lymph drain faster, let's add some **nettles** to
your diet.

Achy: I've never had nettle salad before.

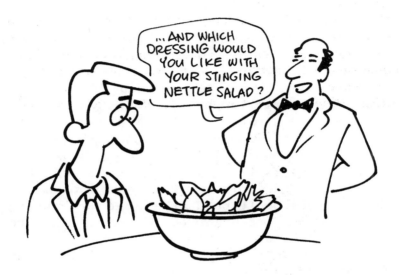

Docque: I wouldn't recommend nettles in a salad since
they're *stinging* nettles. But the new shoots on the top don't
have stingers. A little cooking gets rid of the stingers, and then
you get all the benefits of one of the most nutritious plants in
the world and one of the best at draining the lymph. It also
helps to lower uric acid levels, 'though it's not as strong as
birch sap.

The nettles will help soften up and drain your lymph and
when your lymph system has less protein for your immune
system to attack, your allergies will slowly lessen. Eventually
the memory cells that your white blood cells have made against
those protein antigens will die off, and your allergies and
autoimmune problems will fade away.

Three weeks after you stop dumping antigens into your body through the gut or through the space of Disse, you'll still have as many memory B cells. It takes 12 weeks for all of them to die off. As those internal memory cells die off, your reactions to external antigens—like pollens, bees, dust, and chemicals—should decrease considerably, if not completely, as well.

Achy: In the meantime, I'll continue taking my **nonsteroidal antiinflammatory drugs (NSAIDs)**.

Docque: Well, while NSAIDs may relieve the pain of arthritis, they'll also block the regeneration of cartilage which, in the long term, will worsen your arthritis. **Glucosamine sulphate**, on the other hand, stimulates the regeneration of your cartilage. Glucosamine sulphate is an important building block for cartilage and can be built into the larger connective tissue substance **N-acetyl glucosamine (NAG)**. NAG forms a protective layer over the intestinal mucosa, which helps inhibit leaky gut syndrome and protects against lipid peroxidation, free radicals, and damage from parasites, yeast, **E. coli**, and **lectins**. NAG also helps protect the liver against peroxidation. In addition, NAG is used to build up the larger chondroitin proteoglycans. Since NAG and chondroitins are too large to be absorbed well, the smaller glucosamine sulphate is more absorbable, and your body builds NAG and chondroitins from it. **Shark cartilage** is a good natural source of glucosamine sulphate.The conversion of glucosamine sulphate to NAG, however, is inhibited by alcohol use, NSAIDs, and poor absorption due to inflammatory bowel disease.

There are also specific foods you can use to help relieve pain. Foods high in **copper** help to dull pain somewhat, which is why so many people with arthritis wear **copper bracelets**. Foods highest in copper are oysters—famous for their zinc, which is important for many things, including sex organs—liver juice, nuts, seeds—remember to get ones that aren't rancid—and green olives. We'll give you ginger tea between meals, because it's relatively antiinflammatory.

Spacey: Were you talking about my Auntie Flo?

Docque: No, **Spacey**, that's a-n-t-i-i-n-f-l-a-m-m-a-t-o-r-y.

Spacey: Oh! I don't think that *she's* a relative of mine.

Docque: No, **Spacey**. It's relative to being healthy. The first thing we want to do with *you* is reduce the amount of carbohydrates you're eating, and get more salt and protein into you to get your blood pressure up and stabilize your blood sugar.

In addition, all those refined carbohydrates have flushed out most of your chromium, so your insulin's up, but it's not being bound to the receptors. That ineffective insulin is causing a craving for sweets that are being converted to fats, and that fat is being stored between your chin and your pelvis. One way to reduce the production of fat from sugar is to start eating carbohydrates that release their sugars less rapidly.

Spacey: Oh, good! I like to eat lots of complex carbohydrates like French bread, potatoes, yams, corn, and pasta.

Docque: Well, those complex carbohydrates may be exactly the wrong ones for you. You see, all carbohydrates are made of sugars bound together in different ways and in various combinations. For a long period of time, people believed that starches released their sugars slowly because of the complex way in which their sugars are bound together; they believed it would take a while for the sugars to be broken up and released by the digestive system. Now it's known that starches can release their sugars at extremely different rates. Many starches actually release their sugars into the blood faster than candy. Starches are found mainly in legumes, grains, and tubers.

Many carbohydrates have been assigned a numeral that represents the rate at which each is broken down into sugars that are then absorbed into the bloodstream. These numerals form the **glycemic index**. White bread is assigned the numeral 100; foods that release their sugars more slowly are given lower numbers. Soybeans at 25 are about the slowest to release their sugars, and therefore are one of the best carbohydrates for stabilizing blood sugar. The slower digestion rate of legumes such as soybeans, however, can create problems of gas and bloating for those with weak digestion and/or an overgrowth of Boogy Boys in the small intestine—because their slow digestion can give the bacteria more time to digest their complex sugars, thereby making more gas.

People who want to decrease insulin and lose weight should choose carbohydrates with a glycemic index of 60 or even lower; those who want to gain weight or who are extremely active physically should choose carbohydrates with a glycemic index greater than 60. The effectiveness of the liver and pancreas in stabilizing blood sugar can also be helped by eating foods that contain chromium, such as broccoli, barley, and fish. Refined sugars and high glycemic index refined starches may temporarily satisfy a sugar craving, but they quickly flush out what little chromium you might have. And as your insulin levels increase, your cravings accelerate, and weight gain and moods worsen rapidly. Using licorice root as a tea or in capsules can help to stabilize your blood sugar and thereby reduce your cravings.

Increased chromium and, therefore, more stable blood sugar not only brings stability to your appetite and emotions, it quietly melts down your long-fought fat deposits. Adding fat and protein to carbohydrates helps to moderate the blood sugar, as well.

Spacey: Are you telling me I should eat fat? I can't do that; I'm trying to lose weight! I'm on a low-fat diet.

Docque: Fear of fat. I know—it's an epidemic. Some of this fear is based on reality, but it's mostly based on science fiction. Sure, some fats are bad for you. There's probably nothing harder on your liver than **rancid fats**. Malondialdehyde is produced when fats, mainly animal fats, go bad from exposure to oxygen. Frying fats makes them much harder on your liver, especially if they're **polyunsaturated**, because the oxygen can penetrate them and make them toxic. In fact, your brain is so full of polyunsaturated fats that I've built the blood-brain barrier to protect against your "frying" your brain.

Gaspy: I think it's too late for **Spacey**. Her brain is already scrambled.

Spacey: Huh? I didn't order eggs!

Docque: Your body will tend to recycle "prebuilt" parts. For example, the eggs that you eat are produced by a chicken's ovaries. So *your* ovaries will tend to use the nutrients already assembled for you by the chicken. For example, the deep-orange egg yolks from free-range chickens contain the exact carotenoids that your ovaries need to make a healthy corpus luteum, which is so necessary for fertility. Eating fried eggs on a regular basis, over a long period of time, can "fry" *your* ovaries and make you more prone to ovarian cancer. Poached or soft-boiled eggs are much better for you.

Spacey: Gee, I'm feeling much more sunny-side-up now.

Docque: Fried or rancid fats can jam the liver enzymes, forcing the hormones through the C-16α pathway, which can lead toward cancer. Hormones of this pathway can also cause menstrual cramps and **premenstrual syndrome (PMS)**, with all its mood changes and irritability.

Bitchy: Are you talking about me!!!

Docque: Nothing personal, just a generalization. Let's take a closer look at one of your membranes and how it makes eicosanoids. The fatty acids of your membranes are taken from the fats in your diet. When the fatty acids that make up your membranes are unsaturated, they contain carbon-to-carbon double bonds (C=C) that veer off at a 120 degree angle, putting a "kink" in the fatty acid. This leaves gaps or "dents" in the membrane that can serve as receptors for hormones. If the double bonds are shattered by hydrogenation or peroxidation, the membrane receptors can be affected.

NORMAL CELL MEMBRANE

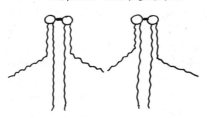

HYDROGENATION or PEROXIDATION

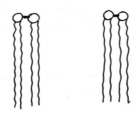

Polyunsaturated fats are often treated with hydrogen to fill those gaps so oxygen can't penetrate, but these **hydrogenated oils** can take on unusual shapes called **trans fats**, which look very similar to the membrane fats that have been damaged by lipid peroxidation. Obviously, over time, this can lead to serious diseases, such as breast cancer.

Your COX and LOX enzymes make their eicosanoids in different ways. COX enzymes use peroxides in making prostaglandins and anything that increases the presence of peroxides along the membrane will increase the production of prostaglandins. These peroxides can be from lipid peroxides that might have snuck past your sleeping conjugation guards in your liver cells or from direct assault by your neutrophils or macrophages, using superoxide radicals that are quickly converted to hydrogen peroxide.

LOX enzymes work similarly to your liver's detoxification enzymes and involve free radical production that can generate peroxides, which can then stimulate COX enzymes.

Anything that's effective in reducing peroxides will also inhibit peroxide production from LOX enzymes, which will directly inhibit COX enzymes. The most important enzyme for reducing peroxides is, of course, your Great Gladiator: glutathione peroxidase. Just as Superman may lose his mighty powers from exposure to just a small amount of kryptonite, so too can your mighty giant, glutathione, be felled by a steady, insidious flow of sugar.

You already know that too much sugar puts your Gladiator defender to sleep, while milk thistle and green tea stimulate it in your intestine and liver. Well, **taurine** helps to increase its activity throughout your body. Taurine can especially help **angina** or a **foggy brain**. The most important thing to remember is that excess sugar will likely offset any benefits you might hope to get from milk thistle, green tea, or taurine.

The drugs **acetasalicylic acid (aspirin)** and **ibuprofen** both inhibit COX enzymes and can thereby reduce the eicosanoids that create pain. Since they don't block LOX enzymes, however, these drugs can result in more arachidonic acid being turned into leukotrienes and make you more prone to asthma, allergies, and anaphylactic shock.

Your adrenal glands make steroid hormones called **corticosteroids** that, when docked in membrane receptors, can block off both COX and LOX enzymes due to their strong antioxidant properties. Of course, long-term suppression of eicosanoid production can have serious side effects, since eicosanoids do have important jobs to do.

Also, virtually any antioxidant can reduce symptoms if it inhibits COX, LOX, and phospholipase A_2 enzymes. **Turmeric** and its extract **curcumin**, ginger, green tea, vitamin E, and the bioflavonoid quercetin are a few of the antioxidants that can inhibit these enzymes. And don't forget the glutathione enzymes—they can also help out here. While milk thistle can increase glutathione activity in the intestine and liver, taurine can increase glutathione activity *beyond* the digestive system.

Some herbs can also help the adrenal glands work better— like ginseng, licorice, and **ribes** (also known as black currant). Since your adrenals are only programmed to run until about three o'clock in the afternoon, these herbs can get you through the afternoon blood-sugar slump. They won't damage your liver enzyme function like sugar, chocolate, coffee, or alcohol will. Licorice inhibits 5α-reductase enzyme, which breaks down **cortisone**, thus extending the lifespan of cortisone.

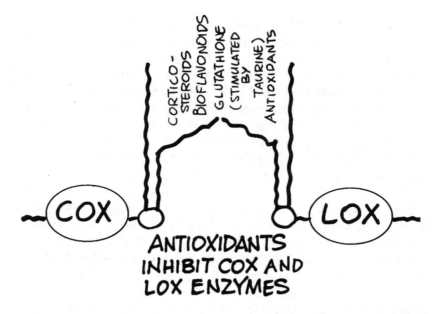

The dosage taken of any antioxidant is crucial; one dose will inhibit these enzymes, while a higher dose will stimulate them. In other words, you can get just as sick from too many supplements as too few—'though it's hard to imagine that with an autoimmune disease, you could take *enough* natural antioxidants to counter the tremendous quantity of free radicals generated by your white blood cells.

Achy: Once war has been declared by your immune system, you're not going to stop my soldiers with a few antioxidants. They're born to kill and trained to kill and they're determined to kill. Once they start killing, they're not easy to shut off. Antioxidants might make your membranes a little more resistant to their superoxy radical bullets and slow down the membranes whining for help with all those PG_2 and LT_4 distress calls, but none of that's going to *end* the war between your immune system and your battered membranes. It's when your white blood cells make PGE_1 that a truce is finally declared; then the shooting, screaming, and bloodshed ends and the healing of the injured, burial of the dead, and a sense of calm and well-being returns to this ravaged land. Dammit! I don't want to suppress "feeling bad" and I'm not content with "feeling good." I want to *"feel great"*! *I want PGE₁*! Give me drugs, if that's what it takes!

Docque: Well spoken, **Achy**. I can see why you're such a renowned general. You're a man with great vision and immense passion. I'm sure that you're well aware of just how elusive PGE_1 can be. It's this PGE_1 state of well-being that drives people to drink and take drugs—just to get that fleeting sense of freedom for a few hours. But the very things they use to get there will soon drive them out of "feel great" and further into "feel bad" as the liver enzymes' function gets twisted out of shape.

You could take evening primrose seed oil to make PGE_1, but you know that insulin can turn it away from "feel great" to "feel bad" by stimulating delta 5 enzyme. It's important to lower your insulin levels when you take evening primrose seed oil or borage seed oil so that it doesn't get turned into arachidonic acid.

Cutting back on high glycemic index foods will help, in the long run, to lower your insulin levels. Taking GTF chromium with your borage or evening primrose seed oil will help you to "feel great" even faster by further lowering your insulin levels. The nicotinic acid in chromium GTF is also important in stopping autoimmune diseases. In addition, eating lots of fish will help your borage oil to be converted to PGE_1 because the EPA in fish also inhibits delta 5 enzyme. Yet it's still going to take many weeks for all of this to work.

Achy: Is there no quick way for me then to shut off this infernal pain so I can feel great again?

Docque: There *is* another way, but I'm not sure I can tell you. I was sworn to secrecy by the **Liver Dwarf Intelligence Unit (LDIU)**.

Achy: But I've been cleared by LDIU. We all have. You *must* tell everything you know to make us "feel great."

Docque: Okay, but you have to swear not to tell anyone else. Not a word to anyone.

Achy, Bitchy, Bloaty, Burpy, Gaspy, Itchy, Sluggy, Spacey: (*Giving the Liver Dwarf Salute*) On a Dwarf's honour, I swear to tell no one!

Docque: (*Lowering his voice*) A long, long time ago, a very brave **Liver Dwarf Agent** infiltrated the "bad" world of arachidonic acid eicosanoids and bought off one of them for a very considerable price.

Spacey: How much did we pay?

Docque: We had to give up all rights to any raven-haired, ruby-lipped, pale-faced, apple-eating young women who have pretensions of marrying into royalty and living happily ever after.

Bitchy: No White!

(*Spacey faints.*)

Bitchy: I mean: No Way!

Achy: It can't be true. What could we possibly get for such a steep price?

Docque: We got one of the arachidonic acid eicosanoids to turn traitor. While most of them are evil-doers—creating pain, inflammation, and stimulating cancer—this one, when called up, will do the exact opposite. That is, reduce pain, and inflammation, fight against cancer, and make you "feel great."

Achy: That sounds like PGE_1. Who is this potent ally, and how do you call him up?

Bitchy: Or her?

Achy: Or her!

Docque: I can only give you the Secret Agent's code name, which is "**prostacyclin**." To call up Agent Prostacyclin, you use **bromelain**.

Achy: I know bromelain; it's an enzyme made from **pineapple stems**. It breaks up the fibrin net that's put up around a war zone to keep any bad guys from slipping away from justice.

Docque: That's right, **Achy**. Since the fibrin net is put up around injured areas and food, pollen, and chemicals, it's really more of an obstacle to healing because it blocks circulation and creates congestion. Congestion helps viruses, bacteria, and cancer to escape your soldiers, and it also inhibits the flow of soothing antioxidants into the area.

Bromelain enzymes can shatter this fibrin and speed up healing. But it's not the enzyme itself that calls up Agent Prostacyclin. Bromelain also has the ability to activate **plasmin**, which causes a decrease in arachidonic acid eicosanoids in general. And this occurs even if the enzyme activity is removed. Even more important, of all the arachidonic acid eicosanoids that are made, our Agent Prostacyclin is increased by bromelain, while thromboxanes and PGE_2 are decreased.

Achy: If thromboxanes and PGE_2 are decreased, then Agent Prostacyclin can only be one of two things: $PGF_2\alpha$ or PGI_2—and $PGF_2\alpha$ is definitely bad, so the Secret Agent must be PGI_2!

Docque: Shhhhhhh! Not so loud; someone might be listening.

Achy: (*Softly*) Yes, you're right. There are spies everywhere. I won't say another word about it.

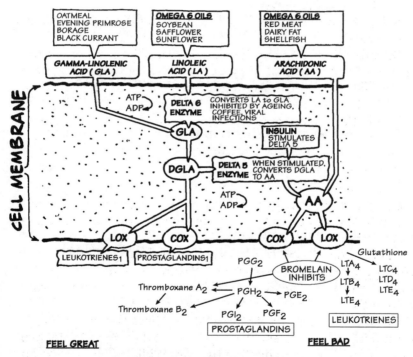

IF YOU CAN IDENTIFY AGENT "PROSTACYCLIN" - THE
"FEEL REAL DARN GOOD" EICOSANOID - THEN KEEP
QUIET OR THE LDIU MAY HAVE TO PAY YOU A VISIT!

Docque: If bromelain doesn't fix you up, **Achy**, I'll mix you up some **cetyl myristoleate**.

Achy: What do you think I am—some kind of rodent? That's only found in mice!

Docque: Mice, sperm whales, and male beavers. It's this oil that circulates in their blood that protects them from autoimmune arthritis. It activates the 1 and 3 Families of eicosanoids, 'though more strongly than fish oil or borage seed oil—thereby neutralizing a wide range of autoimmune diseases.

Bitchy: Won't the mice get a little upset if you take all the protective oil out of their blood?

Docque: Don't worry, I have a recipe to make it from fish oil, cow's butter, or even vegetable oil. But it'll take some time to make you a batch.

Achy: So it's expensive.

Docque: Compared to fish oil, it's very expensive, but for those autoimmune problems that don't respond to cheaper treatments, it can be well worth the expense.

Achy: If it works.

Docque: Yes, if it works. Your immune system is so determined to help that it's not easy to stop it—even if it's killing you.

Spacey: (*Waking up*) Where am I? I was having a dream that a prince came to my house and asked if I had a dark-haired sister. When I said no, he said, "Too bad, I could have turned her into a royal traitor." Does that make any sense?

Achy: It doesn't, **Spacey**, but it's good to see you're back to normal.

Spacey: Did I miss anything?

Achy: **Docque** was just saying that bromelain helps break up congestion and reduces inflammation.

Spacey: Are there any side effects?

Docque: Yes. Weight loss, increased bowel movements, and decreased allergies. Bromelain helps digest proteins, haptens, and lectins and thereby reduces allergies. It's probably best taken between meals. It also helps improve protein digestion and at the same time, reduces fat absorption. Protein helps build your muscle while reducing those fatty "love handles" and cellulite.

Spacey: I like that kind of a side effect from a supplement. Let's get rid of that bad old fat.

Docque: Not all fats are bad, although some fats—like hydrogenated fats—certainly are. Saturated fats don't need to be hydrogenated because they don't have any carbon-to-carbon double bonds. Since saturated fats don't have gaps for oxygen, they don't go rancid as readily and are, in some ways, easier on the liver.

Spacey: You're not going to tell me to eat meat, are you?!

Docque: No. Red meat, with its high levels of arachidonic acid, can cause too many problems, 'though some people do thrive on it—primarily those doing heavy physical work. What I was going to say is that there are fats that aren't saturated but aren't polyunsaturated; they're **monounsaturated fats**—like **olive oil**, which has been used for thousands of years to great advantage throughout the Mediterranean. I first learned about it many centuries ago, while working on a Phoenician trading ship that was carrying amphorae of olive oil. Olive oil doesn't go rancid easily, even under high heat, and therefore it doesn't get **Bloaty** closing down the liver valves.

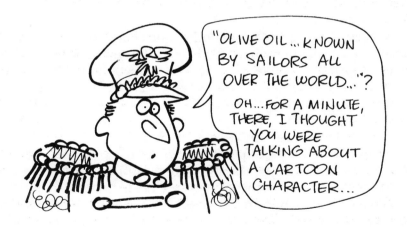

Spacey: But if I live in a colder climate, will it be okay for me?

Docque: It's not as cooling as fruit, so it can be used even in the colder climates, although **canola oil** might be better in a cold climate. In a hotter climate, avocado and macadamia nuts have similar monounsaturated oils. Almonds have very good monounsaturated fats. Nature always provides.

Of course, with indoor heating in cold climates and air conditioning in hot climates, there's more leeway than there was even 50 years ago, when people were buffeted by the extremes of seasonal changes. But just because your market has something for sale, that doesn't mean it's in season and that it'll be ideal for you to eat at that time. It could have travelled half-way around the world to get there. If it's grown out-of-doors locally, it's likely to be closer to what you need.

During winter in a cold climate, most fruit is obviously out of season for you. If you're going to eat fruit, however, note that berries are the most northerly of the fruits. Dried or frozen local berries might be a better choice in the winter than fresh tropical fruit. Plus, when you're buying locally, you've got a better chance to find out who's doing a quality job and using the fewest chemicals. The local fruit would have a less cooling effect on your body than the tropical fruit, and it may even have more nutrition because it was more likely picked in its prime, rather than picked immature and shipped.

Spacey: But if I heat the fruit, won't that make it more warming?

Docque: Heating fruit does add a little energy so it does make it slightly less cooling than eating it raw, but that doesn't change the potassium or sugar level—the two main things that the kidneys use to judge what season you're in. If the kidneys think it's summer, they assume your skin is making lots of vitamin D from the sun so they back off on strong vitamin D activation. High levels of *activated* vitamin D are crucial to *preventing* calcium buildup in fatty deposits in your arteries.

Gaspy: You're going to be shipping me out soon—in a coffin—if you don't hurry up. You sure are long-winded about nothing. I don't need fruits, I need medicine or I'm going to die. Right here, soon!

Bitchy: You've been saying that for 30 years now, **Gaspy**.

Gaspy: Well, I'm not making it up, I could go *just like that*. I've got this squeezing pain in my left chest. Am I blue yet?

Docque: I've got some fruit that might help you out. It's an extract from **Crataegius,** or **hawthorn berry**, and it can relieve mild heart symptoms. This member of the rose family has **proanthocyanidins** that increase the levels of **cyclic AMP** in the heart, which increases its strength. At the same time, hawthorn berry inhibits **angiotensin-converting enzyme (ACE),** which results in lower blood pressure. The dilation of coronary arteries can relieve angina, palpitations, and mild arrythmias. It has a mild diuretic effect and also reduces leg cramps that come from circulation problems.

Gaspy: That sounds good to me. I'm always getting leg cramps.

Docque: Hawthorn berry helps to lower cholesterol as well. Less arachidonic acid from meat and more EPA from fish would also help. The fish that are highest in EPA are the oiliest: sardines, anchovies, and herring.

Gaspy: Now you want me to start eating the bait! What a strange, twisted mind you have. I'll be glad to die just to get away from loonies like you! Eat bait! Why don't you give me a whole bunch of vitamin E, like a normal doctor would do?

Docque: Taking vitamin E, like any other antioxidant, can make you much better or worse, depending on the dose and what other antioxidants you take with it. Vitamin E is stationed at about every 1,000 fat molecules along a membrane, and it's important for intercepting hydroxyl radicals that might come roaring down the membrane—so taking extra vitamin E should help protect your fatty membranes.

The problem with vitamin E supplements is that they only contain **alpha tocopherol**, while *foods* have **alpha, beta, delta,** *and* **gamma tocopherol**. Only gamma tocopherol can intercept the deadly chemical toxin peroxynitrite, which can be at the root of cancer and heart disease in smokers. Too much supplementation with alpha tocopherol can reduce the amount of gamma tocopherol in your membranes. Foods that are high in both are fish, soy, leafy greens, wheat germ, avocados, and mangoes. Wheat germ oil is not only high in tocopherols, but also **octacosenol**, which helps prevent infertility and miscarriage.

There's another side of vitamin E: the four **tocotrienols**—**alpha, beta, delta,** and **gamma tocotrienol**. They're similar to the four tocopherols but they can lower cholesterol by inhibiting the enzyme **HMG CoA reductase**, which is involved in the production of cholesterol. Tocotrienols are especially found in rice bran oil and they also block thromboxane A_2, which is responsible for causing platelet aggregation.

Bitchy: Of course, if the chemical companies hadn't taken the wheat germ and the bran from the rice, we wouldn't need to take them as supplements.

Docque: Using the tocotrienols and the tocopherols together make a better membrane-protecting team. In some situations, alpha tocopherol on its own can bring even more free radicals into the membrane. For example: if there are a lot of free radicals in the fluid part of the cell, the alpha tocopherol can pull them into the membrane and release them there where they could generate even more free radical damage to your membrane.

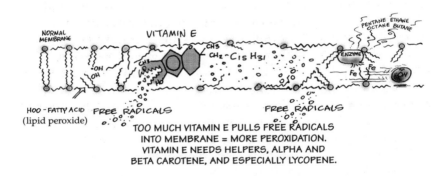

TOO MUCH VITAMIN E PULLS FREE RADICALS INTO MEMBRANE = MORE PEROXIDATION. VITAMIN E NEEDS HELPERS, ALPHA AND BETA CAROTENE, AND ESPECIALLY LYCOPENE.

Alpha and beta carotene from carrots and palm oil, and lycopene from tomatoes can greatly help out vitamin E in the membrane because they're fat-soluble and able to enter the membrane, unlike many of the water-soluble bioflavonoids. They take the free radical from vitamin E, leaving it available to catch another free radical. These bioflavonoid helpers pass the free radical down the membrane to CoQ_{10}, which neutralizes it.

Gaspy: Don't try to get me to take palm oil; I know it's full of saturated fat and that's dangerous for the arteries and heart.

Docque: Well, when I was in the South Pacific where the natives ate large amounts of palm oil, I saw little sign of artery or heart problems. Free radicals, peroxides, and nutrient deficiencies are the main causes of these diseases, not palm oil.

Gaspy: Well, I better take some beta carotene to help my vitamin E neutralize free radicals in my membranes.

Docque: Don't count much on beta carotene to protect you. Alpha carotene is 50 times stronger at quenching free radicals than beta carotene, and lycopene is 100 times stronger than alpha carotene. And alpha carotene inhibits cancer 10 times stronger than beta carotene. So you can see that beta carotene isn't that great. Lycopene is much stronger at protecting the skin from free radicals from the sun, as well as protecting against internal cancers.

So taking extra vitamin E can help if it contains both alpha and gamma tocopherol and if it has a support team of fat-soluble bioflavonoids to help it out. The best of the fat-soluble support team, lycopene, is found in the tomato, a fruit that can easily be salted. Watermelon is another red-fleshed fruit that contains lycopene. But since we don't usually put salt on watermelon like we do tomatoes, watermelon should only be eaten in very hot climates so that you don't decrease your calcium levels and let The Boogy Boys into your small intestine.

You should see by now that plants are your best sources of antioxidants. Because they're packaged with the other members of their team, these antioxidants help each other work better. That's why the antioxidants in vegetables may work more effectively in your body than antioxidants that you take as supplements.

Vitamin C's water-soluble bioflavonoid buddies are quercetin, rutin, and **hesperidin**, to name only three. Taking 500 mg of vitamin C three times a day, over many months, will usually reverse hardening of the arteries—especially if vitamin C is taken with its bioflavonoid assistants. However, while it'll help protect the arteries, more than 60 mg of vitamin C supplements per day can convert harmless **ferric iron** to **ferrous iron**, which can increase oxidation in the body and damage adenine DNA bases.

Remember, antioxidants are used to quench free radicals, and the primary source of free radicals is improper liver function, so your liver is the key to reducing the need to take antioxidant supplements like vitamin C. And since your liver is the filter for your digestive system and your digestive system is at the bottom end of your mouth, what you put into your mouth plays a key role in your health.

Gaspy: Well, I think I'll take some tomatoes with my fish and soy—Ugh!—and maybe some CoQ_{10}, and that'll solve my problem.

Docque: That would probably work well for you, **Gaspy**, because your membranes are in serious need of help and they could use some CoQ_{10}. CoQ_{10} would also help keep your gums strong. Weak gums could allow The Boogy Boy **Bacteroides gingivalus** to get from your mouth into your blood where it can cause heart valve infections.

A younger person who is physically active would probably get worse from taking extra CoQ_{10} because CoQ_{10} in excess would throw out even more free radicals when the body was trying to make ATP.

The way to avoid needing to take extra CoQ_{10} is to get **regular exercise**, especially **aerobic exercise**. When you exercise, all that oxygen flying around in your body is the stimulus to prepare extra antioxidant defences and that gets your liver to make more CoQ_{10}. So regular exercise and a healthy liver are the keys to keeping high natural levels of CoQ_{10} to protect your membranes from free radicals. High levels of CoQ_{10} can even reverse some cancers, especially breast cancer.

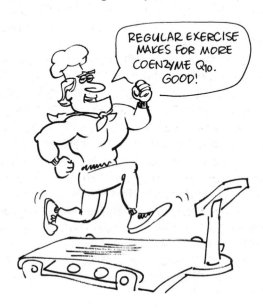

Salmon and mackerel are high in EPA. But the point I was going to make is that these are also high in CoQ_{10}—so important for energy production, especially in the heart, liver, immune system, and nervous system. While the EPA in the fish works for you as an antiinflammatory, the CoQ_{10} will slowly make your heart stronger. One side effect of eating fish is that it will also help to lower your cholesterol levels.

Gaspy: I still don't want to eat fish. I'll take flax seed oil instead, because I know it becomes EPA.

Docque: You're right. Flax seed oil has alpha linolenic acid (ALA), which can become EPA. But flax seed oil becomes rancid very quickly when it's exposed to oxygen. Since the seedcoat of the flax seed protects the oil from oxygen, it's safer to use the actual *seeds* in your cooking, instead of the flax seed *oil*. To release the oil, you need to break the seeds open by grinding, soaking, or boiling them—but be sure to eat them immediately after doing so.

Oatmeal is another food that can help to lower cholesterol, especially oat bran. Oatmeal in the morning is a good way to start the day. It's a starch made up of sugars that can be released too fast if cooked quickly at high temperatures. But *slow-cooking* the *regular* oatmeal—not that instant, precooked stuff—at a lower temperature over a *longer time* is a better way to go, to keep your insulin levels down.

Gaspy: I don't have any time for slow-cooking. I'll be at the Pearly Gates before it's finished!

Docque: When you get there, you may find slow-cooked oatmeal on the menu, since I was once a cook at the Pearly Gates Café. St. Peter was a regular customer. Oatmeal is also one of the few foods that contains GLA—'though only in very small amounts—that can bypass delta 6 enzyme, which tends to weaken with age. As one gets older, and delta 6 enzyme is less capable of creating GLA, then a little evening primrose seed oil or borage seed oil might also be necessary—although high insulin could prevent it from getting past delta 5 enzyme.

Now, back to cholesterol. Grapes—especially the seeds and skins—and apples, berries, grapefruit, and avocados are good at lowering cholesterol. The trick is not to eat so many fruits and vegetables that you cool your kidneys down too much for your particular climate or weather.

Gaspy: Thank you, **Docque**. I'll take my grapes in the liquid form of medicine—wine—because I know that the French prevent hardening of the arteries by drinking lots of wine.

Docque: It *is* true that a *little* alcohol can stimulate your delta 6 enzyme and thereby increase eicosanoids of the 1 Family, which raises serotonin and gives you more self-esteem and social courage. It's also true that a *little* alcohol can have a mild antibiotic effect on bacteria in the intestine. But, it's also true that *more* alcohol can stimulate your P450 enzymes into making epoxides and peroxides strong enough to destroy your liver and create the severe physical, mental, and emotional disturbances that can go along with excess alcohol consumption. Even the French know this, and have greatly reduced their consumption of wine.

Remember that the strong antioxidant properties that can protect the arteries and inhibit cancer are primarily from the grape. Like all seeds, grapes contain phytoalexins. Phytoalexins in legumes and grains have anticancer properties and they're especially predominant in soy and rye. The phytoalexin **resveratrol** is found in peanuts, mulberries, and especially in grapes. It's used by the grape skin to protect itself from fungus infections, but it can also be used by your body to inhibit cancer and protect your arteries.

Resveratrol is a strong antioxidant; it stimulates Phase 2 liver detoxification enzymes and, perhaps most important, it inhibits the activity of the COX enzyme, which makes eicosanoids from arachidonic acid that promote cancer. So you can see that the grape can be a mighty weapon in your struggle to maintain health.

Yet you don't have to drink wine to get the medicinal benefits of grapes. Grape juice will work just fine. Or, in colder climates, perhaps cooking a few raisins—or their smaller cousins, currants—in your cereal will work the same for you. Of course, using raisins and currants that haven't been in contact with pesticides would be the smartest way to go. You should be adding sea salt to your cooked cereal anyway—that's one way you can help reduce the cooling effect of the fruit.

Grape seeds also contain substances that make your blood-brain barrier stronger. This is important because a strong blood-brain barrier helps protect your sensitive nervous system—in diseases like MS—from destructive forces such as your own immune system. Other things that contain these nerve-protecting **anthocyanosides** and **proanthocyanidins** are blue elderberries, blueberries, blackberries, bilberries, cherries, and **pycnogenol** from pine bark. **Bilberry** also increases circulation to the eyes and improves night vision—as was discovered by the RAF in World War II. Proanthocyanidins also inhibit LOX enzymes.

Some other foods that lower cholesterol are less cooling, especially if they're lightly salted. These include carrots, the cabbage family—especially brussels sprouts—and all the legumes, such as beans, lentils, and chickpeas. Soybeans and soy products, such as tofu and soy milk, can dramatically bring down cholesterol. **Sesame seeds**—perhaps in the butter form called **tahini**—also lower cholesterol, and so do **L-carnitine** and **gugulipids**.

Fenugreek seeds also bring down cholesterol and can be used as tea. Some people don't like the body odour that's noticeable when they take fenugreek. A chemical in the seed causes this odour, but if you buy the type of fenugreek that has that chemical extracted from the seed, then you can lower your cholesterol and remain sweet as a rose.

Burpy: Thanks, **Docque**.

Bitchy: I don't think he was referring to you!

Docque: When I was working in Africa, I found the Masai tribe had low cholesterol in their blood, even though they lived on a diet high in cholesterol and animal protein. They made yogurt out of their milk, and because the yogurt actually blocked the production of cholesterol by their adrenal glands—which can be a bigger source of cholesterol than the diet—the Masai had low blood cholesterol and freedom from artery disease. Like most cultures, they also use a lot of bitter herbs as liver tonics. Bitter antidotes sweet, and sweet substances are some of the most destructive for your liver.

Garlic and **raw onions** have powerful oils that can irritate some people's digestive tract; but for those whose system can tolerate them, garlic and raw onions can improve circulation. Garlic is especially effective for killing Boogy Boys and even antibiotic-resistant strains of Helicobacter pylori. Garlic can sometimes reverse hardening of the arteries. Garlic contains **diallyl disulphide**, which inhibits colon and kidney cancer.

Gaspy: It's free radicals that cause hardening of the arteries, I know that.

Bitchy: You've got so many free radicals, you could light up the North Pole at Christmas!

Docque: The most common sources of free radicals are digestion—when your food passes from your mouth to your anus, including its final passage through the mitochondria of your cells—and the P450 enzymes in the liver. The largest, and therefore the most damaging, source of free radicals is your immune system—when it turns its free radical weaponry against enemies, which can be real or presumed invaders. The amount of free radicals generated by your immune system can be many, many times greater than that generated by your liver's P450 enzymes. Of course, a malfunctioning liver will be spilling proteins into your lymph system, and your immune system's attempts to clean up this liver debris can cause the immune system to become chronically overactive.

Fortunately, the plant world is full of natural antioxidants that can neutralize free radicals. My great grandfather was once a **Plant Dwarf**, back in the Olden Days, when the first plant cell gobbled up a Boogy Boy and got him to turn sunlight into food. All the food that we get today originated from this magical ability of those ancient Boogy Boys.

In plants, these captive Boogy Boys are called **chloroplasts**, and their job is to make carbohydrates from water, carbon dioxide, and sunlight. First they pluck a **photon** out of the sky and use it to split H_2O (water) into oxygen and hydrogen. Hydrogen is picked up by NADP to make NADPH. This hydrogen is then used to make ATP, which reacts with a carbon from carbon dioxide gas (CO_2) to form a simple carbohydrate. The oxygen given off by these reactions is released into the atmosphere where we can use it in our mitochondrial energy machines.

The reduction of carbon dioxide and increase of oxygen in the atmosphere also cools our planet down to a temperature we can tolerate. The carbohydrates are the base of the food chain and, along with the oxygen, are two of the plants' great gifts to us. But there's even more good news.

Putting all this energy and oxygen together is like kids playing in the basement with dynamite and matches—the whole thing could blow up. So Great Grandfather and his crew of **Plant Dwarves** worked long hours till they perfected a number of different compounds that could surround the chloroplasts and neutralize different types of free radicals. There got to be so many—over 4,000 of these flavonoids—that he colour-coded the main ones to make it easier to keep track of them.

For example.

- **Beta carotene**, he coloured **orange**.
- **Lutein**, he coloured **green**.
- **Lycopene,** one of the strongest at binding free radicals and inhibiting cancer, he coloured **red**.
- **Quercetin**, he made **yellow**.
- **Malvin** got the **deep blues** and **purples**.

So, to get lutein, you eat green vegetables like Swiss chard; to get lycopene, you eat red tomatoes; for quercetin, you eat yellow onions; for malvin, you eat blueberries.

These multicoloured flavonoids protect the plant from any free radicals that might escape from the chloroplast during its tricky job of converting sunlight into carbohydrate. Since mitochondria in animals do the opposite—by turning food back into energy—with all the same free radical dangers, by eating a rainbow collage of plants, we can recycle these flavonoids and take advantage of the tremendous wisdom that plants have accumulated over millions of years. Of course, the different colours represent the different energy frequencies they work on, so the more colours you eat, the wider the range of antioxidant activity you get.

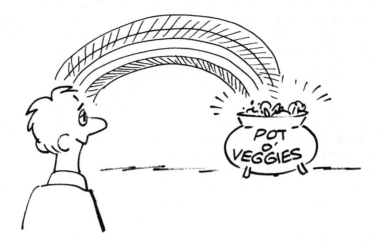

Of course, plants soon found other uses for something as electrically active as the aromatic flavonoids. Some plants—like the legumes: peas, beans, and alfalfa, and even trees like alder— send flavonoids into the soil to invite bacteria called **Rhizobium** over to "play house." The bacteria are stimulated by the flavonoids to make **Nod factor**, which activates the plants' roots to make little rooms for the bacteria, called **nodules**. Then the plant opens small passageways through the root hairs so that the Rhizobium bacteria can enter the root and proceed to the nodules.

Here, the bacteria are fed carbohydrates by the plant until they become so big and round, these now-civilized bacteria develop a unique skill they were unable to perform on their own in the wild. They break apart the tough bonds that hold two nitrogens together. From this atmospheric nitrogen, they make ammonia that the plant can now use as a source of nitrogen to make the precious amino acids *we* are made from!

Gaspy: Uh, wait just a sec there, **Docque**. I know I'm a little slow at times but it seems to me that a while back, you tried to slip something past us about our food coming from *a Boogy Boy living in a plant!?*

Docque: Not only did the first plant chloroplast capture a Boogy Boy and put it to work turning sunlight into food, there's a rumour going around **Liver Dwarf Headquarters** that the organism that does the final stage of our digestion—that is, turning food back into energy so that we can use it—is also a Boogy Boy!

Sluggy: You mean that the mitochondria are Boogy Boys!? That's preposterous!

Docque: I know how you feel. We **Liver Dwarves** have long looked at ourselves as highly advanced, and The Boogy Boys as primitive and crude. But the truth is, they're highly skilled chemists—even magicians, if you will. They pull sunlight out of the sky to make carbohydrates, and nitrogen out of the air to make amino acids. They also make vitamin B_{12}. All the food we eat and even the air we breathe have virtually been built or modified by them.

Many of the metals we use originated from them, living deep in the earth, miles under the bottom of the sea. They would use heat and minerals from volcanoes and turn them into metal compounds that would get deposited in the cracks in the rock. Many of the rocks we walk on today were made by Boogy Boys, millions of years ago.

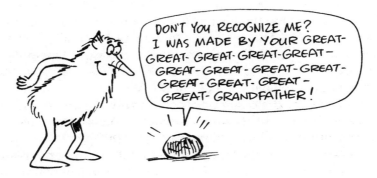

Even the sidewalks we walk on contain limestone made by Boogy Boys. We are totally dependent on them for life. In a sense, we steal our livelihood from them, yet when things go wrong, we blame them for causing our dis-ease.

Burpy: This goes against everything I learned at **Liver Dwarf College**!

Docque: Yes, there have been some big changes in our understanding, some of which might shatter our traditional beliefs. Yes, even mitochondria, our source of energy, were once Boogy Boys. Rumour has it that long ago, one of them was captured and imprisoned in a cell, forced to work as our slave, doing its complicated tricks of turning simple foods into bountiful energy for us to use at our pleasure.

Bitchy: Are you saying that all of us **Liver Dwarves** are slave drivers, keeping oppressed Boogy Boys captive and exploiting them? I couldn't *live* if that were true!

Docque: Well, there is another rumour that The Boogy Boy mitochondria . . .

Bitchy: Perhaps that should be Boogy Girl!

Docque: I stand corrected. The rumour goes that The Boogy *Girl* or Boy mitochondria actually captured us and live safely and peacefully within our cells, buffered from the stresses of life by our sweat and hard work. We toil away at never-ending, menial jobs while they lie back enjoying all the food that our endless labour has bought. Rumour has it that *we* are actually the slaves for the mitochondria, and that we're being used as an easy source of food, and that we're probably the butt of a number of rude jokes when The Boogy Boys—or Girls—gather.

Spacey: Ha! Ha! That's funny, **Docque**, really funny! You *are* kidding, aren't you, **Docque?** Aren't you, **Docque? Docque**— aren't you?

Docque: Let's get back to flavonoids. Vitamin E has its fatty flavonoid friends, the **carotenoids** alpha and beta carotene, and lycopene to help it out. The eye uses the carotenoids lutein and **zeaxanthin** in the **macular pigment** to protect against free radical damage. These flavonoids are found in leafy greens such as swiss chard and spinach. Taking large amounts of beta carotene supplements could disrupt the amount of lutein and zeaxanthin available to your eyes. Supplements can't replace proper diet.

Gaspy: I see.

Docque: **Selenium**, however, is one supplement that's safe to take—up to 200 micrograms per day for an adult—and it can reduce your risk of most cancers by up to 80 percent. And you should know by now that the same things that prevent cancer also prevent heart disease and most other diseases. We know that selenium is crucial for your liver's enzymes to turn deadly peroxides into harmless water, but selenium is also important for protecting your thyroid. When your thyroid adds iodine to your thyroid hormone, hydrogen peroxide is produced, which could "barbecue" your thyroid. To protect your thyroid, it's important that your thyroid's glutathione peroxidase enzymes have adequate selenium. Of course, if your liver is hogging all the selenium, your thyroid could find itself in great distress.

Brazil nuts are very high in selenium. Eating one brazil nut per day is adequate; too much selenium can be toxic. Too much of any nutrient—even water—can be toxic. Remember, nuts can become rancid; of all the nuts, almonds are the least likely to do so because of their monounsaturated oils. Hazelnuts, walnuts, and brazil nuts are the most likely to become rancid.

In the case of people with **Down Syndrome**, their extra chromosome #21 produces extra superoxide dismutase enzyme (SOD)—which as you know, converts superoxide radicals into hydrogen peroxide. This higher production of hydrogen peroxide puts great stress on glutathione and the other antioxidants. When the body is overwhelmed with hydrogen peroxide, supplementing the diet with extra selenium, vitamin E, vitamin C, vitamin A, and zinc can dramatically reduce this damage, even if the problem is rooted in the genes.

Seafood is also high in selenium. In fact, the body does so well on seafood—as opposed to meat—that there's another rumour that our **Liver Dwarf** ancestors were fishermen for a much longer period of time than they were hunters.

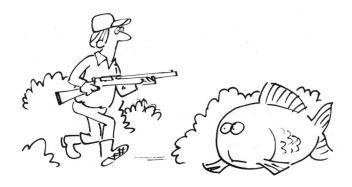

The fact that sea levels have risen since the end of the last Ice Age has concealed much of the archaeological evidence of this, resulting in a bloated exaggeration of the hunter model of human development.

Bloaty: Speaking of bloated, when are you going to get to me?

Docque: Your bloating is a result of spasming of your liver valves due to excess toxins. The quickest way to relieve spasms is with heat—101 degrees F. quickly relaxes the muscles. Fixing the source of the toxins, however, is the longer-term cure. Your liver is the filter for your digestive system, and since your digestive system starts at your mouth, the place to start is with what you put into it. There are actually seven things that can cause you to shut down your liver valves. Excuse me while I use the word "toxins" very broadly to include free radicals, peroxides, and epoxides. Here are the seven things.

1. Toxins in your diet
2. Toxins made by your intestinal flora
3. Toxins made by your liver P450 enzymes
4. Toxins made by your immune system
5. Toxins made by your mitochondria
6. Toxins made by COX and LOX enzymes when making eicosanoids
7. Toxins made by your mind when you harbour gloom-and-doom attitudes or negative thought patterns such as not believing in **Liver Dwarves**.

Achy, Bitchy, Bloaty, Burpy, Gaspy, Itchy, Sluggy, Spacey: Ha! Ha! Ha!

Bitchy: That number 7 is funny, **Docque**. Who'd ever get stuck in that one!

Docque: The obvious liver irritant in your diet is rancid fat. Highly refined carbohydrates like sucrose and alcohol can cause rapid destruction of liver cells, so those two should be minimized, as well.

The next step is to help out your conjugation enzymes. They need a wide range of nutrients, especially protein, so a meal should have adequate protein. And **Bloaty**, you could try eating grapefruit to slow down your P450 enzymes for now. This will help to take a load off your conjugation enzymes.

Bloaty: Citrus bothers my stomach; it's too acidic!

Docque: You could try foods high in ellagic acid, which also slows down the P450 enzymes. These would include strawberries, raspberries, grapes, pomegranates, sprouted wheat, walnuts, and green tea.

Most chemicals, including pesticides and drugs, are fat-soluble and have to be run through the P450 enzymes to be made water-soluble before the conjugation enzymes can deactivate them. The fewer chemicals in your diet, the better. Rancid fats, trans fats from hydrogenation of oils, and fried fats are also going to put more stress on your liver enzymes.

Fish provides EPA, an excellent inhibitor of delta 5 enzymes and therefore of eicosanoids made from arachidonic acid. But fish is also susceptible to rancidity and bacterial contamination and must be handled with care.

Monounsaturated vegetable oils, such as those found in olives and almonds, are the least likely to be rancid, which is part of the success of the diets of the Mediterranean.

Achy: I remember now. In a past life, I was in a Roman villa. I was waited on hand and foot. Yes, I was a mighty Caesar. I was constantly eating and drinking. Every food was brought to me on a platter and I didn't have to lift a finger. What a nightmare! Boy, did my liver ache!

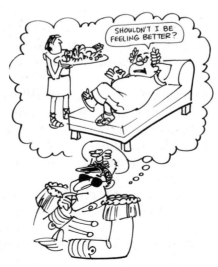

Docque: The liver doesn't work in isolation from the rest of the organs; it gets "pumped" in the same way that the lymph and veins get pumped—not by the heart, like the arteries, but by the act of **breathing**. In fact, the P450 and conjugation enzymes can only be made *partially* effective by using a proper diet. To maximize your liver function, you also have to maximize the pumping of your liver. And remember, oxygen is not only crucial for your mitochondria to work, it also is a key ingredient for efficient liver detoxification.

The lungs are pumped by the muscles between your ribs and by the diaphragm beneath the lungs. During inhalation, some of the muscles between your ribs—the **external intercostals**—contract to pull the rib cage upward and increase its width. At the same time, the diaphragm contracts and flattens, pulling the lower surfaces of the lungs downward. The liver is situated directly below the diaphragm, so this downward pressure of breathing pushes against your liver. During exhalation, these muscles relax and compress the lungs so that air is forced out.

During forced exhalation or heavier breathing, other muscles become active. The **internal intercostals** contract and pull the rib cage downward while the abdominal muscles contract and push the diaphragm upward; this speeds up the expulsion of air. Contraction of the abdominal muscles also "squeezes" your liver.

When your diaphragm and abdominal muscles are working together, they "pump" your liver, and play an important role in its functioning. Obviously, the deeper your breathing is, the greater the pumping action will be on your liver. People who exercise regularly push their hormones toward the C-2 liver pathway by actively pumping their liver, and that can help reduce their cancer risks in a world full of chemicals that are trying to push those same hormones through the C-16α pathway. Women who do <u>active</u> exercise at least four hours per week greatly reduce breast cancer risk.

Sedentary living can lead to insulin resistance, which means you'll have higher levels of insulin and resulting calcium loss and increase in fat deposits. Having a big layer of abdominal fat is going to interfere a lot with abdominal breathing and liver function, and make you much more prone to heart disease, high blood pressure, and diabetes.

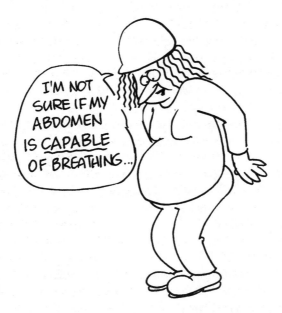

A completely sedentary lifestyle will negate a considerable portion of your liver function by reducing the pumping action of deep breathing—but so will stress and worry. When people are under stress, deep abdominal breathing disappears and breathing moves to the upper chest in the form of shallow breaths. This does nothing to help the liver perform its complex list of jobs. Of course, a sedentary worrier is going to have the least pumping of the liver enzymes and therefore a greater likelihood of poor health, and the greatest difficulty regaining health once it is lost. Prayer, meditation, yoga, martial arts, regular exercise, or even a short nap can greatly help liver detoxification by at least reducing the **emotional constrictions** that inhibit full breathing.

Those who have **gusto** and **joy for life** will be the deepest breathers. Of course, laughter *is* the best medicine, because it helps expel exaggerated fear and opens up deep abdominal breathing.

Burpy: (*Belch*) Sounds good to me, **Docque**. I like to breathe deep.

Bitchy: Whew, what a stink. With sewage breath like yours, nobody would want to share air with you.

Burpy: What can I do, **Docque**? Is there any hope for me?

Docque: Well, **Burpy**, it's good that you're last, because you're maybe the most important of all the **Liver Dwarves**.

Burpy: (*Smiling*) See, I told you so! I told you I was the most important!

Achy, Bitchy, Bloaty, Gaspy, Itchy, Sluggy (*all together*): I thought that **I** was the most important!

Spacey: I knew I wasn't.

Docque: It's okay, **Spacey**. Your serotonin levels are down again. Bright light and active movement are two things that will help to increase your serotonin levels, so exercising in the bright early morning sunshine will shoot your serotonin levels up even faster. Until we can get The Boogy Boys out of your small intestine, where they've been stealing your tryptophan—which is supposed to be going into serotonin production—we'll use some of the herb called **St. John's Wort**. It contains **hypericin, pseudohypericin, xanthones**, and flavonoids. St. John's Wort can inhibit **catechol-o-methyltransferase**—the enzyme that breaks down serotonin—so that serotonin is more readily available for use by your brain.

The advantage of St. John's Wort is that it gently enhances serotonin, norepinephrine, dopamine, and at the same time, it inhibits interleukin-6 (IL-6), which is often high in people who suffer from depression.

Achy: Oooh—St. John's Wort reduces IL-6?! That'll calm the adrenal glands down.

Docque: Yes, St. John's Wort is a wonderful herb, as I explained to Hippocrates just a few centuries ago. He named it **Hypericum**—which means "over an apparition"—because of its ability to chase away evil spirits. Those evil spirits are of viral origin, such as Epstein-Barr, influenza A and B, HSV-1, and HSV-2. Chronic viral infections can deactivate delta 6 enzyme, and the deactivation of this enzyme will weaken your immune system and lower your serotonin receptors' function.

Most people have adapted somewhat to viruses to which they've been exposed for long periods of time. For example, Europeans, because of their cattle-raising background, developed some resistance to viruses that originated from cows, while indigenous peoples of North America and Australia, who had no immunity to these viruses, suffered much more severely when suddenly exposed.

Flu viruses originate in birds and these viruses carry RNA but not DNA. To reproduce, the viruses need to tap into your DNA. To do that, they must gain entry to a cell in your body. They start by locking onto a receptor on the outside of your cell and then they sneak in through your cell's doorway, as if they were an invited guest. Flu viruses in birds generally can't be passed to humans directly because the cell receptors of man and bird are too different. A wild duck, however, can land in a farm pond and pass a recently initiated virus to a domestic duck, who can then pass it on to a pig wallowing in the mud next to the pond. If the virus then goes through another mutation or two, it might be passed from the pig to the farmer through a sneeze. The farmer might pass it on to others at the village market, and this new virus, to which few humans would have resistance, would quickly spread around the world.

Achy: There's an obvious answer to this problem that my creative military mind can grasp. Kill all the ducks or all the pigs. End of the problem. One quick surgical strike worldwide could end flu forever.

Bitchy: Why not kill all the farmers?

Achy: I never thought of that. You might have something there, **Bitchy**. I'll draft you into my army right this minute, complete with a flashy uniform and the appropriate rank—say captain, or major?

Bitchy: Nothing less than Commander-in-Chief!

Achy: Oh, I couldn't do that; that's a higher rank than mine!

Docque: While you two are negotiating World War III, I'll continue. Once a human's upper respiratory system has picked up a new strain of influenza A or B virus, it can be spread to other humans, either by direct contact or through the air on dust or water particles. Since ultraviolet rays from the sun quickly kill them, viruses are usually transmittable only a short distance. But, the darker, cloudier weather of winter permits viruses to spread much further—and therefore, much faster—creating fever, sore throats, headache, muscle pain, fatigue, depression, and even death. This is why phospholipase A_2 enzyme is more reactive in cold, wet weather—to keep your immune system prepared for this expected viral onslaught.

Achy: I've got it! Kill the ducks, pigs, <u>and</u> the farmers!!! Then you'll see results!

Docque: Now hold on, **Achy**. The **Liver Dwarf Code of Ethics** states: "First, do no harm to other people's livers," so your solutions wouldn't be acceptable.

I think **Spacey** should take St. John's Wort. It can chase out these tiny viral demons and give you a giant step toward great health. Since viruses increase with the darker days of winter, that's an especially good time for St. John's Wort to recycle your serotonin and make even the darkest days seem a little brighter. It's best to take St. John's Wort during darker weather because it makes some people more prone to sunburn. An average dose would be 900 mg (or more) of 0.3 percent hypericin a day—one to two capsules of 300 mg, three times a day.

But don't expect St. John's Wort to cure a severe depression on its own since the real causes are likely to be found in the gut/brain interconnections or unresolved spiritual issues. No herb is strong enough to cure a major disease if the root cause remains uncorrected.

Other plants that carry immune-enhancing polysaccharides are **aloe vera, astragalus, reishi mushrooms** and **shitake mushrooms,** as well as **shark cartilage**. Food processing and digestion can destroy some of the activity of a few of the larger molecules. Ginseng is one herb that also has some smaller oligosaccharides that are absorbed intact and still active. I particularly like the **GII333** oligosaccharide preparation from American ginseng, which stimulates your lymphocytes to reproduce more than 100 times faster. I call this my "cold fixer," 'though it also works well on chronic viruses that can make you achy and lay you flat physically and emotionally.

Spacey: Thank you, Spock.

Docque: Uh, that's "**Docque**." Where were we? Oh yes, **Burpy**. Good, quick, effective digestion is the one thing that's as important to liver health as deep breathing is. The more slowly you digest your food, the more chance The Boogy Boys will have to horn in on the process and make toxins, and the more likelihood that there'll be an overloading of the liver's detoxification system, which creates the myriad of problems that the other **Liver Dwarves** are suffering from.

First, you want to minimize putting things into your body that are already toxic—such as toxic fats, sugar, coffee, and alcohol. Plus, you don't want to overeat. When you eat more than you can readily digest, any extra is likely to put The Boogy Boys into a feeding frenzy that your liver may end up having to deal with. Extra food that gets absorbed is likely to be stored as fat or pushed through the mitochondria as fuel that could set off fireworks of free radical activity, particularly as you get older. If your digestion is very weak, it's better to eat frequent small meals rather than several large ones.

Don't eat large, heavy meals late in the day because digestion decreases at night, allowing The Boogy Boys to have a rip-roaring, all-night party, which means less sleep for you. Even melatonin may not help you sleep if your liver's jammed up with toxins. You'll probably awaken between 1 A.M. and 3 A.M. when toxins such as homocysteine are most likely to sneak past **Bloaty**'s outlet liver valves—while she's napping—thus causing irritation to your heart and brain, which can set off a horror show of bad dreams.

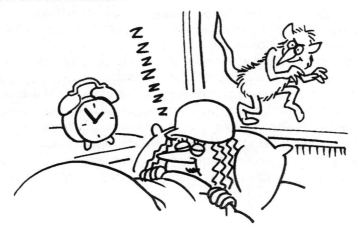

If you're having sleep problems, eat your main meal at lunch and enjoy a lighter vegetarian meal in the late afternoon. Vegetable protein contains only half as much methionine as animal protein, which means there'll be less homocysteine to irritate your brain during the night.

Having your main meal at lunch and a lighter vegetarian meal in the evening will also help with weight loss. Heavy meals eaten late at night can result in increased fat deposits as your body struggles to deal with all those excess calories.

Certain foods are hard to digest quickly, especially legumes, and also grains. They're often not completely digested, and some complex sugars pass into the large intestine where bacteria can make phenomenal amounts of gas from them. Sugars like lactose and fructose can also add to this gastric symphony of bubbles. Now in **Burpy's** case, things are even worse. Worse because his cold kidneys have weakened the ileocecal valve by lowering his calcium levels, allowing the bacteria into the small intestine—so the bacteria get even more opportunity to make gas.

Itchy: How'd you get such cold kidneys?

Burpy: I dunno. Wouldn't be from **juice fasting**, would it?

Docque: When did you do that?

Burpy: Oh, I've done it for years—every spring and fall. And every summer.

Docque: How about winter?

Burpy: Of course. A guy's got to stay healthy, you know.

Docque: Bacteria that get into the small intestine may only become a mild problem if they don't go far. But, the small intestine is about 10 feet long and the further up they go, the more problems they can create.

Burpy: I know, I know; then they start stealing the vitamin B_{12} and tryptophan and making all sorts of toxins.

Docque: They can also methylate relatively harmless **mercury vapours** that might be coming from **mercury amalgam fillings** in your teeth, making the vapours very toxic. This toxic mercury can aggravate the nervous and immune systems and can also be stored in connective tissue. Caution should be used when taking **EDTA** or **citrates** such as **calcium citrate**; they can stir up the mercury and cause more aggravation.

One advantage of having yeast in the intestine is that they tend to attract toxic metals that have found their way into your body. Since toxic metals are even more strongly attracted to algae than to yeast, taking algae will actually strip the toxic metals from the yeast and then remove these metals from your body. So, it's better to pull the metals out of your body with algae before killing the yeast; this will make it easier on your liver.

Itchy: Bring on the algae—let's flush out those metals.

Docque: Algae—especially green algae—should be used with caution if you have ileocecal valve problems, because algae can be cooling.

While it's low calcium that allows the bacteria through the ileocecal valve into the small intestine, the main deterrent to their progress up the small intestine is the secretion of hydrochloric acid by your stomach.

Proteins, especially the animal proteins, are the main stimulus for hydrochloric acid (HCl) production. Carbohydrates are the main inhibitors of HCl and the sweeter the carbohydrate is, the more likely it's going to inhibit HCl. Obviously, mixing sweets and proteins is going to create a conflict in the stomach—a conflict of whether to make acid, or not. The combination of sweets and proteins results in a slower rate of digestion, giving The Boogy Boys in your small intestine more time to party.

Many of the symptoms of acid indigestion that people experience are not due to an excess of hydrochloric acid being made. They're due to the fact that the acid is escaping through the top valve of the stomach into the esophagus, which is much more vulnerable to acid irritation than the tougher stomach.

Taking **antacids** in these situations may relieve some of the symptoms of acid indigestion, but antacids may drive the stomach acid levels much lower than what they should be for proper absorption of minerals. The optimal pH of the stomach is about 1.5 to 3.5. Antacids can raise the pH above 5, which will interfere with mineral absorption and inhibit the conversion of inactive pepsinogen into the very active pepsin—so crucial for protein digestion—and of course, if the pH gets high, The Boogy Boys . . .

Bitchy: Careful there, **Docque**!

Docque: Oh, yes, The Boogy *Girls* . . . when the stomach pH gets to 5, there's not much to stop The Boogy Girls or Boys from stampeding up the small intestine all the way to the stomach, or even further.

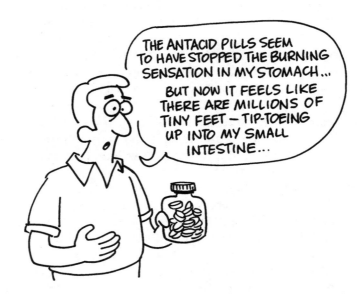

The low acid also allows hitchhikers—like bacteria or parasites—to come in with the food and it gives yeast and Helicobacter a much greater chance to get established in the duodenum or stomach. The **aluminum** in antacids can be absorbed even more if taken with fruit or sodas that contain **citric acid**. If your liver's conjugation enzymes—especially the glutathione-based ones—can't handle the incoming aluminum, it can contribute, over a period of time, to damage to your nervous system.

The cause of stomach acid refluxing up into the esophagus is irritation of the digestive muscles—the duodenum, stomach, and even the esophagus—by toxic bile, for which **Burpy** is so world-renowned.

Burpy: (*Beaming*) Gosh, thanks **Docque**.

Docque: Taking some extra bioflavonoids and zinc will help protect the irritated duodenum from Helicobacter pylori until we can get your bile settled down. The bioflavonoids that are most protective are those found in the herb licorice. If you're prone to high blood pressure, you could take licorice that has been deglycyrrizinated. The herb that has the most damaging effect on your membranes is coffee—it makes you more susceptible to infection, especially from Helicobacter.

Some people make very little hydrochloric acid, and this is called **hypochlorydia**. This can be caused by extreme damage to the stomach from chronic gastritis, but often it's reversible by correcting the underlying lack of T_3 thyroid hormone.

You see, any cell that works hard needs a lot of T_3 to power its protein synthesis and make hydrochloric acid (HCl). To convert T_4 (the more common but less active hormone made by the thyroid) into the much stronger T_3 requires zinc. And then for the T_3 to bind to the DNA receptors of a stomach cell takes even *more* zinc.

Low zinc = low T_3 = low HCl = low zinc absorption. So even if **Burpy** added more foods that contain zinc to his diet—like oysters, cod and other fish, kidney beans, and turkey—it could take months to years before his zinc, T_3 activity, and HCl were back up to normal. So, for a few weeks to several months, we're going to use hydrochloric acid supplements with each meal as well as small doses of **chelated zinc** to dramatically speed up his improvement.

Some people can't take HCl in supplement form because it's just too strong for them, but **bitter herbs** and **homeopathics** can be used to give the stomach a little jump-start until it starts running on its own.

There are also some mild herbs that can help the digestion. **Fennel seed tea** works well even for babies with **colic**, as it's quite soothing to the whole digestive system. **Chamomile tea** is more specific for digestive problems from **nerve irritation**, such as **teething problems**. **Peppermint** can be very soothing to some people, yet could irritate others. **Ginger** is a very good herb for digestive problems and nausea, and is also warming, which is important for **Burpy**.

Most of the digestion is done by the enzymes made by your pancreas. Only one hormone stimulates the pancreas to make digestive enzymes, and that's cholecystokinin from the small intestine. Only two things stimulate cholecystokinin—fat and protein, especially protein. Carbohydrates provide little stimulation for the production of digestive enzymes.

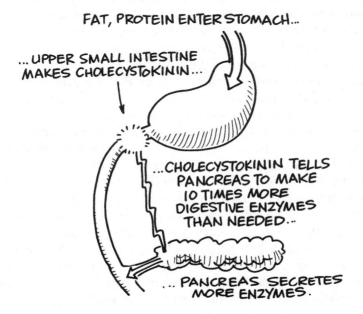

Burpy: That's okay. I can get lots of enzymes from all the juices and raw fruits and salads that I've been taking.

Docque: That's true, raw foods can provide enzymes that can aid digestion a little. The main problem is, if you eat large quantities of high potassium raw fruits and raw vegetables, or their extracts—such as juices or green powder supplements—to get those enzymes, you may end up with overcooled kidneys, low calcium, and a weakened ileocecal valve that allows The Boogy Boys to stampede into your small intestine, particularly in a cool or cold climate. A few raw fruits and vegetables are fine, especially in hot weather when the kidneys would like to be cooled down, but it's more important to eat enough protein and fat with each meal to stimulate cholecystokinin. If cholecystokinin is being made, the pancreas will usually make up to 10 times the amount of digestive enzymes needed for each meal. Surplus enzymes are recycled back to the pancreas for reuse.

With **Burpy**, we may use a **digestive enzyme supplement** for a month or two, until your digestion begins to function better. If there's a perforation in the stomach or intestine—such as a **duodenal ulcer, Crohn's disease**, or **ulcerative colitis**— enzymes that digest protein can't be used since they could make the hole in the membrane bigger.

Hydrochloric acid could also irritate these conditions. Licorice could be very helpful in these cases, and maybe **aloe vera gel**. **Cabbage juice** taken a few times a day can actually heal ulcers within a few weeks to a few months.

Cholecystokinin not only stimulates pancreatic enzyme production, it also stimulates the release of bile. This could be a bit of a problem at the start, because **Burpy**'s bile is obviously toxic and flushing it out too fast could aggravate the bile ducts and the duodenum for a while.

We'll make you a **herbal tonic** of **artichokes** and turmeric— and certainly some milk thistle—to intercept epoxides and free radicals that might be making your bile toxic. Some **Spanish black radish** with every meal will quickly settle down your ileocecal valve symptoms until your calcium levels come up. Spanish black radish helps to "flush" your bile out of your gallbladder, and the bile will gently nudge the bacteria out of your small intestine, back toward the large intestine where they belong. But you have to go slowly, because moving toxic bile too fast could create more indigestion, nausea, and even vomiting.

Spanish black radish is also a member of the cruciferous family that can stimulate the liver's P450 enzymes to eliminate chemicals and break down hormones via the angelic C-2 pathway. Because many of the other members of the cruciferous family are too gassy for people with ileocecal valve problems, black radish's dual action on your liver and small intestine can be of great benefit.

If black radish isn't strong enough to get the bacteria out of your small intestine, we'll use a herbal formula containing

turkey rhubarb, which is stronger. Since some of The Boogy Boys, like E. coli and Bacteroides, aren't really bad guys—just good guys in the wrong place—we don't have to kill them. We can just slowly nudge them out of the small intestine with small doses of black radish or turkey rhubarb, back into the large intestine where they belong, never to return, as long as the ileocecal valve is kept strong with calcium—right, **Burpy**?

Burpy: (*Belch*) Hope so, **Docque**.

Docque: If The Boogy Boys in the small intestine have already damaged the disaccharide-digesting enzymes of the microvilli, you'll have quick relief if you stay off foods high in disaccharides—such as starch and milk—until the intestine can be rebuilt over a few months or longer.

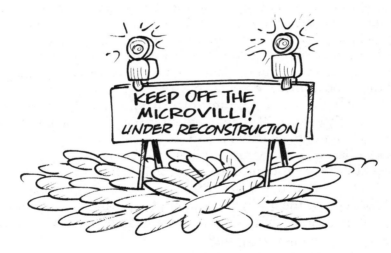

It might not be a bad idea to stay off the grains high in the protein **gluten**.

Burpy: Did you call me a glutton?

Docque: No, I said reduce gluten until we can build up your digestive system. Gluten is a protein found in grains like wheat, rye, barley, and oats. Rice has little gluten.

Bitchy: What about yeast? I bet he's full of yeast.

Docque: Everybody has a small amount of yeast and other fungus lurking in the nooks and crannies of their bodies, just waiting for you to die so they can recycle you like fungus would do to an ailing tree in the forest. Your Boogy Boys make lactic acid, and acid always inhibits yeast; your active white blood cells further control yeast and keep them in their place.

Bitchy: Well, it doesn't seem to be working any more because it seems like everybody has a yeast or fungus problem today.

Docque: Since repeated use of antibiotics kills off the intestinal bacteria, the yeast are free to multiply and take over your intestine, especially if you're eating a lot of those sweets that they thrive on. Often, the good bacteria will battle back and regain control of your intestine unless the yeast make large amounts of **gliotoxin**, which stimulates apoptosis of your white blood cells in your thymus, lymph nodes, spleen, and bone marrow, and interferes with glutathione metabolism.

Achy: So that's why so many of my little soldiers commit suicide after repeated doses of antibiotics.

Docque: And in the last 50 years, millions of pounds of antibiotics have been used in meat, dairy, and poultry farming—not necessarily to protect the animals from infections, but to speed up their growth rates. Those antibiotics end up in *your* body, where they can cause increased yeast growth *and* they can increase the rate of development of drug-resistant bacteria.

Bitchy: They also use synthetic hormones to stimulate growth. Probably stimulates the growth of tumours in me!

Achy: Of course yeast and fungus in the intestines can make toxins that can weaken your immune system.

Bitchy: And then, with the weakened immune system comes yeast overgrowth in the vagina.

Burpy: Or **thrush** in the mouth.

Itchy: Or fungus growth in the skin and the nails! And don't forget that chlorine in the drinking water can not only cause bladder cancer, but it can also inhibit your "good" intestinal bacteria, and cause fungal overgrowth.

Docque: That's just to name a few of the most obvious results of fungal overgrowth. The intestinal overgrowth is the most detrimental because it weakens the immune system enough to allow these other problems to occur. Chronic fungal problems are seen in virtually everyone with chronic immune system problems, including those who have cancer.

Cancer cells use anaerobic fermentation to convert glucose sugar into pyruvic acid, as do The Boogy Boys, yeast, fungus, and your own muscle cells when they're under extreme stress. Your healthy cells normally take the pyruvic acid and, with the use of oxygen, create 36 more ATP plus water and carbon dioxide. Cancer cells alter the pyruvic acid, with the enzyme **lactase dehydrogenase**, to produce 2 ATP and a lot of lactic acid. Anything that slows the lactase dehydrogenase enzyme can slow or block the growth of cancer. These include **oxalates** from herbs such as **sorrel**; fresh **allicin** from garlic; **EDTA**; serotonin; vitamin C (especially with copper); polysaccharides such as from aloe vera; phenols such as flavonoids, lignans, tannins, and saponins; and a wide variety of **alkaloids** from a number of plants. Perhaps the strongest inhibitor is **hydrazine sulphate**.

Since yeast and fungus stimulate lactase dehydrogenase, it's crucial to eliminate them from your body.

Achy: Let's kill them!!!

Spacey: I'd use a bacteria I came across while working in Iceland, called **Bacillus laterosporus**. It's a bacteria found in the soil at the edge of glaciers. That bacteria didn't have much to eat so it acquired a taste for a lot of the bad guys, including yeast and other fungus. You ought to see Icelandic plants thrive when they use laterosporus—it kills the competing fungus in the soil.

Docque: Back when our food came straight from the garden, we used to ingest many soil-based bacteria with our vegetables. Taken internally, they can kill off most of the intestinal bad guys within a few weeks.

The fatty acids **undecylenic acid** and **caprylic acid** can also kill yeast, 'though the oils found in **oregano** herbs are even stronger. **Thyme, cinnamon**, and **cloves** also show strong yeast-killing properties.

Achy: Kill the bad guys, that's my motto! Kill 'em all and kill 'em fast!

Docque: Yeast are quite toxic when they die so you have to kill them slowly. As they die, parts of them can be carried by your portal vein into your liver, so your liver's detoxification ability sets the pace as to how fast you can kill intestinal yeast comfortably. You certainly don't want to get constipated while you're taking a yeast killer, since this could put an extra load on your liver. Using psyllium or even herbal laxatives to keep your bowels working could reduce the load on your liver. Adding **bentonite clay** might pull some of the die-off toxins into your stools and thereby away from your liver.

Burpy: I feel better already.

Achy: I don't!

Docque: The problems of yeast die-off are going to be much greater in your case, **Achy**, because you've been on cortisone (Prednisone) for so long.

Achy: I didn't want to take it, but the pain was just too much. I had to take it.

Docque: As you well know, **Achy**, cortisone reduces the pain from inflammation by reducing the activity of your immune system. Cortisone, however, also reduces the effectiveness of your immune system at guarding the intestinal membranes and both Candida albicans and **Candida tropicalis** can soon translocate through the intestine into the blood system. From here, they can quickly spread . . .

Achy: Yes, I know—quickly spread into the kidneys, liver and spleen, and throughout the body. I know I've let everybody down.

Docque: That's not to say it's too late, **Achy**. Yeast can still be killed when in the bloodstream but you have to be very careful. Yeast dying in the blood could be filtered by the spleen rather than the liver and because of the strong presence of the immune system at the spleen, this could cause a flare-up in immune system activity. Someone with an already overactive immune system, such as in the conditions of rheumatoid arthritis, asthma, eczema, MS, etc., would have to go very slowly. Rather than kill the yeast directly, it might be smarter to use herbs that make yeast too uncomfortable to reproduce and just let them slowly wither away. This would apply to all autoimmune diseases, including cancer.

It's especially important in chronic cases, which are going to take a long time to reverse, to keep a steady supply of fresh good bacteria coming into the intestine. Since the bacteria used in the making of yogurt die off within a few days after production, commercial yogurt is relatively weak at providing a new supply to your gut.

I'll show you how to make yogurt the way I learned in Lebanon. Remember that casein is a stimulant of phospholipase A_2 enzyme and is less abundant in goat's milk than in cow's milk. That means that yogurt made from goat's milk is less likely to aggravate autoimmune disease than yogurt made from cow's milk. If you use fresh yogurt every day or capsules of lively good bacteria, they'll help inhibit the bad guys you've collected in your intestinal zoo. Yogurt also helps the immune system by increasing gamma interferon production.

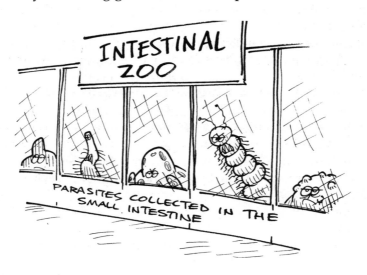

Bitchy: What about **parasites**? I bet **Burpy**'s full of parasites!

Docque: Smaller (single cell) parasites can often be removed with **berberine**, found in a number of herbs. An extract from **grapefruit seeds** is also deadly to parasites. This is very good for people who travel in tropical countries where food can so quickly and easily be contaminated by microorganisms. A few drops taken several times a day can wash them right out of the intestine. Dead.

This grapefruit seed extract works great in water as a gargle. It will work to kill any bacteria, fungus, or virus trying to sneak into the tonsils to take advantage of the fact that **Bloaty** had to shut down your liver valves and the swollen liver dumped protein and fluid into the lymph system. If you need **antibiotics** to treat a dangerous bacterial infection, you should use them. If the infection keeps coming back over and over, you should suspect allergies—that is, your liver dumping toxins into the lymph and the immune system desperately trying to clean up the mess—as being a big part of the problem.

Just improving hydrochloric acid and pancreatic enzyme production is sometimes enough to pass parasites out in bowel movements as your digestion improves. For the tougher ones, a number of herbs—such as **wormwood, black walnut**, and **cloves**—can send them on their way. Cloves are one of the few things—other than your own digestive juices—that are strong enough to kill the eggs of most worms.

Achy: Bye-bye, Boogy Boys' buddies. I think I'm starting to feel better already.

Bitchy, Bloaty, Burpy, Gaspy, Itchy, Sluggy: Me, too!

Spacey: Huh?

Docque: Patience, **Spacey**, your day will come. I've created a handy **three-column food chart** that you can refer to as needed.

DOCQUE'S FOOD CHART

• WARMING

PROTEINS

Recommended
All or most of the time

salmon, sardines, mackerel, trout
cod
bass
sole
halibut
tuna
tempeh
soy yogurt
chicken breast
turkey breast
tofu
soy protein
soy milk

In Moderation

shellfish, herring, anchovies
eggs
lamb
low fat cottage cheese
low fat cheese
quark
veal
beef (low fat)
duck
pork
liver

PROTEIN/CARBOHYDRATE

goat's milk or yogurt
low fat milk or yogurt

• NEUTRAL (if salted with sea salt)

CARBOHYDRATES

Lightly cook: steam or stir-fry.

Recommended

Cruciferous Vegetables

broccoli
cauliflower
brussels sprouts
cabbage
collard greens
kale
kohlrabi
bok choy
turnips/rutabagas
mustard greens
radishes

Other Vegetables

tomatoes
swiss chard, spinach, romaine
nettle
watercress, endive
garlic, onions, leeks
artichoke
asparagus
green/wax beans
eggplant
okra
snow peas
zucchini, yellow squash
celery
fresh herbs
sprouts
cucumber
mushrooms

• COOLING

FRUITS (CARBOHYDRATES)

Fruit should be limited.
Select fruits that are in season for
your growing area.

Approx. glycemic index is shown
in brackets

(n/a) = glycemic index not available

cherries (32)
plums (34)
grapefruit (36)
peaches (40)
apricots, dried (44)
pears (51)
strawberries (n/a)
raspberries (n/a)
blueberries (n/a)
blackberries (n/a)
huckleberries (n/a)
apples (52)
grapes (62)
orange (62)
kiwi (75)
bananas (76)
mangoes (80)
raisins (91)
pineapple (94)
watermelon (103)

FATS

avocado
guacamole

FATS

Recommended
almonds and almond butter
flax seeds
olives and olive oil
sesame oil
tahini
canola oil

In Moderation
mayonnaise (canola)
soybean oil
walnuts
brazil nuts (1 per day)
other legume & nut butters

Use Sparingly
butter
cream
cream cheese
sour cream
nonhydrogenated margarine

OTHER
ginger

• BEVERAGES
water
dandelion/herbal coffee
herbal tea
green tea
vegetable or chicken broth
ginger tea

STARCHES (CARBOHYDRATES)
Approx. glycemic index (in brackets)
soy beans (25)
peas, dried (32)
barley (36)
bean thread (37)
pasta (38 to 131) See ⬆⬆⬆⬆
lentils, dried (41)
kidney beans, dried (42)
black beans (43)
lima beans (46)
chickpeas, dried (47)
oatmeal (slow cooking) (49)
bread (50 to 100+) See ⬆⬆⬆⬆
navy beans (54)
tortillas (54)
chickpeas, canned (60)
pinto beans (55), canned (64)
barley chipati (61)
bulgur (68), frozen peas (68)
kidney beans, canned (74)
lentils, canned (74)
sweet potato (77)
buckwheat (78)
corn (78)
rice: brown or white, long-grain, & basmati (79-83)
new potato (81)
beets (91)
couscous (93)
millet (101)
carrots (101)
potato, baked (121)
parsnips (139)

Examples of PASTAS
protein-enriched spaghetti (38)
egg-enriched fettucine (46)
white spaghetti (52 to 59)
whole meal (53)
durum (78)
brown rice pasta (131)

Examples of BREADS
rye pumpernickel (58)
barley kernel (49 to 66)
oat bran (68)
rye kernel (71)
rye flour (92)
barley flour (95)
whole wheat (99)

Foods Over (100)
bread stuffing
kaiser rolls
melba toast

A balanced diet includes proteins, carbohydrates, and fats.
• **To Lose Weight:**
   Choose carbohydrates from the NEUTRAL column with a glycemic index of less than 60.
• **To Gain Weight:**
   Choose carbohydrates from the NEUTRAL column with a glycemic index higher than 60.

The **right column** consists of cooling foods—foods naturally high in potassium and/or sugar—that tell the kidneys that it's hot outside. The hotter the weather they grow in, the higher they're likely to be in potassium and sugar.

It takes a whole year of very hot weather to build in the extremely high levels of sugar and potassium found in a banana or other tropical fruit. If your kidneys sense these high potassium and sugar levels in your blood, they think you must be surfing in sunny Hawaii—or in a similar latitude—and that your skin must be creating lots of vitamin D directly from the sun, so they stop activating your vitamin D. That only leaves your liver to activate your vitamin D.

Since your liver can only activate your vitamin D very weakly, if you're not *really* enjoying a hot, sunny climate, then you could quickly lose calcium absorption and weaken your ileocecal valve. That would lead to a Boogy Boy stampede into your small intestine to make a great big mess.

Your intake of cooling foods should be reduced in cool weather so that your kidneys know what latitude you're on. Even in hot weather, too many cooling foods can create problems because your kidneys need both sodium and potassium to run properly.

The **centre column** also consists of cooling foods, but they're grains, legumes, and vegetables. Our ancestors found that by adding sea salt to them, the sodium of the sea salt combined with the potassium of the plants to make them neutral—neither cooling nor warming.

I've also added the approximate glycemic index to the carbohydrates to show the rate at which sugar is released from them. Since excess sugar stimulates insulin to convert the sugars into fat, individuals wanting to lose weight should eat foods that are below 60 on the glycemic index, while those who need to gain weight may want to eat foods higher than 60. Of course, the more active you are, the less attention you'll need to pay to the glycemic index because you'll be burning off the sugar as fuel.

The **left column** contains warming foods and consists of proteins and fats, which are usually found together. Animal proteins already have the proper sodium/potassium balance, so they don't need to be salted.

In the northern latitudes, during the months with an "r" in their name, you usually need to supplement your diet with vitamin D—such as a capsule of halibut liver oil or cod liver oil per day. These are the same months that few of the cooling foods should be eaten. The fruits that are best used at this time are the dried berries—soaked or stewed—or if constipation is a problem, you could also include raisins and/or prunes.

Even in the summertime, northern climates can experience cold weather, and a warming diet should be immediately resumed—because within days, enough calcium can be lost that The Boogy Boys and . . . uh . . . The Boogy Girls can crash back into your small intestine and start the whole cycle of liver stress all over again.

The foods that most rapidly lower cholesterol are fish, legumes—especially soy—yogurt, oat bran, tahini-sesame butter, and fenugreek seed tea.

The foods with the highest anticancer properties are fish, legumes—especially soy—the cruciferous vegetables, tomatoes, green tea, nettles, greens, garlic, dark rye bread, grapes and raisins, sprouted wheat, grapefruit, and others.

Since insulin is also a cancer stimulator, it's important to use a ratio of carbohydrates-to-protein-to-fat that will minimize the swings of glucagon and insulin. Since protein and fat are found together in vegetable or animal foods, if you get 20 percent of your calories from protein, you'll be getting about 20 percent of your calories from fat, as well, 'though this is a generalization. Just keep in mind that all protein sources contain fat, and that lean sources of protein will have less fat. Each gram of fat has 9 calories, while each gram of protein or carbohydrate has 4 calories.

Burpy: I think 30 percent of calories from protein, and 30 percent from fat, would be better. As you know, it's protein and fat that stimulate the small intestine to make cholecystokinin, which tells the pancreas to make digestive enzymes. Without digestive enzymes, you can't be healthy.

Bloaty: Yeah, 30 percent protein might be best because the liver's conjugation enzymes need a lot of protein to neutralize toxins. Without liver detoxification, I'd be slamming those liver valves shut and you know what kind of a mess that can create.

Itchy: Wait a minute now. If you start taking in too much protein, you'll start burning it as a fuel. Burning amino acids as fuel gives off all those nitrogen and sulphur residues that have to be dealt with by me down at the kidneys. And let me tell you right now that we don't like that, especially if the kidneys are already weak. You can get into big trouble. Carbohydrates are a cleaner-burning fuel and should make up more than 40 percent of the calories in the diet.

Spacey: Yeah! More carbohydrates. Viva la carbohydrates! One hundred percent chocolate bars sounds right to me. My muscles need glucose.

Gaspy: That's why you're so fat, **Spacey**. Insulin is causing all those sugars to be stored as fat and blocking the burning of stored fat.

Spacey: Hey, I have to keep my insulin levels up so I'll have sugar ready to burn if there's danger, right **Docque**?

Docque: Not exactly, **Spacey**. When your muscles are at rest, they prefer to burn fat, not sugar. High insulin at rest will block the burning of fat and increase fat stores. If intense muscle activity occurs, the muscles will automatically become more porous to glucose without insulin being necessary.

A high carbohydrate diet—one in which up to 70 percent of the daily calories comes from carbohydrates—can renew depleted muscle glycogen stores within two days, while a high protein/high fat diet might take five days or longer to do so.

Bloaty: But **Docque**, a diet where 70 percent of the calories come from carbohydrates would mean that only about 15 percent of calories come from protein and 15 percent come from fat. I don't know if that's enough protein to keep the liver's detoxification enzymes running properly.

Docque: Don't forget that anyone doing exercise that's vigorous enough to burn up his or her glycogen stores is going to be breathing very deeply; that's going to pump the liver thoroughly, which will also help improve the function of the liver's detoxification enzymes. In addition, the considerable oxygen flow will aid liver detoxification. A more sedentary person might need more than 15 percent of their calories from protein. Surplus carbohydrates—like any excess calories—will be turned to fat and stored. Of course, the healthier you are, the more options you have. Maybe that's what health is: lots of options.

Bitchy: And wisdom is using those options for the betterment of all.

Docque: Why, thank you, **Bitchy**—that's very profound. Anyway, you can't be healthy for long on only carbohydrates, especially refined ones. Your body needs protein for growth, repair, and detoxification. You won't make many pancreatic digestive enzymes on a really high carbohydrate diet because carbohydrates don't stimulate the production of cholecystokinin. And without cholecystokinin, you won't get the sense of satiation that comes from eating protein and fat. Ten percent of the calories in the diet from protein would be the minimum amount needed, and for people with kidney problems, that would be as high as they should go. People with kidney problems should also be very careful about taking in too much potassium, since excess potassium could interfere with their heart function.

Those with healthy kidneys can go on a much higher protein diet. I remember when I was the cook on the Lewis and Clark expedition. One winter, about all we had to eat was boiled elk and nobody had any problems on that. Of course, the healthier you are, the more leeway you have.

Achy: Lewis and Clark expedition?! Seems to me that in one of my previous lives, I was the leader of the Blackfoot war party that chased you out of . . .

Bitchy, Bloaty, Burpy, Gaspy, Itchy, Sluggy, Spacey: Enough already!

Docque: Your gut-brain knows when you need more protein or carbohydrate or fat, and it will adjust your appetite accordingly. If you have a large protein meal at night, you'll have little appetite for protein the next morning; carbohydrates will have more appeal, and vice versa. Adjusting the amount of protein, carbohydrates, and fat in your meals—so there are minimal changes in your cravings from one meal to the next—is a sure way of knowing that your glucagon/insulin/ cholecystokonin swings are minimal. Usually this means obtaining 15 to 30 percent of your calories from protein, 15 to 30 percent from fat, and therefore 40 to 70 percent from carbohydrates. This approach is hard to achieve on refined carbohydrates, especially white sugar and white flour, because they're so low in the nutrients needed to stabilize insulin, especially chromium. Eating these foods can lead to wilder and wilder swings in insulin levels, which makes sweets all the more appealing. These processed carbohydrates will quickly reduce the effectiveness of your liver's conjugation enzymes. Of course, once your liver's detoxification enzymes are really jammed up, there may be no appetite at all.

If you've got a small intestine full of fermenters—Boogy Boys and/or yeast—carbohydrates are exactly what they want, especially refined ones, so they can keep their party going. This is where a lower-carbohydrate, higher-protein diet—such as 40 percent of calories from carbohydrates and 30 percent from protein—would work better.

Listen to your body. As you get healthier, it becomes clearer as to what is good and bad for you. And be patient—any changes made too quickly can make you feel worse, since your body probably has been waiting to be detoxified for a long time.

If you're going off things that have been addictive crutches— sugar, coffee, cigarettes, alcohol, **marijuana**, etc.—you may go through a three to four day withdrawal that can include headaches, irritability, and fatigue. There are medicines that a doctor can prescribe to relieve some of these symptoms.

Another thing that can make you feel worse in the beginning is when toxic bile is being flushed out of your liver or gallbladder too quickly. Since it's toxic, it can irritate your duodenum and create gas, burping, nausea, and heartburn. If this happens, reduce the amount of any liver supplements you may be taking.

You can also feel worse if you put more stress on your lymph system, which—because of its close connection to your immune system—can make you more prone to colds, flus, and allergic reactions and can flare up autoimmune diseases. This is particularly likely if you kill yeast too rapidly because the cell walls of yeast can trigger strong immune system reaction. You should try to get your liver and lymph system working better for at least a few weeks before you even consider using a yeast killer.

The tremendous improvement often seen *after* the elimination of yeast is well worth the temporary difficulties you might experience during yeast die-off. Any sign that your lymph, skin, or joints are getting worse means that you should stop or reduce any supplements you're taking until your liver and lymph system catch up to your ambitious start. Of course, if you have any chronic health problem, you should consult with a doctor who understands how overworked you **Liver Dwarves** are, so that some of your tremendous burden might be lifted.

Once you get the liver working smoothly, I'll see that you get some time off, and I'll take you all dancing at this little place I know.

Bitchy, Bloaty, Burpy, Gaspy, Itchy, Sluggy, Spacey: Dancing!!! I haven't had time for dancing in years.

Achy: Dance! I can barely walk after all I've been through! How could I go dancing?

Docque: We'll start real slow and be very patient. When you get your immune system calmed down, you'll be ready for dancing!

Achy: Did I ever tell you what a great dancer I used to be?! I think it was in this life; or was it a previous one??? Hmmmmmmm . . .

Bitchy: Good to have you aboard, **Docque**, but we have to get back to the liver and keep things working. But there's one thing I'd like *you* to know, **Docque**—you're definitely **the most important Liver Dwarf**!

Achy, Bloaty, Burpy, Gaspy, Itchy, Sluggy, Spacey (all together): **That's for sure!!!**

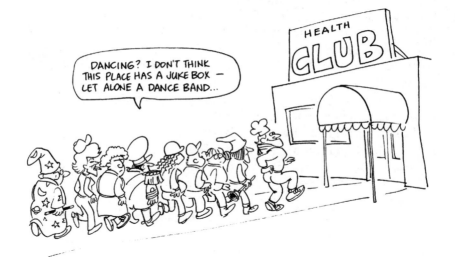

DOCQUE'S MENU SUGGESTIONS AND RECIPES

CONTENTS

MEATLESS MAIN DISHES

MENU SUGGESTIONS

The following menu suggestions will give you an idea of the foods you can eat on this program. Feel free to invent your own, using these as a guideline. Of course, any Lunch and Dinner suggestion may be eaten at breakfast, and vice versa.

Don't go without eating for more than 5 hours; include Snacks to help regulate your blood sugar levels. In addition to the Snack suggestions listed here, many Lunch and Dinner or Breakfast suggestions may be eaten as a Snack—simply use smaller portions.

Menu suggestions in **bold type** indicate recipes that are included in the Recipe section. Many of these recipes also have variations, which will increase your options.

BREAKFAST
- Slow-cooked oatmeal with low-fat milk, soy milk, or rice milk
- Hot cooked cereal with low-fat milk, soy milk, or rice milk (Try different types and combinations of cereals, such as: 1 part buckwheat flakes, 2 parts barley flakes, and 2 parts slow-cooking oats, or use a multiflake cereal, sold in packages in health food stores.)
- Dry packaged cereal with low-fat milk, soy milk, or rice milk (Choose low-sugar varieties and let the cereal soften in the milk before eating.)
- **Scrambled Tofu** and yeast-free rye toast
- **Chicken Vegetable Hash**
- Yeast-free rye toast with smooth almond butter, sesame seed butter, or **Tofu Tahini Spread** (Use nut and seed butters sparingly, since they are high in fat.)
- Soy cheese melted on yeast-free rye toast
- Poached or soft-boiled egg on yeast-free rye toast
- **Steamed Eggs in Spinach "Baskets"** and yeast-free rye toast
- **Zucchini Bread**, muffin, or scone (see Recipes), and low-fat plain yogurt or soy yogurt

SNACKS
- **Oatcakes** with smooth almond butter, sesame seed butter, or **Tofu Tahini Spread**
- **Tofu Bean Dip** and whole wheat tortillas
- **Hummus** and **Dill Scones, Oatcakes**, rye toast, or occasionally, pita bread
- Yeast-free rye bread or rye crackers with **Quark and Herb Spread, Tofu Spread**, or **Yogurt Cheese**
- **Zucchini Bread**, muffin, or scone (See Recipes for options.)
- Low-fat plain yogurt or soy yogurt
- Boiled egg (preferably soft-boiled) and rye toast
- Small bowl of soup (See Recipes for options.)
- **Bean Dip Burrito**
- **Bean Salad**
- Steamed vegetables (such as broccoli, cauliflower, carrots, zucchini, green beans, snow peas, etc.) and any one of the following dips: **Tzatziki, Tofu Bean Dip, Hummus, Yogurt Herb Dip**

LUNCH AND DINNER
- Soup and/or sandwich (Choose from any of those listed in the Recipe section.)
- **Pasta Salad** with sliced, cooked chicken breast or chunks of salmon or tuna, and sliced tomatoes
- Sandwich and steamed vegetables
- Any of the **Wraps** listed in the Recipe section, plus some steamed vegetables
- **Bean Salad**, sliced tomatoes, and yeast-free rye toast
- **Poached Fish Fillets, Broiled Tomatoes**, stir-fried vegetables, and brown rice or lentils
- **Salmon and Spinach Casserole**, steamed broccoli or brussels sprouts with **Yogurt Herb Dip**, and baked butternut squash or sliced tomatoes
- **Broiled Salmon Steaks, Steamed Vegetables with Tofu Parmesan Sauce**, and brown rice or millet
- **Salmon Cakes** with **Yogurt Herb Dip**, steamed asparagus, and **Barley Stew**
- **Tuna Casserole** and steamed green beans, carrots, and cauliflower with **Yogurt Herb Dip**

- **Baked Fish with Black Bean Sauce,** sliced tomatoes, **Sauteed Greens,** and brown rice
- **Breaded Fish Fillets, Stir-Fried Vegetables with Yogurt and Cilantro,** and brown rice or pasta
- **Baked Halibut and Vegetables** and **Barley Stew**
- **Fish Roll-Ups,** sliced tomatoes, steamed broccoli, and lentils
- **Fish Fillets in Foil, Cabbage Casserole,** steamed kale, and brown rice
- Sardines (canned in water) mashed, and mixed with fresh lemon juice and dill, yeast-free rye toast, and steamed vegetables
- **Baked Tofu with Black Bean Sauce,** brown rice, and steamed carrots and Chinese greens
- **Tofu Patty** or **Turkey Burger** with sliced tomato, sprouts, and mayo on rye bread or whole-grain bun, and **Steamed Vegetables with Tofu Parmesan Sauce**
- **Tofu and Veggie Lasagna** and **Sauteed Greens**
- **Tofu and Veggie Stir-Fry** with brown rice, barley, bean thread, or whole-grain pasta
- **Tofu Cabbage Rolls** and steamed vegetables sprinkled with fresh lemon juice and minced fresh herbs
- **Marinated Tofu,** stir-fried vegetables, and brown rice
- **Tofu Chili** or **Turkey Chili,** and **Sauteed Greens**
- **Tofu Bean Casserole** with steamed carrots, brussels sprouts, and green beans
- **Baked Vegetable Frittata,** rye toast, and steamed carrots
- Pizza: choose from **Vegetable Pizza** or **Spinach and Feta Cheese Pizza**
- **Bean Dip Burritos** or **Bean Dip Quesadillas,** and **Sauteed Greens**
- Broiled or baked chicken breast, **Cauliflower Curry,** and brown basmati rice
- **Chicken Vegetable Hash,** poached egg, and steamed broccoli or spinach
- **Chicken, Broccoli, and Rice Casserole** and sliced tomatoes
- **Chicken Kebabs, Tzatziki,** and **Roast Vegetables** or **Greek Salad**
- **Chicken Fajitas** or **Vegetarian Fajitas** and **Sauteed Greens**

- **Chicken Curry**, brown basmati rice, and steamed cauliflower, kale, and peas or **Cauliflower Curry**
- **Breaded Chicken Breasts, Baked Vegetables with Fennel**, and brown rice
- **Chicken with Yogurt and Soy Sauce**, stir-fried vegetables, and whole-grain pasta
- **Chicken with Lemon and Herbs, Barley Stew**, and steamed broccoli and green beans
- **Stuffed Zucchini** and **Steamed Vegetables with Tofu Parmesan Sauce**

In hotter weather, you can add more cooling foods to your diet—in moderation, of course. For example, a serving of fruit grown in season can be eaten as a snack; just make sure that you eat it at least 1 hour before, or 3 to 5 hours after, eating protein foods. (Heavier proteins, such as chicken and fish, will take longer to digest, compared to lighter proteins such as tofu.) Also, steamed or stir-fried vegetables can occasionally be replaced by raw vegetables or **Greek Salad**, and **Sauteed Greens** can sometimes be replaced with green salads.

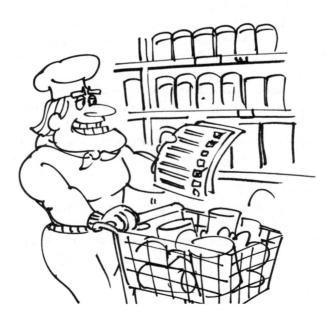

BUT WHAT IF YOU HATE TO COOK
OR DON'T HAVE THE TIME?

Although it's ideal to prepare your own meals using fresh, natural ingredients whenever possible, this isn't practical for everyone, especially those who don't enjoy cooking or don't have the time to cook. Here are some suggestions for foods that require minimal preparation, including foods you can find in health food stores and some grocery stores. When buying these products, be sure to read labels and, as much as possible, avoid those that contain sugar, MSG, and other additives. Better yet, try to find a deli, café, or restaurant that makes healthy soups, sandwiches, and entrees that fit into this eating program.

- Frozen vegetables, if necessary
- Egg sandwich: Mash a hard-boiled egg, add a small amount of mayo and some plain yogurt and sea salt; serve on yeast-free rye bread with sliced tomato, if desired.
- Packaged soup mixes, to which you just add water
- Packaged vegetarian burger or sausage mixes—these contain ingredients such as brown rice, dehydrated vegetables, soy protein, herbs and spices, and grains like barley and oats. You just add water, mix, and sauté.
- Tofu patties and vegetable patties—found in the refrigerated section of grocery and health food stores
- Sauteed tofu or tempeh added to a good quality store-bought tomato or pasta sauce; serve over pasta with steamed vegetables.
- Stir-fried fresh or frozen vegetables with diced firm tofu or chicken; add the sauce that's listed in the **Tofu and Veggie Stir-Fry** recipe.
- **Bean Dip Burritos** or **Bean Dip Quesadillas**, using no-fat refried beans in place of the **Tofu Bean Dip**
- Poached or steamed fish or chicken, steamed vegetables, and rice (Poaching and steaming are fast, easy, and low-fat cooking methods.)
- Store-bought muffins or scones (Choose low-fat, low-sugar varieties.)

EATING OUT

When eating in restaurants, select foods that are cooked with little or no added fat; choose foods that are baked, broiled, poached, steamed, or roasted, and avoid fried and deep-fried foods. For protein choices, select chicken breast, fish, or tofu, served with vegetables (lightly cooked in colder weather, raw or salads occasionally in warmer weather), and a moderate amount of pasta, rice, or potatoes.

The following is by no means a complete list; it's just meant to show that you can eat out and still follow this program fairly closely.

- **Greek**
  Chicken (or lamb) souvlaki, tzatziki, cooked vegetables, and a small amount of roast potatoes
- **Japanese**
  Sushi, miso soup, and soybeans steamed in the pod
- **Mexican**
  Chicken or bean tortilla or soft taco. (Go easy on the cheese and avocado, and use mild salsa.)
- **Italian**
  Protein, such as chicken or fish, with steamed vegetables and a small portion of pasta.
- **Indian**
  Mild chicken curry and vegetables, with basmati rice or chapatis

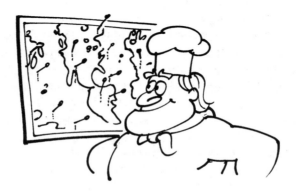

HELPFUL HINTS

Arrowroot Powder
Found in health food stores, it can be substituted for cornstarch as a thickening agent.

Baking Powder
Use nonalum (aluminum-free) baking powder instead of regular, if possible. It's available at health food stores.

Buttermilk
If you'd like to use buttermilk, but don't have any on hand, you can make your own. For each cup of buttermilk that you need, place 1 tablespoon (15 mL) lemon juice or vinegar in a measuring cup. Fill the measuring cup with milk to the 1-cup mark. You can make soy buttermilk in the same way, using soy milk instead of cow's milk.

Fats and Oils
Although it's necessary to have some fat in our diet, too much fat isn't good for us. There are a number of ways you can avoid adding excess fats when preparing meals. When sauteing or stir-frying vegetables, use water instead of oil, or start with a just small amount of oil, then add water as needed to prevent food from sticking. In sandwich spreads and casseroles, replace some or all of the mayonnaise that you would normally use with low-fat plain yogurt. When baking muffins, replace some of the oil the recipe calls for with unsweetened applesauce or pureed prunes (baby food); this will also provide natural sweetness and decrease the need for adding sugar.

When fats and oils are heated to high temperatures, their chemical composition is altered and many toxic substances are created. To protect the oil from overheating when sauteeing or stir-frying—and thereby minimize the formation of toxic substances—do the following: cook at a low temperature, put water into the saucepan, skillet, or wok first, before adding the vegetables and oil, then put the vegetables into the heated pan before adding any oil. Extra virgin olive oil is a suitable oil to use for light sauteing and stir-frying. Or better yet, omit the oil and use water or stock instead; then you can sauté or stir-fry at a slightly higher temperature. Butter is a suitable fat to use in baked goods such as muffins, and to line baking pans and dishes.

Fish
Measure at the thickest portion, and cook for 10 minutes per inch (2.5 cm) of thickness.

Ginger and Garlic
Use only *fresh* garlic and ginger; the dried forms do not compare in taste. Powdered or dried ginger should only be used in baking.

Ground Turkey or Chicken
Make sure these are ground from skinless breast only, to ensure they're low in fat.

Herbs
For the sake of convenience, dried herbs have been used in these recipes, unless otherwise specified. The exceptions are parsley and cilantro; rosemary is another herb that is best used fresh. Use fresh herbs if you have them. When substituting fresh for dried, use 3 times as much fresh herbs; for example, 1 teaspoon (5 mL) of dried herbs is roughly equivalent to 1 tablespoon (15 mL) of chopped fresh herbs. Many different types of fresh herbs are available year-round. They can be found in packages in the produce section of many grocery stores.

Lemon Juice
Use the juice of fresh lemons, whenever possible, or use 100% pure lemon juice from concentrate, available in plastic bottles in the freezer section of some grocery stores.

Mayonnaise
Use canola oil-based mayonnaise or the **Tofu Mayonnaise** recipe.

Miso
Miso is a rich-tasting fermented bean paste made from soybeans and grains, such as wheat, barley, or rice. Use it to flavour soups, sauces, and salad dressings.

Mushrooms
Some of the recipes in the Recipe section call for mushrooms. If you know that you have—or if you suspect that you have—an overgrowth of intestinal yeast, omit the mushrooms.

Organic Foods
Use organically grown foods, whenever possible.

Rice
Brown rice takes longer to cook, but it's more nutritious than white rice. When you're cooking brown rice, make extra for use in the following recipes that call for cooked brown rice: **Salmon Loaf, Fish Roll-Ups, Tofu Patties, Tofu Cabbage Rolls, Tofu Bean Casserole**, and **Chicken, Broccoli, and Rice Casserole**.

Sea Salt
Use unprocessed sea salt, and add it at the end of the cooking time (except in baked products like muffins), to retain the valuable minerals.

Spinach
Use fresh, whenever possible. A large bunch of fresh spinach weighs about 10 ounces (300 g). To cook spinach, wash it well and remove the stems. Place the spinach leaves in a pot, cover, and cook over medium heat for just a few minutes, until wilted. There's no need to add any water to the pot—there'll be enough water clinging to the spinach leaves.

You can also buy 10 ounce (300 g) plastic bags of *prewashed* spinach in many grocery stores; these cost a little more but save a lot of time since you don't have to wash it. A 10 ounce (300 g) package of frozen spinach, thawed and well drained, can often be substituted for fresh spinach, such as in the **Salmon and Spinach Casserole, Fish Roll-Ups, Tofu and Veggie Lasagna, Tofu Bean Casserole,** and **Spinach and Feta Cheese Pizza**.

Tamari Soy Sauce

The recipes in this book call for tamari soy sauce, a Japanese soy sauce that tends to have a richer taste and that's thicker and less salty than Chinese soy sauces. Please use whichever type of soy sauce you prefer.

Tempeh

Tempeh is a bean cake or patty made from fermented soybeans. Usually sold in 8 ounce (250 g) packages, it can be found in the freezer section in some health food stores. Tempeh has a chewy texture and a slightly nutty, smoky flavour.

Tofu

Tofu or soybean curd is high in protein, low in saturated fat, and a good source of calcium. It's also inexpensive and versatile. Many people complain that tofu is bland-tasting but that's the nice thing about it; it'll take on the flavour of the dish in which it's being used. Tofu can be used to replace other protein sources such as eggs, cottage cheese, chicken, or beef. Use firm or extra-firm tofu in stir-fries, burgers, stews, or casseroles, or as a substitute for ground beef or poultry in chili, spaghetti sauce, etc. Silken and soft tofu can be used in dips, dressings, sauces, and soups.

Once the package has been opened, submerge the tofu in fresh water, cover, and store it in the refrigerator for a maximum of 5 days. The water should be changed every day. Tofu can also be frozen for up to 5 months; just drain and wrap well. When thawed, drained, and crumbled, it has a texture similar to ground meat. To drain tofu, press it between 2 pieces of paper towel.

If you aren't accustomed to eating tofu, try introducing it into your meals slowly. For example, replace half the amount of ground turkey in **Turkey Chili** or **Turkey Cabbage Rolls** with tofu. (See the tofu variations of these recipes and add half the amount of tofu called for.) Many people won't even notice that these dishes contain some tofu! Or replace half the tofu with chicken when making **Tofu and Veggie Stir-Fry**.

Note: Processed soy products (for example, some soy cheeses) may contain casein, one of the main proteins found in cow's milk. Casein can be allergy-inducing in some people.

Tomatoes
Use fresh, if possible. When fresh tomatoes aren't in season, canned tomatoes can be used in some recipes, such as soups, **Tomato Sauce**, and **Tofu Chili**.

Tortillas
Try to find whole-wheat tortillas that aren't made with yeast, hydrogenated oils, and/or other additives; these are often available in health food stores. Or use the recipe for **Tortillas** in the Recipe section. If you're sensitive to wheat, try substituting other types of flour.

HOW TO COOK BEANS

Besides being low in fat, beans are an excellent source of vegetable protein, B vitamins, fibre, iron, calcium, and other minerals. When cooked beans are listed in a recipe, use dried beans and soak and cook them yourself whenever possible. The beans will be more nutritious, tastier, and less expensive than canned beans. Although the process takes longer than using canned beans, it's really quite easy to soak and cook dried beans; it just takes some planning. Also keep in mind that once cooked, the beans can be stored in the refrigerator for up to 5 days or frozen for up to 6 months. One cup (250 mL) of dried beans will yield 2 to 2½ cups (500 to 625 mL) of cooked beans.

To Cook Dried Beans

First remove any broken or discoloured beans. Place the beans in a sieve and rinse under cold water. Soak them in water using a 3-to-1 ratio: for every cup of beans, add 3 cups of fresh water. Cover and refrigerate overnight for 6 to 10 hours. Drain off the soaking water, place the beans in a sieve or colander, and rinse well under cold running water. This will help to eliminate much of the indigestible sugars that can cause gas. Place the rinsed beans in a large pot and cover with water, again on a 3-to-1 ratio. Add a piece of dried seaweed, such as nori or kombu, if you have it; this will help to degas the beans as well as add flavour. Bring the water to a boil and skim off any foam that rises to the top. Reduce the heat and cover with the lid slightly ajar. Simmer gently—stirring occasionally and skimming off any foam—until the beans are just tender. This will take anywhere from 45 minutes to 1½ hours, depending on the type of bean. Once cooked, drain off the cooking water and rinse the beans thoroughly; drain well.

Quick-Soak Method

If you don't have time to soak the beans overnight, use the following quick-soak method. Sort through and rinse the dried beans, as directed above. Put the beans into a large pot with 3 times as much water as beans and bring the water to a boil; cook for 2 to 3 minutes. Remove from the heat, cover, and let sit for 1 hour. Drain off the soaking water and rinse the beans well; follow the remaining steps for cooking, as directed above.

The following recipes call for cooked beans (including chickpeas), so if you're cooking some for one recipe, make extra to use in another recipe: **Tofu Bean Dip, Hummus, Minestrone, Bean and Tomato Soup, Bean Salad, Black Bean and Rice Wraps, Tofu Chili,** and **Tofu Bean Casserole.**

To help reduce the intestinal gas that's often caused by eating beans, when you're cooking dried beans, be sure to drain and discard the water in which the beans are soaked or cooked, and always rinse the beans with fresh water after soaking or cooking them. Also, if you're not accustomed to eating beans, be sure to introduce them into your diet slowly; eat small amounts at first and slowly increase. Beans are less likely to cause gas when they're eaten on a regular basis.

If you must use canned beans, be sure to read the label; try to avoid those that contain sugar, MSG, and other additives. Most brands contain salt, but some use seaweed (like kombu) instead. Always drain and rinse canned beans well to help reduce gas. A 14 ounce (398 mL) can is approximately equal to 1½ cups (375 mL) and a 19 ounce (540 mL) can is approximately equal to 2 cups of beans.

HOW TO MAKE YOGURT

In the production of yogurt, bacteria eat the lactose sugar in the milk; that makes it easier for your body to digest the yogurt. Yogurt helps reduce the production of cholesterol in your body.

You can use whole, low-fat, or skim milk to make yogurt. Heat 2 cups (500 mL) milk to just below the boiling point, but do not boil. Remove the pot from the heat and place on a thick towel. Let the milk cool until it's lukewarm. If the milk is too hot when adding the yogurt, it may kill the bacterial culture. Add 1 tablespoon (15 mL) of plain yogurt and stir gently. Use a commercial yogurt that contains only milk ingredients and bacterial culture. Cover the pot with a lid and wrap two more thick towels around and on top of the pot. Leave to sit and ferment for several hours, until thickened; this will take anywhere from 8 to 24 hours. The longer you leave it to ferment, the more of the lactose sugar the bacteria will eat. Homemade yogurt will keep in the refrigerator for 7 to 10 days.

It's important that the temperature stay between 80 and 110 F (27 and 45 C) during the fermentation period. If your kitchen is too cool or drafty, you may find that the above method doesn't work for you. Instead, heat the milk as directed above, then cool until it's lukewarm. Place 1 tablespoon (15 mL) plain yogurt in a large, clean jar and pour in the warm milk; stir gently. Cover and keep warm in an oven that is turned on very low (as low as possible) or in an oven with just the light on. Or, wrap the jar in a heating pad set on the lowest setting. Whichever method you decide to use, be sure to check the temperature with a thermometer first to make sure it's close to, but not over, 110 F (45 C).

Strained Yogurt

Homemade yogurt is not as thick as many of the commercial yogurts. If you like a thicker yogurt, place the yogurt in a sieve lined with about 4 layers of cheesecloth; place the sieve over a bowl. Wrap the cheesecloth around the yogurt and give it a slight squeeze. Place a plate over the bowl and sieve and place them in the refrigerator. Let the yogurt drain for 2 to 3 hours, then discard the liquid. One cup (250 mL) yogurt will yield about ¾ cup (175 mL) strained yogurt. You can strain the yogurt even longer to make **Yogurt Cheese** (see Recipes). If you don't have any cheesecloth, you can use a clean tea towel instead; the draining time will be shorter because the tea towel tends to absorb more of the liquid. Small amounts of yogurt can be drained in a coffee filter.

Uses for Yogurt
Low-fat plain yogurt can be used to replace some or all of the mayonnaise in sandwiches, salads, spreads, and casseroles. It can also be used to replace sour cream. If you or your family aren't accustomed to the taste of yogurt, substitute yogurt for *some* of the mayo or sour cream that you would normally use, and gradually increase the amount of yogurt, while decreasing the amount of mayo or sour cream.

RECIPES

I've created many tasty recipes to help you eat your way to better health. Some you'll love—some, you may not. Give them a try and see what your stomach likes the most. Taste buds can change with time.

As you get healthier, you'll notice how added sugar and chemicals can affect the flavour of food and your mental and physical well-being. Individuals can have reactions to virtually any food. Your goal should be to <u>reduce</u> the number of food sensitivities by gradually improving the function of your digestive organs and lymph system. Combine new eating habits with a regular exercise program, and you're going to feel great soon.

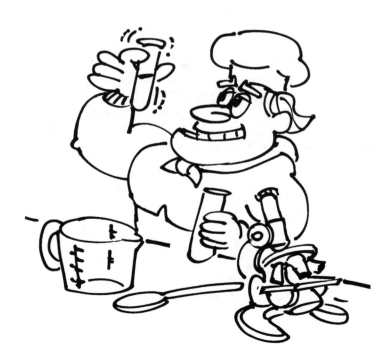

DIPS, SPREADS, AND SAUCES

Tzatziki

1 large cucumber
2 cups (500 mL) low-fat plain yogurt (see Note)
2 garlic cloves, finely minced
1 teaspoon (5 mL) or more, minced fresh dill (optional)
sea salt, to taste

Peel the cucumber, cut it in half, and remove the seeds; grate it and then drain it in a sieve. Combine the grated cucumber, yogurt, garlic, and dill, if using. Season to taste with sea salt. Mix well and refrigerate. Serve with warm pita bread or tortillas, steamed vegetables, fish, chicken, beef, or lamb.

Note
For a thicker sauce, buy an extra-thick variety of yogurt or strain regular yogurt to make it thicker. Place 3 cups (750 mL) of yogurt into a sieve lined with cheesecloth, and set it over a bowl; cover and refrigerate. Let it drain for 2 to 3 hours, or until you have 2 cups (500 mL) of strained yogurt. If you don't have cheesecloth, you can use a clean tea towel and decrease the amount of time that you drain the yogurt. For smaller amounts of yogurt, you can drain it in a coffee filter.

Tofu Bean Dip

1½ cups (375 mL) cooked Romano or pinto beans, or a
    14 ounce (398 mL) can, rinsed and drained
½ cup (125 mL) drained and mashed firm tofu
1 to 2 garlic cloves, minced
2 green onions, chopped
¼ cup (50 mL) chopped fresh cilantro (or parsley or a
    combination)
juice of half a lime (or half a small lemon)
1 teaspoon (5 mL) ground cumin
½ teaspoon (2 mL) sea salt
2 to 4 tablespoons (30 to 60 mL) water

Combine the beans, tofu, 1 of the garlic cloves, green onions,
cilantro and/or parsley, lime or lemon juice, cumin, sea salt, and
2 tablespoons of the water in a food processor. Process until
smooth, stopping to scrape down the sides, if necessary. Add
more of the water, ½ tablespoon (7 mL) at a time, until you
achieve the desired consistency. Taste and adjust the seasonings
and add the other clove of garlic, if desired. Serve with warmed
tortillas or cold steamed vegetables such as broccoli and
cauliflower, or use in **Bean Dip Burritos**, **Bean Dip
Quesadillas**, or **Tortilla Pinwheels**. Makes about 1½ cups
(375 mL).

Tortilla Pinwheels

Spread a thin layer of **Tofu Bean Dip** on whole-wheat tortillas
and sprinkle with diced sweet red pepper. Top with grated soy
cheese, reduced-fat Monterey Jack cheese, and/or Cheddar
cheese. Roll the tortillas up tightly, then wrap them in foil or
plastic wrap and refrigerate for about 1 hour. Cut into ½ inch (1
cm) slices and arrange on a baking sheet. Bake at 350 F (180 C)
for about 10 minutes or until the cheese melts. Serve as an
appetizer with low-fat plain yogurt and mild salsa.

Hummus

2 cups (500 mL) cooked chickpeas, or a 19 ounce (540 mL)
    can, rinsed and drained
2 tablespoons (30 mL) tahini (sesame seed paste)
2 large garlic cloves, minced
¼ cup (50 mL) chopped fresh parsley
1 teaspoon (5 mL) ground cumin
¼ teaspoon (1 mL) sea salt .
1 tablespoon (15 mL) extra virgin olive oil
3 to 4 tablespoons (45 to 60 mL) fresh lemon juice
2 to 3 tablespoons (30 to 45 mL) water

Combine the chickpeas, tahini, garlic, parsley, cumin, sea salt, oil, 3 tablespoons (45 mL) of the lemon juice, and 2 tablespoons of the water in a blender. Process until smooth, stopping to scrape down the sides, if necessary. If the mixture is too dry, add more water, ½ tablespoon (7 mL) at a time, while processing. Taste and adjust the seasonings, and add the rest of the lemon juice, if desired. Serve with warm pita bread or tortillas, on **Dill Scones** or toasted rye bread, with steamed vegetables, or in a sandwich with sliced tomatoes and broccoli sprouts.

Roasted Eggplant Dip

*The seasonings in this dip are similar to those in the **Hummus** recipe, except the quantities have been adjusted slightly.*

1 large or 2 small eggplants
2 tablespoons (30 mL) tahini (sesame seed paste)
1 large clove garlic, minced
¼ cup (50 mL) chopped fresh parsley
½ teaspoon (2 mL) ground cumin
¼ teaspoon (1 mL) sea salt
3 tablespoons (45 mL) fresh lemon juice

Pierce the eggplant in several places with a fork and place on a baking sheet. Bake at 400 F (200 C) for 25 minutes; turn the eggplant over, and bake for 20 to 30 minutes more, until very tender. Split the eggplant in half and drain in a colander until cool. Scoop out the pulp and discard the skin. Add the remaining ingredients to the pulp and mash well, or process in a food processor until smooth. Use as you would **Hummus**. Makes about 2 cups (500 mL).

Yogurt Herb Dip

½ cup (125 mL) low-fat plain yogurt
½ teaspoon (2 mL) chopped fresh dill, cilantro, or basil
pinch sea salt

Combine all the ingredients and mix well. Serve with fish or chicken, or with steamed vegetables such as green beans, broccoli, cauliflower, brussels sprouts, zucchini, snow peas, potatoes, or carrots.

Notes
- For a thicker dip, use strained yogurt.
- Add Dijon mustard, to taste.
- Omit the fresh herbs and add ground cumin or cumin seeds, to taste.

VARIATION
Tofu Herb Dip
Substitute well-drained silken or soft tofu for the yogurt. Add ½ teaspoon (2 mL) lemon juice and ½ teaspoon (2 mL) mayonnaise (optional). Process in a blender for a smoother sauce.

Tofu Tahini Spread

¼ cup (50 mL) well-drained soft or silken tofu
1 tablespoon (15 mL) tahini (sesame seed paste)

Combine the tofu and tahini and mix well, either by hand or in a blender. Use in place of sesame seed spread on toasted, yeast-free rye bread, for breakfast or a snack

Tofu Mayonnaise

1 cup (250 mL) drained and mashed firm tofu
2 teaspoons (10 mL) extra virgin olive oil
1 to 2 teaspoons (5 to 10 mL) lemon juice
1 teaspoon (5 mL) rice vinegar
¼ teaspoon (1 mL) finely minced garlic
½ teaspoon (2 mL) Dijon mustard
2 to 3 tablespoons (30 to 45 mL) water
sea salt, to taste

Combine the tofu, oil, lemon juice, vinegar, garlic, mustard, and
1 tablespoon (15 mL) of the water in a blender; process until
smooth. Add more water, ½ tablespoon (7 mL) at a time, to
achieve the desired consistency. Season to taste with sea salt.
Add some finely minced fresh herbs, such as dill or parsley, if
desired. Keeps in the refrigerator for up to 3 days. Makes about
1 cup (250 mL).

Note
You can substitute 1 cup (250 mL) of well-drained soft tofu for
the firm tofu; this will have a thinner consistency.

Tofu Spread

1 cup (250 mL) drained and mashed firm tofu
1 tablespoon (15 mL) mayonnaise (canola-based mayonnaise
  or **Tofu Mayonnaise**)
1 small garlic clove, finely minced (optional)
2 teaspoons (10 mL) lemon juice
2 teaspoons (10 mL) minced green onion
1 tablespoon (15 mL) minced fresh parsley
¼ teaspoon (1 mL) turmeric
sea salt, to taste

Combine all the ingredients and mix well. Use as a sandwich
spread or to stuff tomatoes. Makes 2 servings.

Note
Add minced fresh herbs such as basil, cilantro, marjoram, or
dill, if you have them.

Yogurt Cheese

Yogurt Cheese *is a soft, rich-tasting spreadable cheese you can use in
sandwiches and on crackers. To make 1 cup (250 mL) of* **Yogurt
Cheese***, start with 2 cups (500 mL) yogurt.*

Place low-fat plain yogurt in a sieve lined with a clean tea towel
or with about 4 layers of cheesecloth; place the sieve over a
bowl. Wrap the tea towel or cheesecloth around the yogurt and
give it a slight squeeze. Put a light weight (such as a bag of rice
or beans) on top, cover with a plate, and leave to drain in the
refrigerator for 6 to 8 hours. For a thicker cheese, you can drain
the yogurt for up to 24 hours.

Yogurt Cheese and Herb Spread

1 cup (250 mL) **Yogurt Cheese**
1 tablespoon (15 mL) minced green onion
1 tablespoon (15 mL) minced fresh parsley
sea salt, to taste

Combine all the ingredients and mix well. Use as a sandwich
spread with tomatoes and sprouts; on baked potatoes instead of
sour cream and butter; on rye toast or crackers; or on hot,
cooked pasta or steamed veggies. Makes 1 cup (250 mL).

VARIATIONS
Yogurt Cheese and Feta Spread
Add 1 cup (250 mL) finely crumbled feta cheese and 1 small
garlic clove, finely minced; mix well. Serve on rye toast, rye
crackers, or toasted whole-grain bagels. Or serve as an
appetizer by spreading it on a plate that has a rim, to contain it.
Garnish the spread with diced fresh tomato, chopped green
onion, diced cucumber, diced sweet red and/or green pepper,
and sliced black olives; serve with whole-grain crackers or pita
bread wedges.

Quark and Herb Spread
Substitute quark for the **Yogurt Cheese** in the **Yogurt Cheese
and Herb Spread** recipe. Quark is a soft, spreadable cheese
available in some grocery stores.

Quark and Feta Spread
Substitute quark for the **Yogurt Cheese** in the **Yogurt Cheese
and Feta Spread** recipe.

Yogurt Cheese and Salmon Spread

For those who like the taste of smoked salmon-flavoured cream cheese, use this recipe instead. It tastes similar but has a lower fat content and doesn't contain the nitrates found in smoked salmon.

¼ cup (50 mL) cooked salmon
⅓ cup (75 mL) **Yogurt Cheese**
1 teaspoon (1 mL) minced fresh dill

In a small bowl, flake the salmon well. Add the **Yogurt Cheese** and dill and mix well. Serve on rye crackers, rye or whole-grain toast, or occasionally, on whole-grain bagels.

VARIATION
Quark and Salmon Spread
Substitute quark for the **Yogurt Cheese**.

Tomato Sauce

Tomatoes are high in lycopene, a bioflavonoid that helps protect your membranes from free radicals made from the sun or by your immune system. Cooked tomatoes—such as tomato sauces, tomato paste, and pizza sauce—are a good source of lycopene because the cooking process causes the lycopene to be released.

You can use large, fresh tomatoes (3 to 4) or Roma tomatoes (6 to 8) to make this sauce. Peel the tomatoes only if the skins are tough; this isn't usually necessary with Roma tomatoes. When tomatoes are not in season, substitute a 28 ounce (796 mL) can of tomatoes, and reduce the amount of water to ½ cup (125 mL).

> 2 teaspoons (10 mL) extra virgin olive oil
> 1 small onion, chopped, about ½ cup (125 mL)
> 1 to 2 garlic cloves, minced
> 3½ cups (875 mL) chopped peeled tomatoes (see Note)
> 5½ ounce (156 mL) can tomato paste
> 1 tablespoon (15 mL) chopped fresh basil or 1 teaspoon
>   (5 mL) dried
> ½ teaspoon (2 mL) oregano
> ½ teaspoon (2 mL) sea salt
> 1 bay leaf
> 1 cup (250 mL) water

Heat a large saucepan over medium-low heat. Add the oil, onion, and garlic and cook until the onion is tender. Add the remaining ingredients; bring to a boil, then reduce the heat and simmer, uncovered, for at least 1 hour. Remove the bay leaf. For a smoother sauce, transfer to a blender or food processor. Process with just a few short pulses until the sauce is smooth (do not overprocess). Use in **Tofu and Veggie Lasagna** or **Tofu Cabbage Rolls,** or puree the sauce slightly and use it in **Stuffed Zucchini, Lasagna Roll-Ups,** or in **Pizza Sauce.** Makes about 4 cups (1 L).

Note

To peel and seed the tomatoes, put them in boiling water until the skins start to split, up to a maximum of 1 minute. Remove the tomatoes from the water with a slotted spoon and immerse in cold water to stop the cooking process. When they're cool enough to handle, cut out the cores and then remove the skins; they should come off easily. Cut the tomatoes in half and squeeze them gently to remove most of the seeds.

VARIATION

Pasta Sauce

Add some protein to the sauce—such as tofu, tempeh, chicken, or turkey—and serve over cooked pasta. When sauteing the onion and garlic, just add some crumbled tofu or tempeh or lean ground chicken or turkey breast. Tofu or tempeh should be cooked for about 10 minutes before adding the remaining ingredients; ground chicken or turkey should be cooked until no longer pink, then any fat should be drained off before adding the remaining ingredients.

Tofu Sauce

1 teaspoon (5 mL) extra virgin olive oil
¼ cup (50 mL) chopped onion
1 garlic clove, minced
1 cup (250 mL) mashed firm or medium-firm tofu
¼ teaspoon (1 mL) oregano
½ teaspoon (2 mL) basil
sea salt, to taste

Heat a skillet or saucepan over medium-low heat. Add the oil, onion, and garlic, and sauté until the onion is tender. Add the tofu, oregano, and basil. Cook over medium-low heat for 20 minutes, stirring occasionally and adding a small amount of water, if necessary. Add sea salt, to taste. Use in **Tofu Bean Casserole**, or double the recipe to use in **Tofu and Veggie Lasagna**.

Basil Pesto Sauce

Use small portions of this flavourful sauce on cooked pasta, rice, or vegetables or stir into soups such as **Minestrone**. *It can also be used on pizza or spread over fish fillets before steaming. To freeze, place a tablespoon of* **Basil Pesto Sauce** *into each portion of an ice cube tray; once they're frozen solid, remove and store the cubes in a plastic freezer bag.*

2 cups (500 mL) fresh basil leaves
2 to 3 garlic cloves, minced
¼ cup (50 mL) pine nuts
½ cup (125 mL) freshly grated Parmesan cheese
3 tablespoons (45 mL) extra virgin olive oil
¼ cup (50 mL) water
½ teaspoon (2 mL) sea salt

Place all the ingredients in a blender. Process until smooth, stopping to scrape down the sides, if necessary. Makes about 1 cup (250 mL).

VARIATION
Parsley Pesto Sauce
If fresh basil is unavailable, use 2 cups (500 mL) fresh parsley, stems removed, plus 2 tablespoons (30 mL) dried basil.

SOUPS

Most of the soup recipes call for stock or water. You can use either **Vegetable Stock** or **Chicken Stock**—these are easy to make and will give the soup much more flavour than if you use water. Stock can be made in advance and frozen for later use. Freeze in 2 cup (500 mL) portions to defrost as needed, or freeze in ice cube trays, then store the cubes in plastic freezer bags to use when stir-frying or sauteing.

Vegetable Stock

10 cups (2.5 L) water
1 large onion, quartered
1 leek, white part only, washed and chopped
2 medium tomatoes, quartered
1 head green leaf or butter lettuce, washed and torn
3 celery stalks with leaves, chopped
2 carrots, chopped
1 bay leaf
1 sprig fresh thyme or ½ teaspoon (2 mL) dried
6 to 8 sprigs fresh parsley, chopped
sea salt, to taste

Combine all the ingredients in a large pot and bring to a boil. Reduce the heat to low and simmer, partially covered, for 1 hour. Strain the stock, and refrigerate for up to 3 days or freeze for later use. Makes about 10 cups (2.5 L).

Chicken Stock

3 to 4 pound (1.5 to 2 kg) chicken or chicken parts (backs,
    wings, necks, etc.)
12 cups (3 L) cold water
2 celery stalks with leaves, chopped
2 carrots, chopped
1 onion, chopped
1 leek, white part only, washed and chopped
1 garlic clove, halved
4 sprigs fresh thyme or 1 teaspoon (5 mL) dried
4 sprigs fresh parsley
1 bay leaf
1 teaspoon (5 mL) sea salt

Place the chicken in a large pot with the water. Bring just to a
simmer over medium heat and cover partially. Do not boil or
stir; this will give a clearer stock. Skim off any foam that rises to
the top. Add more water to replace any liquid that may have
been removed when skimming the foam. Reduce the heat and
add the remaining ingredients. Simmer, partially covered, for 3
to 4 hours.

Remove the pot from the heat and remove the chicken pieces;
set aside. Strain the stock, then cover and refrigerate it until a
layer of fat forms on the top. Remove the fat by carefully
scooping it off with a spoon, by dragging a clean paper towel
over top of it, or by placing a large piece of wax paper on the
fat; the fat will stick to the paper towel or wax paper. The stock
may be refrigerated for up to 3 days or it can be frozen for later
use. Freeze some of the stock in ice cube trays and store the
cubes in a plastic bag in the freezer; use for sauteing and stir-
frying. Recipe makes 10 to 12 cups (2.5 to 3 L) stock.

Remove the meat from the chicken bones. Use the meat on
pizza, in sandwiches, in soups (such as **Chicken Rice Soup**), or
in recipes that call for cooked chicken (such as **Chicken Salad,
Chicken Vegetable Hash**, and **Chicken and Veggie Pesto Wraps**).

VARIATION
Turkey Stock
Substitute the leftover carcass of a roast turkey for the chicken.

Cabbage Soup

8 cups (2 L) **Vegetable Stock** or water
half a small head of cabbage, chopped, approximately
    4 cups (1 L)
2 onions, diced
2 garlic cloves, minced
4 celery stalks, sliced
2 carrots, sliced
2 cups (500 mL) chopped green beans
1 leek, white part only, washed and sliced
5½ ounce (156 mL) can tomato paste
28 ounce (796 mL) can tomatoes, chopped
1 teaspoon (5 mL) basil
2 teaspoons (10 mL) oregano
½ teaspoon (2 mL) kelp powder
2 tablespoons (30 mL) chopped fresh parsley (optional)
1 tomato, chopped (optional)
sea salt, to taste

Combine all the ingredients, except the sea salt, in a large pot
and bring to a boil. Reduce the heat, cover, and simmer until the
vegetables are tender. Season to taste with sea salt. Makes 8 to
10 servings.

Creamy Broccoli Soup

2 cups (500 mL) **Chicken Stock, Vegetable Stock,** or water
1 small onion, chopped
1 garlic clove, minced
1 carrot, sliced
1 celery stalk, sliced
1 tablespoon (15 mL) chopped fresh parsley (optional)
4 cups (1 L) chopped broccoli
1 cup (250 mL) low-fat milk, soy milk, or rice milk
sea salt, to taste
grated reduced-fat Cheddar cheese (optional)

Combine the stock or water, onion, garlic, carrot, celery, and
parsley in a large saucepan. Bring to a boil, then reduce the heat
to medium-low. Cover and cook for 10 minutes, stirring
occasionally. Add the broccoli and stir well. Continue cooking,
stirring occasionally, for 10 to 15 minutes, or until the vegetables
are tender. Puree the soup, in batches, in a blender or food
processor until smooth. Return the soup to the saucepan and
stir in the milk (For a thicker soup, use less milk or omit it
altogether, if you wish.) Cook over medium-low heat just until
heated through; add sea salt. Optional: add a small amount of
grated reduced-fat Cheddar cheese just before serving. Makes
4 servings.

Linda's Lentil Spinach Soup

1 tablespoon (15 mL) extra virgin olive oil
2 onions, chopped
3 garlic cloves, chopped
1½ cups (375 mL) red lentils
7 cups (1.75 L) **Chicken Stock, Vegetable Stock,** or water
1 to 3 teaspoons (5 to 15 mL) chili powder, to taste
1 to 3 teaspoons (5 to 15 mL) ground cumin, to taste
½ to 1 teaspoon (2 to 5 mL) cinnamon, to taste
5½ ounce (156 mL) can tomato paste
1 bunch fresh spinach, washed, stems removed, and torn,
    about 8 cups (2 L)
a few sprigs of fresh parsley, chopped
sea salt, to taste

Heat a large saucepan over medium-low heat. Add the oil, onion, and garlic, and sauté until the onion is tender. Add the lentils, stock or water, chili powder, cumin, and cinnamon. Bring to a boil, then reduce the heat to low. Cover and simmer until the lentils are tender, about 40 minutes. Add the tomato paste, spinach, and parsley, and simmer for 10 minutes more. Season to taste with sea salt. Makes 8 to 10 servings.

Note
Leftover tomato paste can be frozen for later use. Put 1 tablespoon (15 mL) tomato paste into each section of an ice cube tray, cover, and place in the freezer. Once they're frozen, transfer the cubes to a plastic freezer bag and seal. Use the cubes to flavour soups (like this recipe and **Turkey Barley Soup**) and other dishes (such as **Tofu Chili** and **Pizza Sauce**).

Turkey Barley Soup

When buying ground turkey (or chicken), make sure it's ground from skinless breast to ensure it's low in fat.

2 teaspoons (10 mL) extra virgin olive oil
1 small onion, chopped
1 garlic clove, minced
2 celery stalks, diced
2 carrots, diced
1 pound (500 g) lean ground turkey breast
5 cups (1.25 L) **Chicken Stock, Vegetable Stock,** or water
½ cup (125 mL) pot barley
19 ounce (540 mL) can tomatoes, chopped
3 tablespoons (45 mL) tomato paste
1 bay leaf
½ teaspoon (2 mL) celery seed
½ teaspoon (2 mL) sea salt

Heat a skillet over medium-low heat. Add the oil, onion, garlic, celery, and carrots, and cook for 5 minutes. Transfer the cooked vegetables to a large soup pot and return the skillet to the heat. Add the ground turkey to the skillet and cook until it's no longer pink, breaking it up with a fork. Drain off any fat, then add the turkey to the soup pot. Add the stock or water, barley, tomatoes, tomato paste, bay leaf, and celery seed to the pot. Bring to a boil, then reduce the heat to low. Cover and simmer for about 1 hour, until the barley is cooked. Remove the bay leaf and add the sea salt. Makes about 8 servings.

VARIATION
Chicken Barley Soup
Substitute lean ground chicken breast for the ground turkey.

Minestrone

2 teaspoons (10 mL) extra virgin olive oil
1 small onion, chopped
2 garlic cloves, minced
½ cup (125 mL) diced celery
½ cup (125 mL) diced carrots
1 cup (250 mL) chopped peeled tomatoes
4 cups (1 L) **Chicken Stock**, **Vegetable Stock**, or water
½ cup (125 mL) diced zucchini
½ teaspoon (2 mL) basil
½ teaspoon (2 mL) oregano
3 tablespoons (45 mL) chopped fresh parsley
½ cup (125 mL) uncooked short whole-grain pasta
1 cup (250 mL) cooked kidney beans (red or white)
3 cups (750 mL) fresh spinach leaves, washed, stems
    removed, and torn
sea salt, to taste
freshly grated Parmesan cheese (optional)
Pesto Sauce (optional)

Heat a large saucepan over medium-low heat. Add the oil,
onion, garlic, celery, and carrots, and sauté until the onion is
tender. Add the tomatoes, stock or water, zucchini, basil,
oregano, and parsley, and bring to a boil. Reduce the heat to
low, add the pasta, and cook for 5 minutes. Add the beans and
spinach and cook 5 minutes more, or until the spinach is
softened. Season to taste with sea salt. Top each serving with
freshly grated Parmesan cheese and/or a dollop of **Basil Pesto
Sauce** or **Parsley Pesto Sauce**, if desired. Makes 6 servings.

Chicken Rice Soup

2 teaspoons (10 mL) extra virgin olive oil
1 leek, white part only, washed and chopped, or 1 small
   onion, chopped
1 carrot, chopped
1 celery stalk, chopped
4 cups (1 L) **Chicken Stock** or **Vegetable Stock**
⅓ cup (75 mL) uncooked brown rice
½ teaspoon (2 mL) EACH basil, thyme, and marjoram
⅛ teaspoon (0.5 mL) ground sage
1 bay leaf
1½ cups (375 mL) chopped cooked chicken
¼ cup (50 mL) chopped fresh parsley
sea salt, to taste

Heat a large saucepan over medium-low heat. Add the oil, leek
or onion, carrot, and celery, and sauté until the onion is tender,
about 5 minutes. Add the stock, rice, herbs, and bay leaf. Bring
to a boil, then reduce the heat to low. Cover and simmer for 30
minutes. Add the chicken and simmer for another 10 minutes,
or until the rice is done. Remove the bay leaf, add the parsley,
and season to taste with the sea salt. Makes 4 servings.

Note
For a quicker version, omit the uncooked rice and simmer the
stock and seasonings for 10 minutes instead of 30 minutes. Add
1 cup (250 mL) cooked rice or ½ cup (125 mL) uncooked pasta,
when adding the chicken.

Miso Soup

This soup is very quick and easy to make. The amounts of miso, tofu, green onion, and ginger can be adjusted according to taste. Wakame seaweed can be found in the dried form in health food stores. It contains calcium, B vitamins, and minerals, and it adds a nice flavour to this soup. Wakame expands quite a bit, so cut it into very small pieces. Firm tofu can be substituted for soft or silken tofu.

4 inch (10 cm) piece of wakame seaweed (optional)
4 cups (1 L) water
4 tablespoons (60 mL) miso
½ cup (125 mL) finely cubed silken or soft tofu
2 green onions, sliced
½ teaspoon (2 mL) finely minced or grated fresh ginger
  (optional)

Cut the seaweed into small pieces using scissors. In a medium saucepan, combine the seaweed and water. Bring to a boil, then reduce the heat to low. Remove ½ cup (125 mL) of the water from the saucepan and combine with the miso in a small bowl; mix with a fork until the miso is dissolved. Pour the miso mixture back into the saucepan and add the tofu, green onion, and ginger, if using. Simmer for a few minutes until heated through, but do not boil. Makes 4 servings.

VARIATION
Miso Vegetable Soup
When the water comes to a boil, add ½ cup (125 mL) EACH sliced snow peas, and finely sliced bok choy and carrots. Reduce the heat to medium, and simmer for about 5 minutes or until the vegetables are just tender. Add the remaining ingredients, as described above.

Bean and Tomato Soup

2 teaspoons (10 mL) extra virgin olive oil
1 onion, chopped
1 garlic clove, minced
1 celery stalk, chopped
1 teaspoon (5 mL) ground cumin
½ teaspoon (2 mL) ground coriander
2 cups (500 mL) **Chicken Stock**, **Vegetable Stock**, or water
3 cups (750 mL) chopped peeled tomatoes, or a 28 ounce
    (796 mL) can
1½ cups (375 mL) cooked red kidney beans, or a 14 ounce
    (398 mL) can
1½ cups (375 mL) cooked pinto beans or white kidney beans,
    or a 14 ounce (398 mL) can
4 cups (1 L) fresh spinach leaves, washed, stems removed,
    and torn
1 tablespoon (15 mL) fresh lemon juice (optional)
½ teaspoon (2 mL) sea salt

Heat a saucepan over medium-low heat. Add the oil, onion,
garlic, celery, cumin, and coriander, and sauté until the onion is
tender. Add the stock or water and the tomatoes. Bring to a boil,
then reduce the heat to low. Cover, and simmer for 15 minutes.
Add the beans, spinach, and lemon juice, if using, and simmer
for 5 minutes more. Add the sea salt. Makes 6 servings.

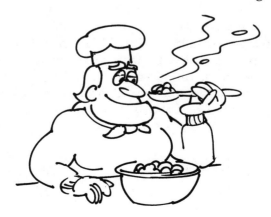

Creamy Vegetable Soup

2 teaspoons (10 mL) extra virgin olive oil
1 onion, chopped
1 garlic clove, minced
1 carrot, chopped
1 celery stalk, chopped
2 cups (500 mL) **Chicken Stock, Vegetable Stock,** or water
1 cup (250 mL) cauliflower florets
1 cup (250 mL) chopped tomatoes
2 tablespoons (30 mL) chopped fresh parsley, divided
½ teaspoon (2 mL) oregano
½ teaspoon (2 mL) ground cumin
¼ teaspoon (1 mL) thyme
2 cups (500 mL) packed fresh spinach leaves, washed, stems
     removed, and torn
1 cup (250 mL) soft or silken tofu
½ teaspoon (2 mL) sea salt

Heat a large saucepan over medium-low heat. Add the oil,
onion, garlic, carrot, and celery; sauté until the onion is tender,
about 5 minutes. Add the stock or water, cauliflower, tomatoes,
1 tablespoon (15 mL) of the parsley, oregano, cumin, and thyme.
Bring to a boil, then reduce the heat to low. Cover and simmer
for 20 minutes. Add the spinach and continue simmering until
the vegetables are tender, about 5 to 10 minutes. Puree the soup,
in batches, in a blender or food processor until smooth. Return
the soup to the saucepan. Puree the tofu until smooth, then stir
slowly into the soup. Heat through, then add the sea salt.
Garnish with the remaining 1 tablespoon (15 mL) parsley.
Makes 4 servings.

Tomato Soup

When tomatoes aren't in season, use three 14 ounce (398 mL) cans of good plum tomatoes.

2 teaspoons (10 mL) extra virgin olive oil
1 small onion, chopped
1 garlic clove, minced
1 celery stalk, chopped
1 carrot, chopped
6 medium tomatoes, peeled, seeded, and chopped, about
   5 cups (1.25 L) (see Note)
1 tablespoon (15 mL) chopped fresh basil
1 tablespoon (15 mL) chopped fresh parsley
1 bay leaf
1 cup (250 mL) **Chicken Stock, Vegetable Stock**, or water
¼ teaspoon (1 mL) sea salt

Heat a large saucepan over medium-low heat. Add the oil, onion, garlic, celery, and carrot, and sauté until the onion is tender, about 5 minutes. Add the tomatoes, basil, parsley, bay leaf, and stock or water. Bring to a boil, then reduce the heat to low. Cover and simmer for 20 to 30 minutes, or until the carrots are tender. Remove the bay leaf and add the sea salt. Use a blender to puree the soup, in batches, until smooth. Makes about 4 servings.

Note
To peel and seed the tomatoes, put them in boiling water until the skins start to split, up to a maximum of 1 minute. Remove from the water with a slotted spoon and immerse the tomatoes in cold water to stop the cooking process. When they're cool enough to handle, cut out the cores and then remove the skins; they should come off easily. Cut the tomatoes in half and squeeze them gently to remove most of the seeds.

SALADS

Ah, finally the dark, cold days of winter have passed. First, the days grow longer and brighter, and now heat is building up in the air; the warm soil is coming alive with green. It's time to enjoy the occasional fresh salad with its bounty of minerals and vitamins and its natural ability to cool down your body.

Salads that contain raw vegetables, like green salads, **Coleslaw**, and **Greek Salad**, should be eaten in moderation, and in warm weather only. Cooked salads, such as **Bean Salad**, **Potato Salad**, **Salmon Salad**, **Tuna Salad**, **Chicken Salad**, and **Egg Salad**, can be eaten in cool weather. The **Pasta Salad** can also be eaten in cool weather, if you lightly cook the broccoli and cauliflower called for in this recipe; steam them for about 3 minutes, then rinse under cold water to stop the cooking process.

Greek Salad

Dressing
¼ cup (50 mL) extra virgin olive oil
1 tablespoon (15 mL) lemon juice
1 tablespoon (15 mL) apple cider vinegar or red wine vinegar
1 garlic clove, minced
½ teaspoon (2 mL) oregano
¼ teaspoon (1 mL) sea salt

2 large or 3 medium tomatoes
1 cucumber (peeled, unless using long English cucumber)
2 small sweet green and/or red peppers
half a red onion
½ cup (125 mL) crumbled feta cheese
Calamata olives

Combine all the dressing ingredients and mix well. Cover and let stand at room temperature for at least 1 hour before serving the salad, to allow the flavours to blend.

Cut the tomatoes, cucumber, peppers, and red onion into bite-size pieces. Toss gently with the feta and olives in a large glass bowl. Add the dressing just before serving, and toss well. You may not need to use all of the dressing, as the chopped vegetables create a lot of juice. Any leftover dressing can be refrigerated for a few days. Makes 6 to 8 servings.

Potato Salad

1 pound (500 g) small new potatoes, white or red (about 10 to 12 potatoes)
½ cup (125 mL) low-fat plain yogurt (use extra-thick or strained yogurt)
1 teaspoon (5 mL) Dijon mustard
1 teaspoon (5 mL) minced fresh dill
1 teaspoon (5 mL) minced fresh parsley
¼ teaspoon (1 mL) sea salt
1 small celery stalk, diced
3 radishes, diced
3 green onions, sliced

Cut the potatoes in quarters and boil them until just tender, but not mushy. Drain and rinse under cold water; drain well and set aside.

While the potatoes are cooking, combine the yogurt, mustard, dill, parsley, and sea salt; set aside.

Combine the potatoes, yogurt mixture, celery, radishes, and green onions. Mix gently and refrigerate for at least 1 hour before serving. Makes 4 to 6 servings.

Note
Add chopped hard-boiled egg, if desired.

Bean Salad

1½ cups (375 mL) fresh green beans, cut into 1 inch (2.5 cm)
    pieces
1½ cups (375 mL) fresh wax beans, cut into 1 inch (2.5 cm)
    pieces
2 cups (500 mL) cooked red kidney beans, or a 19 ounce (540
    mL) can, rinsed and drained
2 cups (500 mL) cooked chickpeas, or 19 ounce (540 mL) can,
    rinsed and drained
¾ cup (175 mL) diced red onion
1 small sweet green pepper, diced
1 celery stalk, diced

Dressing
¼ cup (50 mL) apple cider vinegar
¼ cup (50 mL) fresh lemon juice
⅓ cup (75 mL) canola oil
1 teaspoon (5 mL) Dijon mustard
1 tablespoon (15 mL) chopped fresh parsley
1 garlic clove, minced
½ teaspoon (2 mL) oregano
½ teaspoon (2 mL) basil
½ teaspoon (2 mL) celery seed
½ teaspoon (2 mL) sea salt

Blanch the green beans and the wax beans in boiling water for 4
minutes. Rinse thoroughly in cold water to stop the cooking
process. Drain well and place in a large bowl; add the kidney
beans, chickpeas, red onion, green pepper, and celery.

For the dressing, combine all the dressing ingredients and
pour over the bean mixture; mix well. Cover and refrigerate for
several hours or overnight, stirring occasionally. Makes about
10 servings.

Pasta Salad

Dressing
⅓ cup (75 mL) extra virgin olive oil
2 tablespoons (30 mL) apple cider vinegar
1 tablespoon (15 mL) fresh lemon juice
1 large garlic clove, minced
1 teaspoon (5 mL) basil
¼ teaspoon (1 mL) sea salt

3 cups (875 mL) rotini pasta, uncooked (preferably whole-grain)
½ cup (125 mL) grated carrot
1 cup (250 mL) broccoli florets
1 cup (250 mL) cauliflower florets
1 small sweet red pepper, chopped
1 cup (250 mL) artichoke hearts, drained and chopped
4½ ounce (125 mL) can sliced black olives
½ to 1 cup (125 to 250 mL) crumbled feta cheese
2 tablespoons (30 mL) chopped fresh dill

Mix together all the dressing ingredients and let stand at room temperature for at least 2 hours before serving the salad.

Cook the rotini according to package directions, until just tender. Rinse under cold water and drain well, then toss with a small amount of the dressing to keep it from sticking together. In a large bowl, combine the pasta with the remaining ingredients. Add the dressing just before serving and mix well. Makes 8 to 10 servings.

Note
To add more protein, gently stir in chunks of salmon, cooked chicken, or cubed firm tofu (marinate the tofu in some of the dressing before adding it to the salad).

Coleslaw

Indole-3-carbinol is the most active ingredient of the cruciferous vegetables; it's found in especially high quantities in broccoli, cabbage, and brussels sprouts. Its ability to stimulate the liver enzymes to break down your steroid hormones and eliminate chemicals gives it strong anticancer properties. Cabbage juice also has very strong antiulcer properties.

4 cups (1 L) finely shredded green cabbage
2 cups (500 mL) finely shredded red cabbage
½ cup (125 mL) shredded carrot
½ cup (125 mL) minced red onion or sweet Bermuda onion

Dressing
½ cup (125 mL) canola oil
⅓ cup (75 mL) apple cider vinegar
1 teaspoon (5 mL) Dijon mustard
½ teaspoon (2 mL) celery seed
½ teaspoon (2 mL) sea salt

In a large salad bowl, combine the cabbage, carrot, and onion. Combine all the dressing ingredients and mix well. Pour over the cabbage mixture, stir well, and refrigerate for a few hours before serving, stirring occasionally. Makes 6 to 8 servings.

Cabbage Juice

This recipe requires a juicer. It's important to use only very fresh cabbage and carrots when making this juice.

½ cup (125 mL) cabbage juice (approximately half a small head)
¼ to ½ cup (50 to 125 mL) carrot juice (approximately 2 to 4 carrots)

Combine cabbage and carrot juices, to taste. Serve immediately, and sip slowly.

Sauerkraut Salad

2 cups (500 mL) chopped sauerkraut
¼ cup (50 mL) grated carrot
3 tablespoons (45 mL) finely chopped sweet red pepper
2 to 3 tablespoons (30 to 45 mL) grated or finely chopped red
  or white onion, to taste
¼ teaspoon (1 mL) paprika
sliced green onions (optional)

Place the sauerkraut in a sieve and rinse with cold water to
remove some of the salt; this step is optional as you may wish
to use the sauerkraut as is. Drain off some of the liquid and
place in a large glass bowl. Add the remaining ingredients and
mix well. Makes 4 servings.

MORE SALADS

The following salad recipes use low-fat plain yogurt to replace much of the mayonnaise that's traditionally used in these recipes. Those who cannot eat yogurt can substitute **Tofu Mayonnaise**. These salads can be served with **Pasta Salad** or as sandwich fillings; or in hot weather, these salads can occasionally be served on lettuce leaves as part of a salad plate, with raw and/or steamed veggies.

Salmon Salad

6 ounces (170 g) cooked salmon, about 1 cup (250 mL), or a
7½ ounce (213 g) can, drained
1 tablespoon (15 mL) chopped green onion
2 teaspoons (10 mL) chopped fresh dill or 1 teaspoon (5 mL)
dried
2 teaspoons (10 mL) mayonnaise
1 tablespoon (15 mL) low-fat plain yogurt
1 to 2 teaspoons (5 to 10 mL) lemon juice

Flake the salmon, then add the remaining ingredients and mix well. Use as a sandwich spread on yeast-free whole-grain bread, rye crackers, or tortillas, or stuff into pita bread with broccoli sprouts. Makes 2 servings.

VARIATION
Tuna Salad
Substitute a can of water-packed tuna for the salmon.

Chicken Salad

You can poach 1 whole chicken breast (see recipe for **Poached Chicken Breasts**) *to use in this recipe.*

1 cup (250 mL) diced cooked chicken (approximately 1 whole chicken breast)
1 tablespoon (15 mL) finely chopped celery
1 tablespoon (15 mL) chopped green onion
1 tablespoon (15 mL) minced fresh parsley
2 teaspoons (10 mL) mayonnaise
2 tablespoons (30 mL) low-fat plain yogurt
pinch sea salt

Combine all the ingredients and mix well. Use as a sandwich spread on yeast-free rye bread, stuff into a pita (yeast-free variety, if you have yeast problems), wrap in a warmed whole-wheat tortilla, or use the salad to stuff tomatoes. Makes 2 servings.

VARIATION
Turkey Salad
Substitute turkey for the chicken.

Curried Chicken Salad

1 cup (250 mL) cubed cooked chicken
1 tablespoon (15 mL) finely chopped celery
1 tablespoon (15 mL) chopped green onion
1 tablespoon (15 mL) minced fresh cilantro
2 teaspoons (10 mL) mayonnaise
2 tablespoons (30 mL) low-fat plain yogurt
¼ to ½ teaspoon (1 to 2 mL) curry powder, to taste
pinch ground cumin
pinch sea salt

Combine all the ingredients and mix well. Use as a sandwich spread. Makes 2 servings.

Egg Salad

4 hard-boiled eggs
1 tablespoon (15 mL) finely chopped celery
1 tablespoon (15 mL) chopped green onion
2 teaspoons (10 mL) mayonnaise
3 to 4 teaspoons (15 to 20 mL) low-fat plain yogurt
½ teaspoon (2 mL) Dijon mustard
sea salt, to taste

Peel and mash the eggs. Add the remaining ingredients and mix well. Use as a sandwich spread. Makes 2 to 3 servings.

Note
Optional: discard 2 of the yolks to reduce the fat content of this recipe.

SANDWICHES AND WRAPS

Sandwiches

Here's a list of suggestions for sandwich fillings; serve on yeast-free rye or whole-grain bread. Add sliced tomatoes and/or sprouts (try broccoli sprouts), if desired. For smaller appetites, or for those wishing to reduce the amount of bread they eat, serve open-face on 1 slice of bread. Many of these sandwich fillings can also be served in pita bread (if you don't have yeast problems), or rolled up in whole-wheat tortillas.

Fillings (Those in **bold type** indicate recipes included in this book.)
- **Hummus**
- **Tofu Spread**
- **Yogurt Cheese and Herb Spread; Quark and Herb Spread**
- **Salmon Salad; Tuna Salad**
- **Chicken Salad; Turkey Salad**
- **Curried Chicken Salad**
- **Egg Salad**
- Slices of **Marinated Tofu**
- Sliced cooked chicken or turkey breast (not the processed kind!), with a small amount of mayo mixed with yogurt

Wraps

Wraps make a nice change from sandwiches. To assemble the wraps, place the listed ingredients in the middle of a whole-wheat tortilla, fold one end over the filling, then fold both sides over and wrap tightly. The amount of each ingredient will depend on personal taste and on the number of servings you wish to make. If you're taking the wrap for lunch at work, package the tortilla separately from the filling ingredients, and assemble the wrap just before eating.

If possible, use whole-wheat tortillas that aren't made with yeast or hydrogenated oils; be sure to read labels. Or make your own, using the **Tortillas** *recipe. To warm the tortillas, wrap them tightly in foil and place in a 350 F (180 C) oven for 10 to 15 minutes.*

Black Bean and Rice Wraps

In a small baking dish, mix together basmati rice (preferably brown basmati), black beans, ground cumin, and lime juice. Cover and place in the oven for 15 minutes with the tortilla(s). Place the rice/bean mixture on the tortilla(s) and add diced tomato, chopped green and/or red onion, minced fresh cilantro, mild salsa, and low-fat plain yogurt. Additional toppings include cooked chicken, sliced avocado, and grated reduced-fat cheese (such as Cheddar and/or Monterey Jack) or soy cheese.

Chili and Feta Wraps

Wrap up warmed **Tofu Chili** (or **Turkey Chili** or **Tempeh Chili**), feta or goat cheese, diced tomato, and brown rice.

Chicken and Veggie Pesto Wraps

Sauté sliced chicken breast plus some sweet green and/or red pepper until the chicken is no longer pink inside; add torn, fresh spinach, cover, and continue cooking until the spinach is wilted (about 2 minutes). Combine with brown rice and a small amount of **Basil Pesto Sauce** or **Parsley Pesto Sauce** in a whole-wheat tortilla.

Chicken Souvlaki Wraps

Wrap up **Chicken Kebabs** (remove the skewer!), **Tzatziki**, diced tomato, and any of the following optional toppings: feta cheese or goat cheese, diced onion, steamed or sauteed greens (such as spinach or kale).

Roast Vegetable Wraps

Follow the recipe for **Roast Vegetables** using eggplant instead of the carrots, the rutabaga, and the potatoes (see VARIATION). Combine the **Roast Vegetables** with feta cheese or goat cheese, **Tzatziki**, and steamed or sauteed greens (optional).

FISH

Salmon and Spinach Casserole

Salmon is one of the many fish that are high in EPA, which helps inhibit many chronic diseases by making eicosanoids of the 3 Family. EPA also inhibits eicosanoids made from arachidonic acid. Fish also contain DHA, which aids memory.

    1 cup (250 mL) short whole-grain pasta, such as small shells
        or rotini
    6 ounces (170 g) cooked salmon, about 1 cup (250 mL), or a
        7½ ounce (213 g) can, drained
    half a bunch fresh spinach, washed, steamed, well drained,
        and chopped
    2 tablespoons (30 mL) finely minced red onion
    ¼ teaspoon (1 mL) sea salt
    ½ cup (125 mL) rice milk
    2 teaspoons (10 mL) cornstarch or arrowroot powder
    ¼ teaspoon (1 mL) dry mustard powder
    1 garlic clove, finely minced

Cook the pasta according to the package directions, but undercook it slightly. Drain and rinse under cold water; drain again and set aside.

In a large bowl, flake the salmon. Add the pasta, spinach, red onion, and sea salt; set aside.

In a small saucepan, whisk together the rice milk, cornstarch or arrowroot powder, dry mustard powder, and garlic. Bring the mixture just to a boil, stirring constantly. Remove from the heat and add to the pasta/salmon mixture. Mix gently, then press into a small, lightly buttered baking dish. Cover and bake at 350 F (180 C) for about 20 minutes, until hot. Makes 2 to 3 servings.

Broiled Salmon Steaks

2 tablespoons (30 mL) lemon juice
1 tablespoon (15 mL) Tamari soy sauce
1 teaspoon (5 mL) minced or grated fresh ginger
1 garlic clove, minced
2 salmon steaks

Mix together the lemon juice, soy sauce, ginger, and garlic. Pour over the salmon steaks and marinate in the refrigerator for 20 minutes, turning the steaks over after 10 minutes.

Place the salmon on a lightly buttered broiler pan. Measure steaks at their thickest portion, and broil for 10 minutes per inch (2.5 cm) of thickness, or until the salmon flakes easily when tested with a fork. Turn the steaks over halfway through the cooking time, basting with the marinade. Good hot or cold. Makes 2 servings.

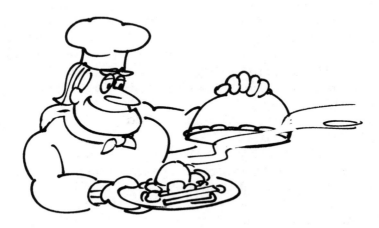

Salmon Cakes

6 ounces (170 g) cooked salmon, about 1 cup (250 mL), or a
    7½ ounce (213 g) can, drained
1 egg
3 tablespoons (45 mL) fine dried whole-grain bread crumbs
1 tablespoon (15 mL) minced green onion
1 tablespoon (15 mL) minced red onion
1 tablespoon (15 mL) minced sweet red pepper
1 tablespoon (15 mL) minced fresh parsley
1 tablespoon (15 mL) minced fresh dill or 1 teaspoon (5 mL)
    dried
1 teaspoon (5 mL) lemon juice
¼ teaspoon (1 mL) sea salt
1 teaspoon (5 mL) extra virgin olive oil

Combine all the ingredients except the oil, and mix well. On a
plate, shape the mixture into 4 small or 2 large patties, about ½
inch (1 cm) thick.

Heat a skillet over medium-low heat. Add the oil, then add
the patties (use a lifter as they will be quite moist). Cook for 3 to
4 minutes per side, or until lightly browned. Alternatively, place
the salmon cakes on a lightly buttered baking sheet and broil
for 3 to 4 minutes per side. Good served with lemon juice and
low-fat plain yogurt, or with **Yogurt Herb Dip** (made with dill).
Makes 2 to 4 servings.

VARIATION
Tuna Cakes
Substitute a can of water-packed tuna for the salmon.

Salmon Loaf

6 ounces (170 g) cooked salmon, about 1 cup (250 mL), or a
7½ ounce (213 g) can, drained
1 cup (250 mL) cooked brown rice
½ cup (125 mL) grated low-fat cheese or soy cheese
2 tablespoons (30 mL) chopped green onion
2 tablespoons (30 mL) chopped celery
1 egg
¼ cup (50 mL) chopped fresh parsley
1 tablespoon (15 mL) minced fresh dill or 1 teaspoon (5 mL)
dried
¼ teaspoon (1 mL) sea salt

Flake the salmon, then add the remaining ingredients and mix
well. Press into a lightly buttered small loaf pan and bake at 350
F (180 C) for 25 to 30 minutes, or until firm. This tastes good
served with **Yogurt Herb Dip** or with low-fat plain yogurt.
Serve hot or cold. Makes 2 to 4 servings.

VARIATION
Tuna Loaf
Substitute a can of water-packed tuna for the salmon.

Tuna Casserole

Try using pasta made from spelt, quinoa, kamut, soy, or whole-wheat flour.

¾ cup (175 mL) short whole-grain pasta, such as macaroni or
  rotini
2 cups (500 mL) broccoli florets
6½ ounce (184 g) can water-packed tuna, drained
3 tablespoons (45 mL) sliced green onion
¼ cup (50 mL) finely chopped celery
½ cup (125 mL) low-fat plain yogurt
2 tablespoons (30 mL) mayonnaise
1 teaspoon (5 mL) lemon juice
1 tablespoon (15 mL) chopped fresh parsley
¼ teaspoon (1 mL) thyme
¼ teaspoon (1 mL) sea salt
1 tomato, sliced
½ cup (125 mL) grated reduced-fat cheese (optional)

Cook the pasta according to the package directions, but
undercook it slightly; add the broccoli during the last 2 minutes
of cooking time. Drain and rinse under cold water; drain again
and set aside.

In a large bowl, flake the tuna. Add the green onion, celery,
yogurt, mayonnaise, lemon juice, parsley, thyme, and sea salt;
mix well. Gently stir in the pasta and broccoli. Spoon the
mixture into a lightly buttered baking dish, arrange the tomato
slices on top, and sprinkle with the cheese, if using. Cover and
bake at 350 F (180 C) for 30 minutes, until hot. Makes 2 large or
4 small servings.

Poached Fish Fillets

Poaching is a quick, low-fat method for cooking chicken as well as fish. Other vegetables—such as onion, celery, tomato, sweet green pepper— and herbs such as thyme, bay leaf, etc., can be substituted or added to the poaching liquid.

    2 firm fish fillets, about 4 ounces (125 g) each
    water
    juice of half a lemon
    1 garlic clove, cut in half
    1 carrot, chopped
    2 sprigs fresh parsley
    1 sprig fresh dill or fennel

Fill a deep skillet or wok with enough water to cover the fish (but don't add the fish yet). Add the lemon juice, garlic, carrot, parsley, and dill or fennel; bring just to a boil. Reduce the heat to a very gentle simmer, and using a slotted spatula, add the fish. Cover and cook for 5 to 10 minutes, until the fish flakes easily when tested with a fork. Carefully remove the fillets with a slotted spatula and drain before serving. Discard the poaching liquid and other ingredients. Makes 2 servings.

Baked Fish with Black Bean Sauce

2 fish fillets, about 4 ounces (125 g) each (use snapper, cod, halibut, sole, etc.)
¼ cup (50 mL) water
1 garlic clove, minced
2 teaspoons (10 mL) minced fresh ginger
2 tablespoons (30 mL) Chinese salted black beans, rinsed, drained, and chopped
1 tablespoon (15 mL) Tamari soy sauce
2 green onions, sliced
½ to 1 teaspoon (2 to 5 mL) sesame oil, to taste (optional)

Place the fish in a baking dish and set aside.

Heat a small saucepan or skillet over medium heat. Add 1 to 2 tablespoons (15 to 30 mL) of the water, plus the garlic, ginger, and black beans; sauté until fragrant, about 1 minute. Add the remaining water and the soy sauce, reduce the heat, and simmer for 3 minutes. Spread the sauce over the fish fillets, then sprinkle the green onions over top. Bake at 425 F (210 C) for 7 to 10 minutes or until the fish flakes easily when tested with a fork. Drizzle with sesame oil, if using, and serve. Makes 2 servings.

VARIATIONS
Baked Tofu with Black Bean Sauce
Substitute half a 12 ounce (350 g) package of firm tofu for the fish fillets. Cut the tofu into ½ inch (1 cm) slices and arrange in a single layer in a baking dish.

Baked Tempeh with Black Bean Sauce
Substitute an 8 ounce (250 g) package of tempeh for the fish fillets. Cut the tempeh in half, crosswise, then into ½ inch (1 cm) slices lengthwise; arrange in a single layer in a baking dish.

Stir-Fry Tofu and Veggies in Black Bean Sauce
Substitute half a 12 ounce (350 g) package of firm tofu for the fish fillets. Cut the tofu into ½ inch (1 cm) cubes and set aside. Heat a wok or skillet over medium-high heat. Sauté the garlic,

ginger, and black beans in the water as instructed above. Add the remaining water and the soy sauce, plus 2 thinly sliced small carrots, 1 cup trimmed snow peas, and 1 small bunch broccoli, cut into bite-size pieces. Cover and cook for 2 minutes, stirring occasionally and adding more water to prevent sticking, if necessary. Remove the cover and add the cubed tofu and green onion. Gently stir-fry for 3 minutes, or until the vegetables are tender-crisp. Drizzle with sesame oil, if using, before serving.

Breaded Fish Fillets

½ cup (125 mL) **Oat and Whole-Grain Coating** (see
  following recipe) or ½ cup (125 mL) fine whole-wheat
  bread crumbs
1 tablespoon (15 mL) freshly grated Parmesan cheese, rice
  cheese, or soy cheese (optional)
1 tablespoon (15 mL) minced fresh parsley
¼ teaspoon (1 mL) basil
1 teaspoon (5 mL) finely grated lemon rind
pinch sea salt
1 egg
¼ cup (50 mL) low-fat plain yogurt
4 skinless, boneless fish fillets, about 4 ounces (125 g) each
  (use any type of white fish)

Combine the **Oat and Whole-Grain Coating** or bread crumbs
with the cheese, parsley, basil, lemon rind, and sea salt in a
shallow dish or pie plate. In a separate dish, beat together the
egg and yogurt. Dip each fillet into the yogurt mixture, then
into the bread crumb mixture. Place the coated fillets in a lightly
buttered baking dish. Bake at 425 F (210 C) for 8 to 10 minutes,
or until the fish flakes easily when tested with a fork. Makes 4
servings.

Oat and Whole-Grain Coating

⅓ cup (75 mL) oats
⅔ cup (150 mL) fresh whole-grain bread crumbs (use whole-
  wheat bread, rye bread, etc.)
1 teaspoon (5 mL) dry mustard powder

In an ungreased skillet, cook the oats, stirring frequently, over
medium-low heat for 5 to 10 minutes, until lightly toasted. Set
aside to cool.

Combine the oats, bread crumbs, and mustard powder. Use
in **Breaded Fish Fillets** or **Breaded Chicken Breasts**. The
Coating can be stored in the refrigerator in a tightly closed jar
for about 1 week.

Note
To make the bread crumbs, finely chop or grate (by hand or in a food processor) 1 slice of bread.

Baked Halibut and Vegetables

You can substitute other types of fish (snapper, cod, etc.) for the halibut and/or you can use fillets instead of steaks. Just remember to cook the fish for approximately 10 minutes per inch (2.5 cm) of thickness (measure the thickest portion of the fish), adding the vegetables and seasoning during the last 5 minutes.

1 pound (500 g) halibut steaks
water or stock
1 small zucchini, cut into ¼ inch (6 mm) slices
1 tomato, chopped
1 cup (250 mL) snow peas, trimmed
2 green onions, chopped
½ teaspoon (2 mL) basil or 2 teaspoons (10 mL) minced fresh
   dill
¼ teaspoon (1 mL) sea salt

Place the fish in a single layer in a baking dish. Add just enough water or stock to cover the bottom of the dish, about ¼ cup (50 mL). Cover and bake at 450 F (230 C) for 5 minutes. Remove from the oven and arrange the zucchini, tomato, snow peas, and green onion around the fish. Sprinkle with the basil or dill and sea salt. Cover and bake for 5 to 10 minutes more, or until the fish flakes easily when tested with a fork. Makes 4 servings.

Fish Roll-Ups

You can use any type of white fish in this recipe. Choose long, thin fillets suitable for rolling.

4 boneless sole fillets, about 4 ounces (125 g) each
2 teaspoons (10 mL) lemon juice
2 teaspoons (10 mL) extra virgin olive oil
¼ cup (50 mL) diced onion
¼ cup (50 mL) diced celery
half a bunch fresh spinach, washed, steamed, well drained,
    and chopped
½ cup (125 mL) cooked brown rice
¼ cup (50 mL) low-fat plain yogurt
¼ teaspoon (1 mL) sea salt

Sprinkle ½ teaspoon (2 mL) of the lemon juice along the length of each fillet and set the fillets aside.

Heat a small saucepan over medium-low heat. Add the oil, onion, and celery and sauté until tender. Add the spinach and cook for 2 minutes more to remove any excess moisture. Remove from the heat and add the rice, yogurt, and sea salt. Spoon an equal amount of the mixture onto each fillet; roll up and secure with toothpicks. Place the fillets in a lightly buttered baking dish. Cover and bake at 375 F (190 C) for about 15 minutes, or until the fish flakes easily when tested with a fork. Serve plain or with lemon wedges and/or **Yogurt Herb Dip** (made with dill). Makes 4 servings.

Note
The roll-ups can be steamed instead of baked in the oven; see **Steamed Fish Fillets** for instructions.

Fish Fillets in Foil

4 fish fillets, about 4 ounces (125 g) each
2 teaspoons (10 mL) **Tofu Mayonnaise** or canola oil-based
   mayonnaise
1½ teaspoon (7 mL) chopped fresh dill or ½ teaspoon (2 mL)
   dried
1 tablespoon (15 mL) chopped fresh parsley
¼ teaspoon (1 mL) sea salt
8 thin slices of onion
8 thin slices of lemon or lime

Place each fillet on a piece of lightly buttered heavy aluminum
foil. Spread each fillet with ½ teaspoon (2 mL) of mayonnaise,
then sprinkle with the dill, parsley, and sea salt. Place 2 onion
slices and 2 lemon slices on top of each fillet. Fold the foil and
seal it tightly—use a double fold so the juices cannot escape.
Place the foil packets on a baking sheet and bake at 375 F (190
C) for 15 to 20 minutes, until the fish flakes easily when tested
with a fork. Alternatively, cook over medium heat on the
barbeque, turning the foil packets a few times during cooking.
Serve with fresh lemon and/or **Yogurt Herb Dip**. Makes 4
servings.

Steamed Fish Fillets

Steaming is a quick, low-fat method for cooking fish and chicken, as well as vegetables. If you don't have a folding metal steaming rack, you can use one of the following: a bamboo steamer, a pasta pot with an accompanying perforated steaming basket, or an electric steamer. Or you can make your own steamer by placing a cooling or roasting rack inside a wok, roasting pan, or electric frying pan; just make sure that whatever container you use has a tight-fitting lid.

To steam fish, set a folding metal steaming rack into a large saucepan so that the rack is fully open. Add about 1 inch (2.5 cm) of water to the saucepan. The water shouldn't touch the fish; add enough water to keep the saucepan from boiling dry. Place each fish fillet (use any type of fish) on a piece of aluminum foil or parchment paper. You can add herbs to the water or you can sprinkle them directly onto the fish. Bring the water in the saucepan to a boil, then place each piece of foil or parchment paper (with the fish) into the steaming rack. Cover with a tight-fitting lid and steam for about 5 minutes (depending on the thickness of the fillet) or until the fish flakes easily when tested with a fork.

VARIATIONS
Steamed Fish with Pesto
Spread a thin layer of **Basil Pesto Sauce** or **Parsley Pesto Sauce** over the fish fillets before steaming.

Steamed Fish with Black Bean Sauce
Follow the recipe for **Baked Fish with Black Bean Sauce**, except steam the fish instead of baking it.

Steamed Fish with Ginger and Soy Sauce
Follow the recipe for **Broiled Salmon Steaks**, substituting salmon fillets for the steaks; steam the salmon instead of baking.

Steamed Fish Roll-Ups
Follow the recipe for **Fish Roll-Ups**, except steam the roll-ups instead of baking them.

MEATLESS MAIN DISHES

Tofu Patties

Tofu is made from soybeans and is called bean curd by some people. It's easily digested, compared to many legumes. Tofu is high in isoflavonoids and therefore has anticancer properties.

1 cup (250 mL) well-drained and mashed firm tofu
1 cup (250 mL) cooked brown rice
2 tablespoons (30 mL) flour
½ cup (125 mL) grated carrot
1 garlic clove, minced
¼ teaspoon (1 mL) sea salt
1 tablespoon (15 mL) Tamari soy sauce
½ teaspoon (2 mL) basil
½ cup (125 mL) grated reduced-fat Cheddar cheese or soy
    cheese (optional)

In a large bowl, mix together all the ingredients. Using your hands, shape the mixture into 4 patties and place them on a lightly buttered baking sheet. Bake at 350 F (180 C) for 15 minutes. Gently turn the patties over and bake for 10 to 15 minutes more, until lightly browned. Makes 2 to 4 servings.

VARIATION
Curried Tofu Patties
Omit the soy sauce, basil, and cheese. Add 1 teaspoon (5 mL) minced fresh ginger and 1 teaspoon (5 mL) curry powder. If the mixture is too dry to form patties, add 1 to 2 tablespoons (15 to 30 mL) water.

Tofu and Veggie Lasagna

This version of lasagna is lower in fat than traditional lasagna recipes—it uses less cheese, and tofu replaces the cottage cheese and ground beef.

1 batch **Tomato Sauce**
2 batches **Tofu Sauce** or 2 cups (500 mL) well-drained and
　　mashed firm tofu
8 lasagna noodles, preferably whole-grain
1 bunch fresh spinach, washed, steamed, well drained, and
　　chopped
2 tablespoons (30 mL) chopped fresh parsley
½ cup (125 mL) freshly grated Parmesan cheese, soy cheese,
　　or rice cheese, divided
1 medium zucchini, cut into ¼ inch (6 mm) slices
1 cup (250 mL) grated reduced-fat Mozzarella cheese

Make the **Tomato Sauce** and the **Tofu Sauce**, if using, then set them aside.

Cook the lasagna noodles until just tender. Do not overcook; it's better to slightly undercook the noodles. Drain and rinse under cold water to stop the cooking process; drain again and set aside.

In a large bowl, combine the **Tofu Sauce** or tofu, spinach, parsley, and ¼ cup (50 mL) of the cheese; mix well and set aside.

Spread ½ cup (125 mL) **Tomato Sauce** on the bottom of a 9 x 13 inch (23 x 33 cm) baking dish. Top with 4 lasagna noodles, ½ the tofu mixture, ½ the sliced zucchini, ½ the Mozzarella cheese, and ½ the remaining **Tomato Sauce**. Repeat the layers and sprinkle the remaining cheese on top. Bake at 325 F (160 C) for 40 to 45 minutes, until hot and bubbly. Remove from the oven and let stand for 10 minutes before serving. Makes 6 to 8 servings.

Notes
- Half-a-pound (250 g) lean ground turkey or chicken breast can be added to the **Tomato Sauce** recipe when sauteing the onion and garlic. Drain off any fat before adding the remaining ingredients.
- For those who don't have yeast problems, add 1 cup (250 mL) sliced fresh mushrooms to the **Tomato Sauce** recipe.
- Replace half or all of the zucchini with sliced eggplant.
- Replace the Parmesan cheese that goes on the top with ¼ cup (50 mL) grated reduced-fat Cheddar cheese.
- For those who are sensitive to dairy products, replace the Parmesan and Mozzarella cheeses with soy cheese and/or rice cheese.

VARIATION
Quick Tofu and Veggie Lasagna
Shorten the preparation time by using any combination of the following.
- A good quality tomato sauce instead of the **Tomato Sauce** recipe
- Well-drained and mashed firm tofu instead of the **Tofu Sauce** recipe
- A 10 ounce (300 g) package of frozen spinach, thawed and well drained, instead of the fresh spinach
- Fresh or "no-cook" lasagna noodles instead of the dried variety. When using "no-cook" noodles, adjust the cooking time and add extra water, if called for on the package.

Scrambled Tofu

1 to 2 teaspoons (5 to 10 mL) extra virgin olive oil
¼ cup (50 mL) chopped onion
¼ cup (50 mL) chopped sweet green or red pepper
1 cup (250 mL) well-drained and mashed firm tofu
¼ teaspoon (1 mL) turmeric
½ teaspoon (2 mL) oregano
1 small tomato, diced
sea salt, to taste

Heat a skillet over medium-low heat. Add the oil, onion, and pepper, and sauté until tender. Add the tofu, turmeric, and oregano, and cook for about 5 minutes, or until any extra moisture evaporates. Add the tomato and cook for 2 minutes more. Season to taste with sea salt. Serve with rye toast or rolled up in warmed whole-wheat tortillas. Makes 2 servings.

Tofu Bean Casserole

This is a good recipe for using up any leftover cooked brown rice and/or beans. Use whatever type of beans you have on hand. You can also substitute whatever type of cheese you prefer for the feta, such as soy cheese, rice cheese, or Cheddar.

1 batch **Tofu Sauce**
1 to 1½ cups (250 to 375 mL) cooked beans (Romano, pinto, black beans, etc.)
1 cup (250 mL) cooked brown rice (preferably basmati)
½ cup (125 mL) crumbled feta cheese or goat cheese
half a bunch fresh spinach, washed, steamed, well drained, and chopped
6 canned artichoke hearts, halved (optional)
1 teaspoon (5 mL) Tamari soy sauce
1 tomato, sliced
¼ cup (50 mL) freshly grated Parmesan cheese, soy cheese, or rice cheese (optional)

In a large bowl, combine all the ingredients except the tomatoes and Parmesan cheese; mix well. Press into a lightly buttered casserole. Arrange the tomato slices on top and sprinkle with the cheese, if using. Cover and bake at 350 F (180 C) for 20 to 30 minutes, until heated through. Makes 2 to 4 servings.

Tofu and Veggie Stir-Fry

Stir-frying is usually done over high heat. To reduce the risk of toxic fats, this recipe (like all others that involve sauteing or stir-frying in this book) uses a lower temperature to cook the food. **Chicken Stock,** **Vegetable Stock,** *or water can be used in place of the oil—in which case a slightly higher temperature can be used.*

The following vegetables and amounts are suggestions only. You can use fewer varieties of vegetables than those called for here. Feel free to use others, such as zucchini, celery, onion, cabbage, green beans, asparagus, sweet green pepper, tomato, daikon radish, or spinach and other leafy greens. Just remember that the harder, firmer vegetables should be cooked longer than the softer vegetables. Be sure to have all of the vegetables chopped and ready before you start to cook.

1 tablespoon (15 mL) cornstarch or arrowroot powder
1 tablespoon (15 mL) Tamari soy sauce
2 teaspoons (10 mL) rice vinegar
1½ cups (375 mL) well-drained and cubed firm tofu

Sauce
¼ cup (50 mL) water
1 tablespoon (15 mL) Tamari soy sauce
2 teaspoons (10 mL) cornstarch or arrowroot powder
¼ to ½ teaspoon (1 to 2 mL) sesame oil (optional)

2 teaspoons (10 mL) extra virgin olive oil
½ cup (125 mL) sliced carrots
¾ cup (175 mL) broccoli florets
¾ cup (175 mL) cauliflower florets
¼ cup (50 mL) **Chicken Stock, Vegetable Stock,** or water
1 garlic clove, minced
1 to 2 teaspoons (5 to 10 mL) minced fresh ginger
½ cup (125 mL) snow peas, trimmed
¾ cup (175 mL) bok choy stalks
1 cup (250 mL) bok choy leaves, chopped
½ cup (125 mL) bean sprouts
1 green onion, chopped

In a small bowl, mix together the cornstarch or arrowroot powder, soy sauce, and rice vinegar. Add the tofu and mix well, to coat. Marinate in the refrigerator for 1 hour.

Combine all the sauce ingredients and set aside.

Heat a large skillet or wok over medium-low heat. Add the olive oil, carrots, broccoli, and cauliflower; stir-fry for 1 minute. Add the stock or water, cover, and cook for 1 minute more. Add the garlic, ginger, snow peas, and bok choy stalks; stir-fry for 2 minutes. Small amounts of stock or water may be used at any time to prevent sticking. Add the bok choy leaves, bean sprouts, green onion and tofu; stir-fry for 2 minutes more. Stir the sauce, then pour into the skillet; stir-fry until the sauce thickens. Serve over brown rice, barley, pasta, or bean thread (vermicelli noodles made from beans). Makes 2 to 3 servings.

VARIATIONS

Stir-Fry with Black Bean Sauce
Omit the sauce. When adding the garlic and ginger to the wok, also add 1 tablespoon (15 mL) Chinese salted black beans that have been rinsed, drained, and chopped.

Tempeh and Veggie Stir-Fry
Substitute an 8 ounce (250 g) package of tempeh for the tofu. Use black beans as directed above, if desired.

Chicken and Veggie Stir-Fry
Substitute 1 whole boneless, skinless chicken breast, cut into 1 inch (2.5 cm) pieces, for the tofu. Cook the chicken in the oil first (before adding the carrots and other vegetables), then remove it and set aside. Follow the remaining directions, returning the chicken to the wok just before adding the sauce at the end. Use black beans, if desired.

Tofu Cabbage Rolls

1 large or 2 medium heads green cabbage
1 teaspoon (5 mL) extra virgin olive oil
1 large onion, chopped
2 cups (500 mL) mashed or crumbled firm tofu
2 cups (500 mL) cooked brown rice
1 teaspoon (5 mL) EACH sage, thyme, ground rosemary,
    marjoram, celery seed, and sea salt
2 to 3 cups (500 to 750 mL) tomato sauce (see recipe for
    Tomato Sauce or use canned tomato sauce), or a 28 ounce
    (796 mL) can tomatoes, chopped

Core the cabbage(s) and gently place in a large pot of boiling water. Lower the heat and simmer, removing the leaves as they become soft and pliable (but NOT mushy). This will take about 10 to 15 minutes. You'll need approximately 16 leaves; set them aside to drain well on towels. Remove the cabbage from the water. Set aside a few extra cabbage leaves to place on top of the cabbage rolls. Leftover cabbage can be chopped and used in soups or stir-fries.

Heat a skillet over medium-low heat. Add the oil and onion, and sauté for 2 minutes. Add the tofu and sauté for 5 minutes more. Transfer to a large bowl and add the rice and seasonings; mix well.

Place 2 to 3 spoonfuls of the rice mixture onto each cabbage leaf, depending on the size of the leaf. Roll up from the base, tucking in the sides as you roll. You may need to cut out the centre rib at the base of the leaf to make the cabbage leaf easier to roll. Place the cabbage rolls in a baking dish and pour some tomato sauce or chopped tomatoes over them. Cover the rolls with the extra cabbage leaves; pour the remaining tomato sauce over top. Cover and bake at 350 F (180 C) for about 1 hour. Makes approximately 16 cabbage rolls.

VARIATION
Turkey Cabbage Rolls
Substitute 1 pound (500 g) lean ground turkey (or chicken) breast for the tofu. Cook until the turkey is no longer pink. Drain off any fat before adding the remaining ingredients.

Quick Cabbage "Rolls"

Use this method if you don't have the time to roll the cabbage leaves. Do not boil the cabbage; instead, carefully remove a few of the outer leaves and set them aside (to place on top of the finished casserole). Chop the rest of the cabbage. In a large casserole dish, put a layer of chopped cabbage, then a layer of rice mixture. Continue alternating layers like this until all of the rice mixture is used. Spread some tomato sauce over top. Cover with the reserved cabbage leaves and pour the remaining tomato sauce over top. Cover and bake at 350 F (180 C) for about 1 hour. Makes 6 to 8 servings.

Tofu Chili

If you don't have time to soak and cook the beans, use canned beans; just be sure to rinse and drain them first. Omit the mushrooms if you have yeast problems.

2 teaspoons (10 mL) extra virgin olive oil
1 onion, chopped
2 garlic cloves, minced
1 celery stalk, chopped
half a sweet green pepper, chopped
12 ounce (350 g) package of firm tofu, mashed or crumbled
   (see Note)
3½ cups (875 mL) chopped peeled tomatoes, or a 28 ounce
   (796 mL) can
2 cups (500 mL) cooked red kidney beans, black beans, or
   pinto beans (or a combination)
6 large mushrooms, sliced (optional)
2 tablespoons (30 mL) tomato paste
1 teaspoon (5 mL) oregano
2 to 3 teaspoons (10 to 15 mL) chili powder, to taste
1 teaspoon (5 mL) ground cumin
½ teaspoon (2 mL) celery seed
1 teaspoon (5 mL) sea salt
1 teaspoon (5 mL) vinegar (optional)
chopped fresh cilantro (optional)

Heat a large saucepan over medium-low heat. Add the oil, onion, garlic, celery, and green pepper, and sauté for 2 minutes. Add the tofu and sauté for 5 minutes. Add the remaining ingredients, except the sea salt, vinegar, and cilantro. Bring to a boil, then reduce the heat to low, cover, and simmer for at least 1 hour, stirring occasionally. Add the sea salt and vinegar, if using; taste and adjust the seasonings, if necessary. Sprinkle each serving with chopped fresh cilantro, if desired. Makes 6 to 8 servings.

Note

If you want the tofu to have more of a ground meat texture, freeze it first, then thaw, drain well, and crumble.

VARIATIONS

Tempeh Chili

Substitute an 8 ounce (250 g) package of tempeh for the tofu.

Turkey Chili

Substitute 1 pound (500 g) lean ground turkey or chicken breast for the tofu. Cook until the turkey is no longer pink. Drain off any fat before adding the remaining ingredients.

Stuffed Zucchini

3 medium zucchini, about 7 inches (18 cm long)
2 teaspoons (10 mL) extra virgin olive oil
half a 12 ounce (350 g) package of firm tofu, well drained and
    mashed
1 small onion, diced
1 garlic clove, minced
half a bunch fresh spinach, washed, steamed, well drained,
    and chopped
¼ to ½ cup (50 to 125 mL) freshly grated Parmesan cheese,
    soy cheese, or rice cheese (optional)
2 cups (500 mL) tomato sauce (see recipe for **Tomato Sauce**
    or use canned tomato sauce), divided
½ teaspoon (2 mL) basil
½ teaspoon (2 mL) oregano
¼ teaspoon (1 mL) sea salt
½ cup (125 mL) grated low-fat cheese (optional)

Slice the ends off each zucchini and cut in half lengthwise.
Scoop out the centres, leaving a shell at least ¼ inch (6 mm)
thick. Chop the scooped-out zucchini and set aside. Place the
zucchini shells in boiling water for 2 to 3 minutes, just until they
are slightly tender. Remove from the water and drain on paper
towels.

Heat a skillet over medium-low heat. Add the oil, tofu, onion,
garlic, and chopped zucchini. Cook until the vegetables are
tender. Add the spinach, cheese (if using), 1 cup (250 mL) of the
tomato sauce, and the basil, oregano, and sea salt; mix well.
Spoon some of the mixture into each zucchini shell.

Spread the remaining 1 cup (250 mL) tomato sauce onto the
bottom of shallow baking dish(es). Place the stuffed zucchini
shells on top of the sauce and bake at 350 F (180 C) for 20 to 30
minutes, until heated through. Sprinkle with cheese, if using,
and cook for 5 minutes more. Spoon some tomato sauce from
the baking dish over the stuffed zucchini and serve. Makes 3
large servings or 6 small servings.

VARIATIONS
Stuffed Eggplant
Use 1 large eggplant instead of the zucchini. Increase the baking time to 35 to 45 minutes, or until the eggplant is tender.

Stuffed Green Peppers
Use 3 medium sweet green peppers instead of the zucchini. Cut each one in half lengthwise, and remove the seeds and membranes.

Turkey Stuffed Vegetables
Use ½ pound (250 g) lean ground turkey breast instead of the tofu. Drain off any fat after sauteing, if necessary.

Lasagna Roll-Ups

Follow the recipe for **Stuffed Zucchini**, omitting the zucchini. The stuffing mixture can then be rolled up in lasagna noodles. Cook 8 lasagna noodles until *al dente*. Spread an equal amount of the stuffing mixture along the length of each lasagna noodle, leaving the last ¼ section bare; roll up. Spread ½ cup (125 mL) of the tomato sauce on the bottom of a baking dish. Arrange the lasagna roll-ups on top of the sauce and cover with the remaining tomato sauce. Cover and bake at 350 F (180 C) for 20 to 30 minutes, until hot and bubbly. If using the cheese, sprinkle it on top of the roll-ups during the last 5 minutes of baking time. Makes about 4 servings.

Notes
- Follow the recipe for **Stuffed Zucchini**, using only half the zucchini called for in the recipe. Use the leftover stuffing to make half a batch of **Lasagna Roll-Ups** for the next day's lunch or dinner.
- Use ½ pound (250 g) lean ground turkey, instead of tofu.

Marinated Tofu

12 ounce (350 g) package of firm tofu, cut into ½ inch (1 cm)
  slices
¼ cup (50 mL) Tamari soy sauce
1 tablespoon (15 mL) water
1 tablespoon (15 mL) minced or grated fresh ginger
1 garlic clove, minced

Arrange the tofu slices in a single layer in a baking dish.
Combine the soy sauce, water, ginger, and garlic, and pour over
the tofu. Cover and marinate in the refrigerator for 30 minutes
or longer. (If possible, marinate for several hours or overnight;
the longer it marinates, the more flavourful it'll be.) Turn the
slices over at least once while marinating. Cover and bake at
350 F (180 C) for 10 minutes. Turn the tofu slices over and bake,
uncovered, for 10 minutes more. Serve with stir-fried vegetables
and brown rice, or use in sandwiches. Good hot or cold. Makes
2 to 4 servings.

Curried Lentils and Rice

2 teaspoons (10 mL) extra virgin olive oil
1 small onion, diced
1 garlic clove, minced
1 teaspoon (5 mL) minced fresh ginger
½ teaspoon (2 mL) curry powder
¼ teaspoon (1 mL) ground cumin
2 cups (500 mL) **Chicken Stock, Vegetable Stock**, or water
½ cup (125 mL) brown basmati rice, rinsed and drained
½ cup (125 mL) brown lentils, sorted, rinsed, and drained
2 tablespoons (30 mL) chopped fresh cilantro
¼ teaspoon (1 mL) sea salt

Heat a saucepan over medium-low heat. Add the oil, onion, garlic, and ginger, and sauté until the onion is tender. Add the curry powder and cumin and cook for 1 minute more. Add the stock or water, rice, and lentils. Bring to a boil, then reduce the heat to low. Cover and simmer for about 40 minutes, or until the rice and lentils are cooked. Remove from the heat, and stir in the cilantro and sea salt. Makes 4 main-course servings.

VARIATION
Herbed Lentils and Rice
Omit the ginger, curry powder, and cumin and add 1 teaspoon (5 mL) oregano and 1 teaspoon (5 mL) basil. Substitute parsley for the cilantro and add ¼ cup (50 mL) freshly grated Parmesan cheese, soy cheese, or rice cheese when adding the sea salt and parsley.

Steamed Eggs in Spinach "Baskets"

5 cups (1.25 L) packed fresh spinach leaves, washed and
    stems removed
2 eggs
2 tablespoons (30 mL) finely crumbled feta cheese or goat
    cheese
tomato slices (optional)
sea salt, to taste

Place a folding metal steaming rack in a large saucepan and add
water. The water shouldn't touch the food that will be sitting in
the steaming rack, but add enough water so that the saucepan
doesn't boil dry. Place the spinach in the steaming rack, cover
with a tight-fitting lid, and bring to a boil. Steam the spinach
until it just starts to wilt; this takes about 1 to 2 minutes once
the water has come to a boil. Turn off the heat, and remove the
steaming rack from the saucepan.

Inside the steaming rack, separate the spinach into 2 equal
parts, then form it into 2 small "baskets" by creating sides and
bottoms that won't leak. Carefully crack an egg into each
spinach "basket."

Return the saucepan to the heat and bring to a boil again.
Turn the heat down to medium-high, then place the steaming
rack—with the spinach baskets—inside the saucepan. Cover
and steam until the egg whites are almost set, about 3 minutes.
Place 1 tablespoon (15 mL) of the cheese on top of each egg.
Replace the lid and simmer for 1 minute more, or until the egg
whites are set and the cheese is melted. Sprinkle with sea salt, to
taste. Serve on top of tomato slices and/or yeast-free rye toast.
Makes 1 to 2 servings.

Notes
- If you don't have a folding metal steaming rack, see
  Steamed Fish Fillets for options.
- For additional flavour, use **Chicken Stock** or
  Vegetable Stock as a steaming liquid instead of water,
  and/or add garlic to the steaming liquid.

Baked Vegetable Frittata

Feel free to add or substitute other vegetables such as spinach, sweet red pepper, asparagus, leeks, or mushrooms. Other herbs such as basil, dill, or marjoram can be used instead of, or in combination with, the oregano.

2 whole eggs
2 egg whites
¼ cup (50 mL) low-fat milk
½ cup (125 mL) reduced-fat Mozzarella cheese
2 tablespoons (30 mL) diced onion (use green, white, or red onion)
½ teaspoon (2 mL) oregano
¼ teaspoon (1 mL) sea salt
½ cup (125 mL) water
2 cups (500 mL) chopped broccoli
1 teaspoon (5 mL) extra virgin olive oil
1 garlic clove, minced
1 cup (250 mL) chopped zucchini
1 tomato, diced or sliced

Mix together the eggs, egg whites, milk, cheese, green onion (if using), oregano, and sea salt; set aside.

In a skillet, bring the water to a boil. Reduce the heat slightly and add the broccoli; cover and cook for 2 minutes, stirring occasionally. Add the oil, white or red onion (if using), garlic, and zucchini; cook over medium heat for 2 minutes more. Remove from the heat and stir into the egg mixture. Pour the mixture into a lightly buttered 9 inch (23 cm) pie plate and arrange the tomato on top. Bake at 350 F (180 C) for 20 to 25 minutes, or until the eggs are set. Makes 4 servings.

Vegetable Pizza

Feel free to add or substitute other toppings, such as roasted sweet red pepper, roasted garlic, artichokes, onion, zucchini, sun-dried tomatoes, black olives, or grated carrot. Increase protein by adding chopped cooked chicken, cooked lean ground turkey breast, or sauteed tempeh or tofu. If you have yeast problems, omit the mushrooms. Reduced-fat Cheddar cheese can be substituted for some or all of the Mozzarella cheese.

Pizza Dough (see Note)
   2 cups (500 mL) flour, e.g., 1 cup (250 mL) whole-wheat flour
      + 1 cup (250 mL) unbleached flour
   1 teaspoon (5 mL) nonalum baking powder
   ½ teaspoon (2 mL) baking soda
   ¼ teaspoon (1 mL) sea salt
   2 tablespoons (30 mL) extra virgin olive oil
   1 cup (250 mL) low-fat plain yogurt

Pizza Sauce
   7½ ounce (213 mL) can tomato sauce or 1 cup (250 mL) of the
      Tomato Sauce recipe, slightly blended
   2 tablespoons (30 mL) tomato paste
   1 garlic clove, finely minced
   1 teaspoon (5 mL) basil
   1 teaspoon (5 mL) oregano
   (This makes enough for 2 pizzas; leftover sauce can be frozen
      for later use.)

Toppings
   2 cups (500 mL) broccoli florets, cut into small pieces and
      steamed for 2 minutes
   1 small green or red pepper, sliced or chopped
   1 cup (250 mL) sliced mushrooms
   1 tomato, sliced
   1½ cups (375 mL) grated reduced-fat Mozzarella cheese or
      soy cheese

To make the **Pizza Dough,** combine all the dry ingredients in a large bowl. Stir together the yogurt and oil, then add to the dry ingredients. Mix well, then knead the dough on a lightly floured surface. Roll into a ball, cover, and set aside while preparing the sauce and toppings.

To make the **Pizza Sauce,** mix together all the ingredients and set aside.

Have all the topping ingredients ready before rolling out the dough.

Roll out the dough on a lightly floured surface to fit into a lightly buttered 12 inch (30 cm) pizza pan, or press into a lightly buttered baking sheet. Prick the dough with a fork several times. Prebake at 425 F (210 C) for about 7 minutes or until the crust begins to brown. Remove from the oven and spread ½ the **Pizza Sauce** over the crust. Arrange the broccoli, then the green/red pepper, mushrooms, and tomatoes on top. Sprinkle with the cheese, then bake for 8 to 10 minutes, until the cheese is bubbly and the crust is browned. Makes one 12 inch (30 cm) pizza.

Note
The **Pizza Dough** will make a fairly thick crust. If you prefer a thinner crust, roll out the dough to the desired thickness, then use the leftover dough to make another smaller pizza; just use more toppings.

Alternatively, you can make just half of the **Pizza Dough** (the recipe is easily halved) and roll out the dough to make a 10 or 12 inch (25 to 30 cm) pizza crust.

VARIATION
Tortilla Pizzas
Instead of using **Pizza Dough,** use whole-wheat tortillas as pizza crusts. Place the tortillas on baking sheets; broil for about 1 minute on each side (watch carefully to make sure they don't burn). Preheat the oven to 400 F (200 C) while putting the sauce and toppings on the tortillas. Bake for 10 minutes or until the cheese is melted.

Spinach and Feta Cheese Pizza

1 batch **Pizza Dough** and 1 batch **Pizza Sauce** (see recipe for
    Vegetable Pizza)
1 bunch fresh spinach, washed, steamed, well drained, and
    chopped
1 cup (250 mL) crumbled feta cheese
1 tomato, diced
½ cup (125 mL) grated reduced-fat Mozzarella cheese

Prepare **Pizza Dough** and **Pizza Sauce** according to
instructions.

Prebake the **Pizza Dough** at 425 F (210 C) for about 7 minutes
until the crust begins to brown. Spread half the **Pizza Sauce**
over the crust. Arrange the spinach on top of the sauce, then
sprinkle with the feta cheese and tomatoes. Top with the
Mozzarella cheese and bake for 8 to 10 minutes, until the cheese
is bubbly and the crust is browned. Makes 1 pizza.

Bean Dip Burritos

Place some **Tofu Bean Dip**—about ¼ cup (50 mL)—in the middle of an 8 inch (20 cm) whole-wheat tortilla. Top with some diced fresh tomato and any of the optional toppings listed below. Fold one end of the tortilla over the filling, fold both sides over, and roll up tightly. Repeat with additional tortillas, depending on the number of servings you want to make. Place the tortillas seam-side down in a lightly buttered baking dish. Bake at 350 F (180 C) for 10 to 15 minutes, until heated through.

Optional Toppings
 Plain low-fat yogurt
 Mild salsa
 Grated reduced-fat Cheddar or Mozzarella cheese or soy
  cheese
 Diced mild green chilies (fresh or canned)
 Diced white or green onion
 Mashed or sliced avocado
 Chopped sweet green or red pepper
 Steamed chopped vegetables, such as zucchini, broccoli,
  spinach
 Minced fresh cilantro

VARIATION
Chicken Burritos
Substitute sliced cooked chicken breast for the **Tofu Bean Dip**.

Bean Dip Quesadillas

Place an 8 inch (20 cm) whole-wheat tortilla on a baking sheet. Spread some **Tofu Bean Dip**—about ¼ cup (50 mL)—over the entire tortilla. Top with some diced tomato and any other optional toppings listed in the **Bean Dip Burritos** recipe. Place another tortilla on top and press down firmly. Bake at 425 F (210 C) for about 5 minutes, or until the cheese is melted and the top begins to turn brown. Cut into wedges and serve with low-fat plain yogurt and mild salsa. Makes 1 to 2 servings.

VARIATION
Chicken Quesadillas
Substitute sliced cooked chicken breast for the **Tofu Bean Dip**.

POULTRY

Turkey Burgers

1 pound (500 g) lean ground turkey breast
2 tablespoons (30 mL) oats
1 egg white
2 tablespoons (30 mL) freshly grated Parmesan cheese, soy
   cheese, or rice cheese (optional)
1 green onion, finely chopped
1 small garlic clove, minced
½ teaspoon (2 mL) basil
½ teaspoon (2 mL) oregano
¼ teaspoon (1 mL) sea salt

In a large bowl, combine all the ingredients and mix well. Shape
the mixture into 4 patties and place on a lightly buttered broiler
pan. Broil for 5 to 7 minutes on each side, until cooked. Serve
with **Tzatziki** or on whole-grain buns with tomatoes, sprouts,
and a small amount of mayonnaise. Makes 4 servings.

VARIATIONS
Turkey Loaf
Add 1 more tablespoon (15 mL) oats, plus ¼ cup (50 mL)
packed grated carrot, and a 10 ounce (300 g) package of frozen
chopped spinach, thawed and well drained. Mix well and press
into a lightly buttered loaf pan. Bake at 350 F (180 C) for about
45 minutes, or until no longer pink in the centre. Pour off any
liquid and let stand for a few minutes before serving. Makes
4 servings.

Chicken Burgers
Substitute lean ground chicken breast for the turkey breast.

Poached Chicken Breasts

Chicken Stock, approximately 2 cups (500 mL)
2 teaspoons (10 mL) chopped fresh rosemary
1 garlic clove, quartered
1 whole boneless, skinless chicken breast, cut in half

Fill a deep skillet or wok with just enough **Chicken Stock** to cover the chicken. Add the rosemary and garlic and bring just to a boil. Reduce the heat to a very gentle simmer, and, using tongs or a slotted spatula, add the chicken. Cover and simmer for 12 to 15 minutes, until the chicken is no longer pink inside, turning the chicken over after 6 minutes. Remove the chicken and drain before serving. Discard the poaching liquid and other ingredients. Serve with **Tzatziki** or **Yogurt Herb Dip**. Makes 2 servings.

Notes
- If you don't have **Chicken Stock** on hand, use water instead and add some fresh lemon juice—about 1 tablespoon (15 mL).
- The poached chicken can also be used in sandwiches or in recipes that call for cooked chicken, such as **Chicken Salad, Chicken Rice Soup, Black Bean and Rice Wraps, Chicken and Veggie Pesto Wraps, Chicken Vegetable Hash, Chicken Burritos** and **Chicken Quesadillas**.

Chicken Vegetable Hash

2 teaspoons (10 mL) extra virgin olive oil
½ cup (125 mL) chopped onion
½ cup (125 mL) chopped sweet green and/or red pepper
1 small potato, diced
¼ cup (50 mL) **Chicken Stock, Vegetable Stock,** or water
1 cup (250 mL) cubed cooked chicken (or turkey)
1 tomato, chopped
sea salt, to taste

Heat a large skillet over medium-low heat. Add the oil, onion, and pepper, and sauté until the onion is almost tender. Add the potato and stock or water. Cover and simmer until the potato is tender, about 10 to 15 minutes, stirring occasionally and adding a small amount of water, if necessary. Add the chicken and tomato; sauté for 2 minutes more. Season to taste with sea salt. Serve with poached eggs, if desired. Makes 2 to 3 servings.

Chicken, Broccoli, and Rice Casserole

1 teaspoon (5 mL) extra virgin olive oil
1 whole boneless, skinless chicken breast, cut into 1 inch
    (2.5 cm) pieces
¾ cup (175 mL) rice milk
1 tablespoon (15 mL) cornstarch or arrowroot powder
½ teaspoon (2 mL) curry powder
¼ teaspoon (1 mL) sea salt
1½ cups (375 mL) cooked brown rice (use basmati rice, if you
    have it)
2 cups (500 mL) broccoli florets, cut into bite-size pieces
¼ cup (250 mL) grated reduced-fat Cheddar cheese (optional)

Heat a skillet over medium-low heat. Add the oil and chicken;
sauté for 1 to 2 minutes on each side, adding a small amount of
water to prevent sticking, if necessary. Remove from the heat
and drain off any liquid; set aside.

In a small saucepan, whisk together the rice milk, cornstarch
or arrowroot powder, and curry powder; bring just to a boil,
stirring constantly. Remove from the heat and add the sea salt.

Combine the chicken, sauce, and rice in a small lightly
buttered baking dish. Cover and bake at 350 F (180 C) for 15
minutes. Meanwhile, steam the broccoli for 2 minutes. Once the
casserole has cooked for 15 minutes, remove it from the oven
and gently stir in the steamed broccoli. Top with the cheese, if
using, and bake uncovered for 5 minutes more. Makes
2 servings.

Chicken Kebabs

2 whole boneless, skinless chicken breasts
1 tablespoon (15 mL) extra virgin olive oil
1 tablespoon (15 mL) lemon juice
1 tablespoon (15 mL) apple cider vinegar
1 teaspoon (5 mL) chopped fresh oregano or ½ teaspoon
   (2 mL) dried
1 teaspoon (5 mL) chopped fresh rosemary
1 garlic clove, minced

Cut the chicken into 1 inch (2.5 cm) cubes, place on metal or wooden skewers, and arrange in single layer in a large glass baking dish. Mix the remaining ingredients together and spoon over the chicken. Cover and refrigerate for 1 hour. Place the kebabs on a broiler pan and broil for 3 to 5 minutes. Turn the kebabs over and continue broiling until the chicken is no longer pink inside. Alternatively, cook the kebabs in the baking dish at 350 F (180 C) for 15 to 20 minutes, or until done. Serve with **Tzatziki** or **Yogurt Herb Dip**. Makes 4 servings.

Chicken with Yogurt and Soy Sauce

1 whole boneless, skinless chicken breast, cut in half
½ cup (125 mL) low-fat plain yogurt
1 tablespoon (15 mL) Tamari soy sauce
1 teaspoon (5 mL) Dijon mustard
1 tablespoon (15 mL) chopped fresh parsley

Place the chicken in a baking dish. In a small bowl, combine the yogurt, soy sauce, and mustard; mix well, then spoon over the chicken. Bake uncovered at 350 F (180 C) for 30 to 35 minutes, until the chicken is no longer pink inside. Remove the chicken to a serving plate. Whisk the sauce, then spoon it over the chicken and sprinkle with the parsley. Makes 2 servings.

Chicken Fajitas

8 whole-wheat tortillas
2 teaspoons (10 mL) extra virgin olive oil
1 sweet red pepper and 1 sweet green pepper, cut into thin
     strips
1 red or yellow onion, sliced thin, then cut into halves
2 garlic cloves, minced
½ teaspoon (2 mL) oregano
½ teaspoon (2 mL) ground cumin
pinch cayenne (optional)
2 whole boneless, skinless chicken breasts, cut into thin strips
1 small tomato, chopped
juice of 1 lime
2 tablespoons (30 mL) minced fresh cilantro
¼ teaspoon (1 mL) sea salt

Wrap the tortillas in foil and bake at 300 F (150 C) for 10 to
15 minutes, until warm.

Heat a large skillet over medium-low heat. Add 1 teaspoon
(5 mL) of the oil, plus the peppers, onion, and garlic; sauté for
about 5 minutes, adding water to prevent sticking, if necessary.
Add the oregano, cumin, and cayenne (if using), and sauté for
2 minutes more. Remove the vegetables from the skillet and set
aside. Add the remaining 1 teaspoon (5 mL) of the oil plus the
chicken to the skillet; sauté until the chicken is no longer pink
inside. Drain off any fat. Return the vegetables to the skillet and
add the tomato, lime juice, cilantro, and sea salt. Cook for
2 minutes more.

Place an equal amount of the chicken/vegetable mixture
down the centre of each tortilla. Add optional toppings, if
desired, and roll up the tortillas. Makes 8 fajitas.

Optional Toppings
Chopped tomatoes
Grated reduced-fat cheese
Low-fat plain yogurt
Mild salsa
Sliced or mashed avocado

VARIATION
Vegetarian Fajitas
Omit the chicken and use some **Tofu Bean Dip** as an additional topping, or add sliced tempeh when sauteeing the peppers, onions, and garlic.

Breaded Chicken Breasts

½ cup (125 mL) low-fat plain yogurt
¼ teaspoon (1 mL) sea salt
1 tablespoon (15 mL) minced fresh parsley
1 tablespoon (15 mL) minced fresh herbs (such as basil,
    oregano, thyme, dill, or chives) or 1 teaspoon (5 mL) dried
2 whole chicken breasts, skinned and cut in half
1 cup (250 mL) **Oat and Whole-Grain Coating** (see **Breaded**
    Fish Fillets) or 1 cup fine whole-grain bread crumbs
2 tablespoons (30 mL) freshly grated Parmesan cheese, soy
    cheese, or rice cheese (optional)

Combine the yogurt, sea salt, parsley, and other herbs in a glass bowl and mix well. Add the chicken and toss to coat. Cover and marinate in the refrigerator for 1 hour, if time permits.

On a pie plate, combine the **Oat and Whole-Grain Coating** with the cheese, if using. Coat the chicken with the breading mixture and place on a lightly buttered baking sheet. Bake at 350 F (180 C) for 30 to 35 minutes for boneless, or 40 to 45 minutes for bone-in chicken, until chicken is no longer pink inside. Makes 4 servings.

Chicken Curry

For those with dairy sensitivities, the use of yogurt is optional.

2 teaspoons (10 mL) extra virgin olive oil
2 whole skinless chicken breasts (bone-in), cut into halves
1 large onion, chopped
2 garlic cloves, minced
1 tablespoon (15 mL) minced fresh ginger
1 tablespoon (15 mL) ground cumin
1 tablespoon (15 mL) ground coriander
2 teaspoons (10 mL) turmeric
2 large tomatoes, chopped
¾ cup (175 mL) low-fat plain yogurt (optional)
¼ to ½ teaspoon (1 to 2 mL) garam masala, to taste
½ teaspoon (2 mL) sea salt
chopped fresh cilantro, to taste

Heat a large skillet over medium-low heat. Add the oil and chicken. Sauté for about 5 minutes, until the chicken is lightly browned on both sides, adding a small amount of water to prevent sticking, if necessary. Remove the chicken from the skillet and keep it warm. Add the onion, garlic, and ginger to the skillet. Sauté for about 5 minutes, or until the onion is tender, adding more water, if necessary. Add the cumin, coriander, and turmeric, and sauté for 1 minute. Add the tomatoes and mix well. Return the chicken to the skillet and reduce the heat to low. Cover and simmer for 20 minutes, stirring occasionally. Stir in the yogurt, if using, then cover and simmer for another 5 to 10 minutes, until the chicken is tender and no longer pink inside. Remove from the heat and stir in the garam masala, sea salt, and cilantro. Serve with basmati rice and/or chipatis. Makes 4 servings.

Note
For a smoother sauce, transfer the sauce (in batches, if necessary) to a blender, and process until smooth.

VARIATIONS
Chicken Curry with Spinach
Add 1 to 2 cups (250 to 500 mL) chopped fresh spinach when adding the yogurt. Puree the sauce in a blender, if desired.

Tofu and Chickpea Curry
Omit the chicken and sauté the onion, garlic, and ginger as directed above. Add the cumin, coriander, and turmeric and cook for 1 minute more. Add the tomatoes, then cover and simmer for 5 minutes, stirring often. Stir in the yogurt, if using. (Sauce may be pureed in a blender at this point, then returned to the skillet.) Add a 12 ounce (350 g) package of firm tofu—cut into ½ inch (1 cm cubes)—and 2 cups (500 mL) cooked chickpeas. Cover and simmer 5 minutes more. Remove from the heat and stir in the garam masala, sea salt, and cilantro. Makes 4 to 6 servings.

Chicken with Lemon and Herbs

1 whole skinless chicken breast, cut in half
1 garlic clove, minced
1 teaspoon (5 mL) extra virgin olive oil
1 tablespoon (15 mL) lemon juice
1 tablespoon (15 mL) water
½ teaspoon (2 mL) oregano
½ teaspoon (2 mL) basil
pinch sea salt

Place the chicken in a baking dish. Combine the remaining ingredients and pour over the chicken. Bake uncovered, basting occasionally, at 350 F (180 C) for 30 to 35 minutes for boneless, 40 to 45 minutes for bone-in, or until chicken is no longer pink inside. Makes 2 servings.

VEGETABLES AND SIDE DISHES

All vegetables are high in potassium and therefore have a cooling effect on the body. This can be offset somewhat by cooking and salting them. It's important not to use too many cooling foods, especially in cool weather, or you may weaken your ileocecal valve enough to permit your intestinal bacteria to travel from your large intestine up into your small intestine. The cooking process helps break down the tough fibres of the vegetables and improves the absorption of bioflavonoids, which can be 100 times more powerful free-radical scavengers than vitamin C. Excess cooking, however, can cause a loss of vitamin C and folic acid. Cooking doesn't affect glucosinolates, which are converted by gut bacteria to isothiocyanates.

A quick and easy way to cook many types of vegetables is by steaming them in a steaming rack over boiling water until they're tender-crisp. You can add flavour to the vegetables by adding herbs, ginger, onion, and/or garlic to the steaming water. Instead of butter or margarine, season steamed vegetables with minced fresh herbs and/or a squeeze of fresh lemon juice. Or use **Yogurt Herb Dip**, **Tofu Herb Dip**, **Tzatziki**, or **Tofu Parmesan Sauce**.

Sauteed Greens

Use any combination of greens that you like in this recipe; even some lettuces, such as Romaine, can be used. Some of the sturdier greens, such as collard, mustard, and dandelion greens, may need to be blanched first. To do this, add the greens to a large pot of boiling water, and cook for approximately 3 minutes.

    1 tablespoon (15 mL) extra virgin olive oil
    1 medium shallot or ¼ cup (50 mL) finely chopped onion
    1 to 2 garlic cloves, minced
    2 to 3 teaspoons (10 to 15 mL) minced or grated fresh ginger
    8 to 10 cups (2 to 2.5 L) washed, torn greens with stems
        removed (Choose from swiss chard, spinach, cabbage, bok
        choy, kale, dandelion greens, watercress, broccoli rabe,
        mustard greens, collard greens, or beet greens.)

Chicken Stock, Vegetable Stock, or water
sea salt, to taste
fresh lemon juice, rice vinegar, or soy sauce (optional)

Heat a large skillet or wok over medium-low heat. Add the oil,
shallot or onion, garlic, and ginger, and sauté for about
2 minutes. Add the sturdier greens (cabbage, mustard greens,
kale, collard greens, beet greens, etc.) and toss well. Add a small
amount of water or stock; cover and cook for 2 minutes. Add
the remaining greens (lettuce, spinach, swiss chard, watercress)
and toss well; cover and cook for 3 to 5 minutes more or until
the greens are tender, stirring occasionally and adding more
water or stock, if necessary. Sprinkle with sea salt and lemon
juice, vinegar, or soy sauce, to taste. Makes 4 servings.

Baked Vegetables with Fennel

*Use as much of each vegetable as desired, depending on the number of
servings you wish to make. Add or substitute other vegetables, if you
wish.*

Celery
Carrots
Eggplant
Zucchini
Fennel bulb
Snow peas
Pinch of basil
Water

Cut the celery, carrots, eggplant, zucchini, and fennel bulb into
½ inch (1 cm) pieces and place in a baking dish. Trim the snow
peas and add to the remaining vegetables. Add enough water to
just cover the bottom of the baking dish. Sprinkle with basil.
Cover and bake at 350 F (180 C), stirring occasionally, for
30 minutes, or until the vegetables are tender.

Stir-Fried Vegetables with Yogurt and Cilantro

Use as much of each of the listed ingredients as needed, depending on the number of servings you wish to make. Other greens, such as bok choy, swiss chard, beet greens, collard greens, etc., can be added or substituted for the spinach. If you choose to stir-fry the vegetables using stock or water instead of oil, you can cook them at a higher temperature.

Extra virgin olive oil
Sliced carrots
Cauliflower florets
Minced fresh ginger
Minced garlic
Snow peas
Broccoli florets
Fresh spinach, washed and torn into pieces
Chopped tomato
Chopped fresh cilantro
Low-fat plain yogurt (at room temperature)

Heat a skillet or wok over medium-low heat. Add a small amount of oil and the carrots and cauliflower; stir-fry for 2 minutes, adding water to prevent sticking, if necessary. Add the garlic, ginger, snow peas, and broccoli, and stir-fry for 2 minutes more. Add the spinach and tomatoes; stir until the tomatoes are heated through and the spinach is cooked. Turn the heat down to low, add the cilantro and a few tablespoons of yogurt, and heat through.

Cabbage Casserole

2 teaspoons (10 mL) extra virgin olive oil
1 onion, chopped
1 garlic clove, minced
½ cup (125 mL) **Chicken Stock** or **Vegetable Stock**
2 tablespoons (30 mL) cornstarch or arrowroot powder
19 ounce (540 mL) can tomatoes, chopped
¼ cup (50 mL) chopped fresh parsley
½ teaspoon (2 mL) sea salt
1 medium head green cabbage, chopped
1 carrot, grated

Heat a large skillet over medium-low heat. Add the oil, onion, and garlic, and sauté until the onion is tender. Whisk together the stock and cornstarch or arrowroot powder, and stir into the skillet. Add the tomatoes, parsley, and sea salt and mix well.

Place the cabbage and carrots in a large, lightly buttered casserole. Add the onion/tomato mixture and mix well. Cover and bake at 350 F (180 C) for 1 to 1¼ hours, until tender, stirring every 15 minutes. Makes about 8 servings.

Roast Vegetables

1 teaspoon (5 mL) chopped fresh rosemary
1 teaspoon (5 mL) chopped fresh thyme or ½ teaspoon (2 mL)
    dried
1 tablespoon (15 mL) extra virgin olive oil
¼ teaspoon (1 mL) sea salt
2 carrots, cut into 1 inch (2.5 cm) pieces
½ small rutabaga, cut into 1 inch (2.5 cm) pieces
4 small red or white potatoes, unpeeled and cut in half
1 red onion, cut into 8 wedges
2 garlic cloves, slivered
¼ cup (50 mL) **Chicken Stock, Vegetable Stock,** or water
1 small zucchini, cut into 1 inch (2.5 cm) pieces
1 medium sweet green pepper, cut into 8 wedges

Combine the rosemary, thyme, oil, and sea salt in a roasting pan
or large glass baking dish. Add the carrots, rutabaga, potatoes,
onion, and garlic, and toss well to coat. Add the stock or water.
Cover and bake at 375 F (190 C) for 25 minutes. Remove the
cover and add the zucchini and green pepper. Stir well, adding
a small amount of water, if necessary. Bake uncovered, stirring
occasionally, for 15 to 20 minutes more, until the vegetables are
tender and golden. Makes 4 servings.

VARIATION
Roast Eggplant
Substitute 1 large eggplant, cut into 1 inch (2.5 cm) cubes, for
the carrots, rutabaga, and potatoes. Cook for only 5 minutes
before adding the zucchini and green pepper.

Barley Stew

1 tablespoon (15 mL) extra virgin olive oil
1 small onion, finely chopped
1 garlic clove, minced
1 carrot, grated
1 celery stalk, finely chopped
1 cup (250 mL) pot barley
3 medium tomatoes, peeled and chopped (see Note)
1½ cups (375 mL) **Chicken Stock, Vegetable Stock,** or water
2 tablespoons (30 mL) chopped fresh parsley
¼ teaspoon (1 mL) sea salt

Heat a saucepan over medium-low heat. Add the oil, onion, garlic, carrot, and celery, and sauté until the onion is tender. Rinse the barley, then drain it and add to the saucepan. Cook for 3 minutes, stirring constantly and adding a small amount of stock or water to prevent sticking, if necessary. Add the tomatoes, stock, and parsley. Bring to a boil, then reduce the heat to medium-low. Cover and cook for 40 to 45 minutes, until the liquid is absorbed and the barley is tender. Let sit for 10 minutes, then season with the sea salt. Sprinkle with more chopped fresh parsley before serving, if desired. Makes 6 to 8 servings.

Note

To peel and seed the tomatoes, put them in boiling water until the skins start to split, up to a maximum of 1 minute. Remove the tomatoes from the water with a slotted spoon and immerse in cold water to stop the cooking process. When they're cool enough to handle, cut out the cores and then remove the skins; they should come off easily. Cut the tomatoes in half and squeeze them gently to remove most of the seeds.

Steamed Vegetables with Tofu Parmesan Sauce

The sauce can be used over any steamed vegetables or over rice or pasta.

1 carrot, sliced
¾ cup (175 mL) cauliflower florets
¾ cup (175 mL) broccoli florets
half a small zucchini, cut into ¼ inch (6 mm) slices
¼ cup (50 mL) silken or soft tofu, mashed
2 tablespoons (30 mL) low-fat plain yogurt
2 tablespoons (30 mL) freshly grated Parmesan cheese, soy
    cheese, or rice cheese
pinch sea salt

Steam the vegetables until tender-crisp. (Steam the carrots and cauliflower for about 2 minutes, then add the broccoli and zucchini and steam for 2 minutes more.) Mix together the remaining ingredients and pour over the steamed vegetables. Makes 2 servings.

Note
For a creamier sauce, process the tofu, yogurt, cheese, and sea salt in a blender until smooth.

Broiled Tomatoes

2 large tomatoes
½ cup (125 mL) finely crumbled feta cheese or goat cheese
¼ cup (50 mL) low-fat plain yogurt
1 tablespoon (15 mL) chopped fresh basil or 1 teaspoon
    (5 mL) dried
1 green onion, chopped

Cut the tomatoes in half and scoop out some of the centres. In a small bowl, combine the remaining ingredients; spoon into the tomato halves. Broil for about 5 minutes. Makes 2 to 4 servings.

Cauliflower Curry

1 tablespoon (15 mL) extra virgin olive oil
1 large onion, finely chopped
1 garlic clove, minced
1 teaspoon (5 mL) minced fresh ginger
1 teaspoon (5 mL) curry powder
1 small head cauliflower, cut into bite-size florets
½ cup (125 mL) water
1 cup (250 mL) peas, fresh or frozen
1 teaspoon (5 mL) garam masala
¼ teaspoon (1 mL) sea salt
2 tablespoons (30 mL) chopped fresh cilantro

Heat a large skillet over medium-low heat. Add the oil, onion, garlic, and ginger, and sauté until the onion is tender, about 5 minutes. Add the curry powder; stir well, and sauté for 1 minute. Add the cauliflower and sauté for 2 minutes. Add the water and peas and reduce the heat to low. Cover and cook for 10 to 12 minutes, stirring occasionally, until the cauliflower is tender. Remove from the heat and stir in the garam masala, sea salt, and cilantro. Makes 4 to 6 servings.

QUICK BREADS, MUFFINS, ETC.

Those who wish to lose weight should be mindful of the glycemic index of grains, especially processed grains. The higher the glycemic index number, the faster the starch will be released into your body. Excess sugar will be stored as fat, particularly in the abdominal area. Generally, those who wish to lose weight, or who are having problems with high blood sugar, should use carbohydrates with a glycemic index number of 60 or less.

Use whole-grain flours whenever possible. For those who are sensitive to wheat, a variety of alternate flours can be used, such as barley, rye, oats, rice, soy, millet, bean, etc. Keep in mind, however, that not all of these flours can replace wheat flour on a 1-to-1 ratio; you will need to experiment with different amounts and combinations to find what works best for you. For those who require gluten-free baked goods, try experimenting with soy, bean, rice, or millet flours.

Hearth Bread

1 cup (250 mL) slow-cooking oats
3 cups (750 mL) flour, e.g., 2 cups (500 mL) rye flour + 1 cup
    (250 mL) unbleached flour
2 teaspoons (10 mL) baking soda
1 teaspoon (5 mL) nonalum baking powder
1 teaspoon (5 mL) sea salt
2 tablespoons (30 mL) fructose or molasses (optional)
¼ cup (50 mL) melted butter
1 egg
1½ cups (375 mL) soy milk, buttermilk, low-fat milk, or water

Combine the oats with 1 cup (250 mL) of the milk or water. Mix well and let stand in the refrigerator for 1 hour, or overnight. Mix the dry ingredients together and add to the oat mixture. Mix the wet ingredients together, including the remaining ½ cup (125 mL) of milk or water. Add to the oat/flour mixture, stirring as little as possible. Place in a lightly buttered loaf pan or form into a round shape on a baking sheet. Bake at 375 F (190 C) for 50 to 60 minutes.

Note

If you'd like to use buttermilk, but don't have any on hand, you can make your own. For each cup of buttermilk that you need, place 1 tablespoon (15 mL) lemon juice or vinegar in a measuring cup. Fill the measuring cup with milk to the 1-cup mark. You can make soy buttermilk in the same way, using soy milk instead of cow's milk.

Zucchini Bread

1 cup (250 mL) whole-wheat pastry flour
1 cup (250 mL) unbleached flour
1 cup (250 mL) slow-cooking oats
1 tablespoon (15 mL) nonalum baking powder
1 teaspoon (5 mL) baking soda
1 teaspoon (5 mL) sea salt
1 teaspoon (5 mL) cinnamon
1 teaspoon (5 mL) nutmeg
1 teaspoon (5 mL) powdered ginger
2 eggs
½ cup (125 mL) melted butter
½ cup (125 mL) unsweetened applesauce
¼ cup (50 mL) low-fat milk, soy milk, or rice milk
1½ cups (375 mL) packed grated zucchini
½ cup (125 mL) packed grated carrot

In a bowl, combine the flour, oats, baking powder, baking soda, salt, cinnamon, nutmeg, and ginger. In another large bowl, beat together the eggs and butter. Add the applesauce, milk, zucchini, and carrot, and mix well. Stir into the dry ingredients. Place the batter into 2 buttered 8 x 4 inch (1.5 L) loaf pans. Bake at 350 F (180 C) for 45 to 50 minutes or until a toothpick comes out clean when inserted into the centre. Cool on a wire rack before serving. Makes 2 loaves.

Blueberry Muffins

*Berries are the fruit of the north and are loaded with healthy lignans.
Some can be easily dried for winter use. Cranberries, lingonberries,
and blueberries are the least cooling. Raspberries, strawberries, and
blackberries are a little more cooling. Apples, pears, plums (prunes),
etc., are grown in warmer weather, while peaches, grapes, melons, etc.,
are grown in hotter weather. Oranges, papaya, pineapple, and bananas
are a few of the fruits of the very hot tropics. Eating the fruits in
season in your area is one way to let your kidneys know what climate
you live in so they can help adjust your body's mineral levels to suit
your weather.*

    1 cup (250 mL) slow-cooking oats
    1 cup (250 mL) low-fat buttermilk, soy milk, or rice milk
    3 tablespoons (45 mL) melted butter
    ¼ cup unsweetened applesauce
    2 egg whites
    2 tablespoons (30 mL) molasses
    1 tablespoon (15 mL) finely grated lemon peel (optional)
    1¼ cups (300 mL) whole-wheat pastry flour
    1 tablespoon (15 mL) nonalum baking powder
    ¼ teaspoon (1 mL) sea salt
    1 cup (250 mL) fresh or frozen blueberries

In a large bowl, combine the oats and milk; mix well and let
stand for at least 15 minutes. Add the butter, applesauce, egg
whites, molasses, and lemon peel, if using; mix well. In a
separate bowl, mix together the flour, baking powder, and sea
salt. Pour into the wet ingredients and mix just until moistened.
Gently stir in the berries. Spoon into a lightly buttered or paper-
lined muffin pan. Bake at 375 F (190 C) for 20 to 25 minutes, or
until firm. Place the muffin pan on a wire rack to cool for
10 minutes before removing the muffins. Makes 12 muffins.

Notes
- Substitute other berries such as raspberries,
  blackberries, or cranberries (fresh or dried) for the
  blueberries.

- Whole-wheat pastry flour gives baked goods a lighter texture than regular whole-wheat flour. Whole-wheat pastry flour can be found in some health food stores. If you don't have any, use ¾ cup (175 mL) whole-wheat flour and ½ cup (125 mL) unbleached flour.
- Muffins are best if eaten within 2 days, or they can be frozen for later use.
- If using canned applesauce in this recipe, leftover sauce can be frozen in ¼ cup (50 mL) packages for future batches of muffins, or for use in Zucchini Bread.

VARIATION
Apple Muffins
Omit the lemon peel and add 1½ teaspoon (7 mL) cinnamon to the dry ingredients. Substitute 1 cup (250 mL) of chopped peeled apple for the berries.

Carrot Oat Muffins

1 cup (250 mL) slow-cooking oats
1 cup (250 mL) low-fat buttermilk, soy milk, or rice milk
4½ ounce (128 mL) jar strained prunes (baby food)
½ cup (125 mL) packed grated carrot
3 tablespoons (45 mL) molasses
1 egg white
1¼ cups (300 mL) whole-wheat pastry flour
1 tablespoon (15 mL) nonalum baking powder
1½ teaspoons (7 mL) cinnamon
½ teaspoon (2 mL) nutmeg
½ teaspoon (2 mL) sea salt

In a large bowl, combine the oats and milk; mix well and let stand for at least 15 minutes. Add the prunes, carrot, molasses, and egg white; mix well. In another bowl, combine the flour, baking powder, cinnamon, nutmeg, and sea salt; mix well, then add to the wet ingredients. Mix just until moistened. Spoon into a lightly buttered or paper-lined muffin pan. Bake at 350 F (190 C) for 15 to 18 minutes, or just until a toothpick inserted in the centre of a muffin comes out clean; do not overcook. Place the muffin pan on a wire rack to cool for 10 minutes before removing the muffins. Makes 12 muffins.

VARIATIONS
Zucchini Oat Muffins
Substitute ½ cup (50 mL) packed grated zucchini for the carrot.

Pumpkin Spice Muffins

1 cup (250 mL) slow-cooking oats
¾ cup (175 mL) low-fat buttermilk, soy milk, or rice milk
1 cup (250 mL) mashed cooked pumpkin
3 tablespoons (45 mL) pure maple syrup
3 tablespoons (45 mL) butter, melted
1 egg white
2 cups (500 mL) oat flour
1 tablespoon (15 mL) nonalum baking powder
1 teaspoon (5 mL) cinnamon
½ teaspoon (2 mL) nutmeg
½ teaspoon (2 mL) ground (powdered) ginger
½ teaspoon (2 mL) sea salt

In a large bowl, combine the oats and milk; mix well and let stand for at least 15 minutes. Add the pumpkin, maple syrup, butter, and egg white; mix well. Combine the flour, baking powder, cinnamon, nutmeg, ginger, and sea salt, then add to the other ingredients. Mix just until moistened. Spoon into a lightly buttered or paper-lined muffin pan. Bake at 375 F (190 C) for about 20 minutes, or just until a toothpick inserted in the centre of a muffin comes out clean. Place the muffin pan on a wire rack to cool for 10 minutes before removing the muffins. Makes 12 muffins.

Dill Scones

1 cup (250 mL) flour, e.g., ½ cup (125 mL) whole-wheat flour
+ ½ cup (125 mL) unbleached flour
1 tablespoon (15 mL) nonalum baking powder
¼ teaspoon (1 mL) sea salt
¼ cup (50 mL) soft butter
1 cup (250 mL) slow-cooking oats
3 tablespoons (45 mL) chopped fresh dill or 1 tablespoon
(15 mL) dried
⅔ cup (150 mL) low-fat plain yogurt

Mix together the flour, baking powder, and salt. With a fork,
blend in the butter until the mixture resembles coarse crumbs.
Add the oats and dill; mix well and then stir in the yogurt.
Knead the dough several times on a lightly floured surface,
then shape into a circle about ½ inch (1 cm) thick. Cut into
12 wedges, place on baking sheet, and bake at 425 F (220 C)
for 12 to 15 minutes. Makes 12 scones.

VARIATIONS
Blueberry Scones
Omit the dill and add 1 tablespoon (15 mL) fructose to the flour
mixture. Gently stir ½ cup (125 mL) blueberries (or other
berries) into the mixture, after stirring in the yogurt.

Cheese Scones
Omit the dill and add ¾ cup (175 mL) grated reduced-fat
Cheddar cheese when adding the yogurt (use aged Cheddar, if
you have it).

Oatcakes

Oatcakes are available in some stores, but they are often made with hydrogenated vegetable oil. If you can't find oatcakes in your area, or if you wish to avoid eating hydrogenated oils, use this easy recipe to whip up a batch yourself. Use oatmeal, not oat flakes, available in health food stores and some grocery stores. Alternatively, you can use a coffee grinder to make your own oatmeal; just grind old-fashioned large oat flakes, in batches, until they're the consistency of oatmeal. This takes only about 3 short (1 second) pulses in the coffee grinder— be sure not to grind them too fine.

3 to 4 tablespoons (45 to 60 mL) boiling water
1½ tablespoons (22 mL) butter, softened
1 cup (250 mL) oatmeal (or ground oat flakes)
¼ teaspoon (1 mL) baking powder
¼ teaspoon (1 mL) sea salt

In a cup or small bowl, combine 3 tablespoons (45 mL) of the boiling water with the butter. Stir and let stand until the butter is melted. Meanwhile, combine the oatmeal, baking powder, and sea salt in a large bowl. Add the water/butter mixture and mix well. Add more hot water, a few drops at a time, until you have a stiff dough. Knead the dough, then roll out on a lightly floured surface (use oat flour, if you have it) until very thin, about ⅛ inch (3 mm) thick. Cut the dough into squares or triangles, or use the mouth of a drinking glass to cut the dough into circles. Place on a baking sheet and bake at 350 F (180 C) for about 20 minutes, or until crisp but not brown. Makes 8 to 10 round oatcakes, each about 3 inches (8 cm) in diameter.

Tortillas

½ cup (125 mL) whole-wheat flour
½ cup (125 mL) unbleached flour
¼ teaspoon (1 mL) sea salt
⅓ cup (75 mL) water
1 teaspoon (5 mL) olive oil

Stir together the flour and salt. Add the water and mix well. Knead the dough well, adding extra flour if needed, then divide into 4 equal-size balls. Roll out each ball on a lightly floured surface as thin as possible, about ⅛ inch (3 mm) thick.

Heat a large skillet over medium-high heat. Add ¼ teaspoon (1 mL) of the oil and spread it evenly over the skillet. Add 1 of the tortillas and cook for about 3 minutes per side, until lightly brown. Repeat for remaining tortillas. Use immediately, or cool completely and store in the refrigerator in a tightly sealed plastic bag. Makes 4 tortillas.

Apple Berry Crisp

2 medium apples, sliced
1 tablespoon (15 mL) fresh lemon juice
2 cups (500 mL) blueberries, fresh or frozen
2 cups (500 mL) raspberries, fresh or frozen

Topping
1 cup (250 mL) slow-cooking oats
2 tablespoons (30 mL) flour
1 teaspoon (5 mL) cinnamon
2 tablespoons (30 mL) softened butter

Spread the apple slices in a lightly buttered 9 x 13 inch
(23 x 33 cm) baking dish. Sprinkle the lemon juice over the
apples, then layer the blueberries and raspberries on top. Mix
together the topping ingredients and sprinkle over the
raspberries. Bake at 350 F (180 C) for 25 to 30 minutes, until hot
and bubbly. Makes 6 to 8 servings.

Note
Other fruits such as pears, apricots, and blackberries can be
used.

.

RESEARCH

Reference Articles: Summary of the most important medical health research of the last 100 years

1. Effect of patterns of eating and antacids on faecal urobilinogen excretion

S. L. Malhotra, *Gut*, 9, 1968, pp. 38–41

Chewing food thoroughly may help regulate gallbladder contraction.

2. The bacteria behind ulcers

Martin J. Blaser, *Scientific American*, February 1996, pp. 104–107

In Western cultures, Helicobacter pylori is rare in children but common by 60 years of age. In developing countries, 60 to 70 percent of children have it by age 10, yet 90 percent of people with it never develop any symptoms. It is believed that Helicobacter causes almost all cases of ulcer disease that don't result from medication, and it is usually found in the area of the ulcer.

3. Mechanism of gastric mucosal damage induced by ammonia

Masahiko Tsujii, et al., *Gastroenterology*, 102, 1992, pp. 1881–1888

Ammonia produced by Helicobacter pylori may weaken mitochondrial energy metabolism and weaken mucosal defences.

4. The relationship between Helicobacter pylori and oxygen-derived free radicals in the mechanism of duodenal ulceration

Aws S. Salim, *Internal Medicine*, Vol. 32, No. 5, May 1993, pp. 359–364

Most people over 65 are carriers of Helicobacter pylori, yet they don't develop ulcers. Ulceration likely occurs only after free radicals have damaged the duodenal membrane, allowing penetration by Helicobacter.

5. Effects of flavonoids on parietal cell acid secretion, gastric mucosal prostaglandin production and Helicobacter pylori growth

W. Beil, et al., *Arzneim.-Forsch./Drug Res.* 45 (I), Nr. 6, 1995, pp. 697–700

Flavonoids were tested on Helicobacter pylori bacteria and all inhibited its growth; the strongest was flavone.

6. Gastric analysis in acne rosacea

J. A. Ryle and H. W. Barber, *The Lancet*, December 11, 1920,
pp. 1195–1196

Acne rosacea appears to result from a deficiency of hydrochloric
acid production that may allow fermentation of carbohydrates in the
stomach or small intestine.

7. Vitamin U therapy of peptic ulcer

Garnett Cheney, et al., *Cal. Med.*, Vol. 84, No. 1, January 1956

This study at San Quentin prison with 26 convict ulcer patients had
24 healed in three weeks on cabbage juice, and the other two patients,
with larger ulcers, healed within five weeks.

8. The role of zinc in the development of gastric ulcers in rats

G. Oner, et al., *European Journal of Pharmacology*, 70, 1981,
pp. 241–243

Zinc deficiency was accompanied by a weakening of the stomach
mucosa and many hemorrhages. The stomach was also less able to
make hydrochloric acid due to increased activity of zinc-dependent
carbonic anhydrase enzyme.

9. Indicanuria after gastric surgery

Gerald H. Tomkin and D. G. Weir, *Quarterly Journal of Medicine*,
New Series, XLI, No. 162, April 1972, pp. 191–203

The presence of abnormally high amounts of indican (indoles) in
the urine are directly related to high amounts of bacteria, such as
E. coli, in the upper small intestine.

10. Inhibition of gastric acid secretion reduces zinc absorption in man

G. C. Sturniolo, et al., *Journal of the American College of Nutrition*,
Vol. 10, No. 4, 1991, pp. 372–375

Zinc absorption was reduced after cimetidine administration,
suggesting that gastric pH influences zinc absorption.

11. Normal and abnormal zinc absorption in man and animals: the tryptophan connection

G. W. Evans, *Nutrition Reviews*, Vol. 38, No. 4, April 1980,
pp. 137–141

This review shows that tryptophan is converted by the pancreas to
picolinic acid, which increases zinc absorption. Breast milk contains
15 times the picolinic acid of cow's milk, while the infant formulas
contain almost none.

12. Normal bacterial populations of the intestine and their relation to intestinal function (continued)

Robert M. Donaldson, Jr., *The New England Journal of Medicine*, Vol. 270, No 19, May 7, 1964, pp. 994–1001

Intestinal bacteria can make niacin (vitamin B_3), thiamine (B_1), riboflavin (B_2), pyridoxine (B_6), vitamin B_{12}, folic acid, pantothenic acid, biotin, and vitamin K. Bacteria in the intestine can turn protein into ammonia, which can cause coma if not neutralized by the liver. Bacteria in the small intestine can turn tryptophan into tryptamine, indoles, and indican. Lack of disaccharide enzymes can lead to bacterial fermentation of carbohydrates, which leads to buildup of acids such as lactic, formic, and acetic, which can result in diarrhea.

13. The bacterial content of the small intestine in normal and cirrhotic subjects: relation to methionine toxicity

G. A Martini, et al., Journal unknown, pp. 35–51

In patients with liver disease and in some dyspeptic individuals, free amino acids are completely digested in the small intestine by coliform organisms and converted into ammonia, which can overload a damaged liver. Increased coliform in the ileum may cause increased gas production, which creates intestinal distention.

14. Characterization and quantitation of a zinc-binding ligand in human milk

Gary W. Evans and Phyllis E. Johnson, *Pediatric Research*, 14, 1980, pp. 876–880

The absorption of zinc from human milk is greater than from cow's milk, possibly because picolinic acid in the breast milk improves absorption in the intestine. This is also explained by the fact that children with acrodermatitis (an inherited zinc disorder) improve on breast milk. Digestive enzymes made from pancreas concentrates have also been found to contain picolinic acid.

15. Nutrition, bacteria, and the gut

M. S. Gracey, *Medical Bulletin*, Vol. 37, No. 1, 1981, pp. 71–75

Overgrowth of bacteria in the gut inhibits absorption of carbohydrates, vitamin B_{12}, iron, and water-soluble nutrients such as amino acids and monosaccharides, and also causes diarrhea, lactose intolerance, and anemia. In malnourished children and some others, yeasts, including Candida, may cause clinical disease.

16. Zinc and copper in self-selected diets

Joanne M. Holden, et al., *Journal of the American Dietetic Association*, Vol. 75, July 1979, pp. 23–28

Diets that are adequate in energy and protein may be deficient in zinc and copper.

17. Zinc deficiency, chronic starvation, and hypothalamic-pituitary-thyroid function

J. E. Morley, et al., *The American Journal of Clinical Nutrition*, 33, August 1980, pp. 1767–1770

Zinc deficiency lowers the levels of the active thyroid hormone T_3. It is possible that zinc is necessary for cells to convert T_4 to the more active T_3.

18. Conversion of thyroxine into tri-iodothyronine in zinc deficient rat liver

Shigehiro Fujimoto, et al., *Journal of Pediatric Gastroenterology and Nutrition*, Vol. 5, No. 5, 1986, pp. 799–805

Conversion of T_4 to the more active T_3 hormone in the liver was correlated with the zinc-dependent alcohol dehydrogenase enzyme.

19. Zinc supplementation alters thyroid hormone metabolism in disabled patients with zinc deficiency

Soroku Nishiyama, et al., *Journal of the American College of Nutrition*, Vol. 13, No. 1, 1994, pp. 62–67

Zinc may play a role in thyroid hormone metabolism in patients with low levels of T_3 and may in part contribute to conversion of T_4 to T_3 in humans.

20. Zinc affects the metabolism of thyroid hormones in children with Down's syndrome: normalization of thyroid stimulating hormone and of reversal triiodothyronine plasmic levels by dietary zinc supplementation

Federico Licastro, et al., *Intern. J. Neuroscience*, Vol. 65, 1992, pp. 259–268

Down syndrome children show a mild but important deficiency in zinc, which has been shown to affect the immune system. Down syndrome is also associated with both hyper- and hypothyroidism and antibodies against the thyroid. Abnormal levels of TSH and T_3 hormone are also reported to decrease intellectual functions.

It is speculated that zinc deficiency may inhibit the liver's conversion of T_4 into the more active T_3, and also that low zinc levels may interfere with the binding of T_3 to its receptors. Low levels of zinc may explain many of the thyroid problems seen in Down's syndrome.

21. Hypometabolism in allergy: a review for otolaryngologists

Ben T. Withers, *Laryngoscope*, 84, 1974, pp. 43–52

A highly active person expending 3,500 calories would use a three-foot mound of white powder called ATP. This is enough energy to run 1,500 light bulbs of 100 watts each for 60 seconds. The active thyroid hormone T_3 is necessary to release the energy from ATP. Low T_3 can slow the liver's clearance of cholesterol and the kidney's clearance of uric acid.

22. Discovery of human zinc deficiency and studies in an experimental human model

Ananda S. Prasad, *Am. J. Clin. Nutr.,* 53, 1991, pp. 403–412

Zinc supplementation reduces the enlargement of the liver and spleen in patients with schistosomiasis.

23. The effect of zinc supplementation on pregnancy outcome

Robert L. Goldenberg, et al., *JAMA,* Vol. 274, No. 6, August 9, 1995, pp. 463–468

Zinc is important in many biochemical functions and is highest in seafood, meats, nuts, and milk. Zinc supplementation in early pregnancy increased birth weight.

24. A high-fiber diet does not cause mineral and nutrient deficiencies

Jacob Rattan, et al., *J. Clin. Gastroenterol.,* 3, 1981, pp. 389–393

Diets high in fibre, such as bran, don't prevent absorption of nutrients such as zinc, magnesium, calcium, and iron.

25. Essentiality and toxicity of zinc

Amanda S. Prasad, *Scand. J. Work Environ. Health,* 19 Suppl. 1, 1993, pp. 134–36

Certain factors inhibit the nontoxic antioxidant zinc from being absorbed into the body. They include alcohol, cereals containing organic phosphate compounds, malabsorption disorders, chronic liver and kidney diseases, sickle-cell anemia, and chronic debilitating disorders. Zinc deficiency during growth leads to dwarfism and lack of development of secondary sexual characteristics.

26. Influence of gastric acidity on bacterial and parasitic enteric infections

Ralph A. Giannella, et al., *Annals of Internal Medicine,* 78, 1973, pp. 271–276

Stomach acid can control bacteria that enter the small intestine from the diet, but low stomach acid may lead to proliferation of the bacteria in the small intestine.

27. The human intestinal microflora

Gary L. Simon and Sherwood L. Gorbach, *Digestive Diseases and Sciences,* Vol. 31, No. 9, September 1986 Supplement, pp. 147S–162S

The normal gastrointestinal tract has few bacteria in the stomach and in the small intestine but past the ileocecal valve, the populations rise sharply. There are 1000 times more anaerobic (oxygen-hating) bacteria than aerobic (oxygen-needing). Facultative bacteria (which can live with or without oxygen) moderate the gut environment by using oxygen that would harm anaerobic bacteria. Anaerobic bacteria make short-chain fatty acids and E. coli make colicines, which inhibit other bacteria. Intestinal bacteria play an active role in the breakdown of steroid hormones and this can be dramatically affected by antibiotics.

Slow peristalsis and low hydrochloric acid (worsened by the use of antacids) can allow bacterial overgrowths in the small intestine. Anaerobic bacteria in the small intestine can cause poor fat metabolism, poor absorption of carbohydrate, and poor absorption of vitamins, especially B_{12}. In addition, tryptophan is converted to indoles and indican and disaccharide enzymes are destroyed.

28. Stimulation of IBD-lpmc from inflamed intestine by resident bacterial flora

R. Duchmann, et al., *Gastroenterology*, Vol. 106, No. 4, Part 2, page A674

Bacterial products of the intestinal flora play a direct role in maintaining local inflammation in irritable bowel disease.

29. Spectrum of antibiotic-associated diarrhoea

A. H. Lishman, et al., *Gut*, 22, 1981, pp. 34–37

Clostridium difficile is responsible for diarrhea after antibiotic use, but the range of symptoms indicate that there may be other factors involved.

30. Gut fermentation (or the 'auto-brewery') syndrome: a new clinical test with initial observations and discussion of clinical and biochemical implications

Adrian Hunnisett, et al., *Journal of Nutritional Medicine*, 1, 1990, pp. 33–38

Bacterial and yeast overgrowth in the small intestine can result in fermentation of carbohydrates into alcohol, lactate, acetate, formic acid, and acetaldehyde. Studies of two groups of unwell people showed that over 60 percent were producing alcohol.

31. Gut permeability measured by polyethylene glycol absorption in abnormal gut fermentation as compared with food intolerance

K. K. Eaton, et al., *Journal of the Royal Society of Medicine*, Vol. 88, February 1995, pp. 63–66

A new test has been verified that shows blood alcohol levels rise after carbohydrate administration in people who have abnormal gut fermentation. Gut fermentation normally takes place in the colon where bacteria ferment fibres into short-chain fatty acids. The new test indicates that the bacterial fermentation is taking place in the small intestine and can also cause abnormal gut permeability, food intolerance, abnormal vitamin and mineral absorption, catarrhal, and even psychological symptoms.

32. Effect of oral tetracycline, the microbial flora, and the athymic state on gastrointestinal colonization and infection of BALB/c mice with Candida albicans

Paul B. Helstrom and Edward Balish, *Infection and Immunity,* Vol. 23, No. 3, March 1979, pp. 764–774

A normal intestinal flora protects against Candida albicans, and broad-spectrum antibiotics use can increase levels of intestinal Candida albicans.

33. Candidiasis of the gastrointestinal tract

Ricardo Bolivar and Gerald P. Bodey, *Candidiasis,* pp. 181–201, edited by G. P. Bodey and V. Fainstein, Raven Press, New York © 1985

Candida species are common but the gastrointestinal defence mechanisms are able to keep them under control, unless disrupted. Children entering and leaving hospital were tested and 30 percent cultured positive for yeast on admission, compared to 64 percent after three days of hospitalization.

34. Experimental candidiasis in liver injury

Fumihiko Abe, et al., *Mycopathologia,* 100, 1987, pp. 37–42

This study showed that liver injury promotes Candida yeast infection.

35. Biological and chemical characterization of toxic substances from Candida albicans

Jim E. Cutler, et al., *Infection and Immunity,* Vol. 6, No. 4, October 1972, pp. 616–627

Candida albicans contains at least two different toxic components.

36. Steroid hormone systems found in yeast

Gina Kolata, *Science,* Vol. 25, August 31, 1984, pp. 913–914

Sex steroids and corticosteroids in yeasts may explain their pathogenicity and yield clues to the evolution and function of hormones. Candida yeast have been found to make and to bind a glucocorticoid hormone which may help explain some of their toxicity.

37. Dead fecal yeasts and chronic diarrhea

Michelle Caselli, et al., *Digestion*, 41, 1988, pp. 142–148

Twenty cases of chronic recurrent diarrhea, often with abdominal cramps, were probably caused by dead Candida albicans yeast cells as identified by microscope.

38. Role of enteric microorganisms in malabsorption

Robert M. Donaldson, Jr., *Federation Proceedings*, Vol. 26, No. 5, Sept.–Oct. 1967, pp. 1426–1431

"Normal" bacteria that get into the small intestine can result in malabsorption, particularly of vitamin B_{12} and fats, due to "toxic" bile.

39. Levels of zinc and thymulin in plasma from patients with Crohn's disease

E. Mocchegiani, et al., *J. Clin. Lab. Immunol.*, 32, 1990, pp. 79–84

Crohn's patients showed low levels of zinc and thymulin, the zinc-bound form of thymic hormone. Adding zinc restored thymulin levels.

40. Competition between bacteria and intrinsic factor for vitamin B_{12}: implications for vitamin B_{12} malabsorption in intestinal bacterial overgrowth

R. A. Giannella, et al., *Gastroenterology*, Vol. 62, No. 2, 1972, pp. 255–260

The presence of intrinsic factor protects vitamin B_{12} from being ingested by bacteria in the small intestine, though some bacteria may alter intrinsic factor and bind to B_{12}, thus interfering with its absorption.

41. Lactobacillus acidophilus: natural antibiotics and beyond

Debasis Bagchi and S. K. Dash, *Townsend Letter for Doctors and Patients*, Feb./Mar. 1996, pp. 78–82

Lactobacillus acidophilus is an intestinal bacteria that can produce chemicals that inhibit many other bacteria, including Staphyloccus aureus, Salmonella typhosa, Clostridium perfringens, Shigella dysenteriae, Campylobacter pylori, Helicobacter pylori, Escherichia coli (E. coli), and Candida albicans.

Lactobacillus acidophilus stimulates the synthesis of B vitamins and improves absorption of calcium. Lactobacillus casei stimulates the synthesis of IgA and IgM and it increases activity of T cells and macrophages.

42. Is Crohn's disease caused by antibiotics?

L. Demling, *Hepato-Gastroenterol.*, 41, 1994, pp. 549–551

Crohn's disease has increased dramatically since the 1950s, which is also the same time that antibiotics became normally used in medicine and animal farming. Crohn's disease may be caused by the prolonged use of antibiotics, which alter intestinal flora.

43. Antibody to Saccharomyces cerevisiae (bakers' yeast) in Crohn's disease

Janice Main, et al., *British Medical Journal*, Vol. 297, October 29, 1988, pp. 1105–1106

Patients with Crohn's disease were found to have significantly higher antibody levels (IgG and IgA) to baker's yeast (Saccharomyces cerevisiae) than control patients.

44. Enzymatic and morphometric evidence for Crohn's disease as a diffuse lesion of the gastrointestinal tract

W. T. Dunne, et al., *Gut*, 18, 1977, pp. 290–294

Crohn's disease, a diffuse lesion of the gastrointestinal tract, shows reduction in brush border disaccharidase enzymes but normal dipeptidases, while in ulcerative colitis all enzymes are normal.

45. Abnormalities in the apparently normal bowel mucosa in Crohn's disease

M. J. Goodman, et al., *The Lancet*, February 7, 1976, pp. 275–278

In Crohn's disease, abnormal rectal mucosa is present in unaffected bowel tissue and, even after surgery, Crohn's disease can recur anywhere between the mouth and the anus.

46. The faecal flora of patients with Crohn's disease

F. Wensinck, *Antonie van Leeuwenhoek*, 41, 1975, pp. 214–215

Chronic inflammation of the intestine in patients with Crohn's disease may be due to abnormal flora.

47. Selected bacterial antibodies in Crohn's disease and ulcerative colitis

I. O. Auer, et al., *Scand. J. Gastroenterol.*, 18, 1983, pp. 217–223

The fecal flora of individuals with Crohn's disease contains higher amounts of anaerobic bacteria and a cell-wall-defective organism Pseudomonas maltophilia.

48. Role of glutathione metabolism in the reduction of proteinuria by dimethylthiourea in adriamycin nephrosis

Lawrence S. Milner, et al., *Nephron*, 62, 1992, pp. 192–197

Stimulation of the glutathione peroxidase and transferase enzymes in the kidney resulted in a reduction of protein leaking from the kidneys. This is possibly because the glutathione removes free radical peroxides or inhibits thromboxane A_2 activity.

49. Endotoxaemia in active Crohn's disease. Treatment with whole gut irrigation and 5-aminosalicylic acid

W. Wellmann, et al., *Gut*, 27, 1986, pp. 814–820

This supports the hypothesis that abnormal intestinal flora and a damaged intestinal mucosa allow endotoxins into the portal vein. Large amounts of endotoxin can overload the liver and spill over into the peripheral blood, which can create a number of symptoms, including a decrease in blood (serum) iron.

50. Zuckerarme and faserreiche kost bei morbus Crohn - Summary: Sugar-reduced and fiber-rich diet in Crohn's disease

Von J. F. Riemann and S. Kolb, *Fortschr. Med.* 102. Jg.,1984, Nr. 4, pp. 67–70

Patients with Crohn's disease show a prior history of increased consumption of refined carbohydrates compared to a control group. Therapy with reduced refined carbohydrates and increased fibre has shown some improvement.

51. Increased sugar consumption in Japanese patients with Crohn's disease

Toshiyuki Matsui, et al., *Gastroenterologia Japonica*, Vol. 25, No. 2, 1990, page 271

In developed countries, the rising rate of Crohn's disease has been partly explained by a high intake of carbohydrates, especially refined sugar. This study verifies a similar pattern in Japan.

52. A working hypothesis for the etiology and pathogenesis of nonspecific inflammatory bowel disease

R. G. Shorter, et al., *Digestive Diseases*, Vol. 17, No. 11, November 1972, pp. 1024–1032

Inflammatory bowel disease (ulcerative colitis and Crohn's disease) may result from passage of bacteria from the intestine and recognition of this bacteria by the gut lymphoid tissue, which develops a hypersensitive state and an immune reaction to the bowel wall.

53. Is measles vaccination a risk factor for inflammatory bowel disease?

N. P. Thompson, et al., *The Lancet*, Vol. 345, April 29, 1995, pp. 1071–1074

The rising incidence of Crohn's disease and ulcerative colitis led to a study of people who had received live measles vaccination in 1964. This study showed that this vaccination may have contributed to an increase of these diseases.

54. Measles-mumps-rubella (MMR) vaccine as a potential cause of encephalitis (brain inflammation) in children

Harold E. Buttram, *Townsend Letter for Doctors and Patients,* December 1997, pp. 100–102

Injection of vaccinations bypasses the immune system that guards the mucous membranes, which normally buffers an infection with secretory IgA. This article proposes that autism in children may be a result of immune reactions from the measles-mumps-rubella (MMR) vaccination.

55. A controlled therapeutic trial of various diets in ulcerative colitis

Ralph Wright and S. C. Truelove, *British Medical Journal,* 2, 1965, pp. 138–141

Approximately 20 percent of patients with ulcerative colitis could benefit from a milk-free diet.

56. Ulcerative colitis provoked by milk

S. C. Truelove, *British Medical Journal,* January 21, 1961, pp. 154–160

Milk and protein milk-products, such as cheese, aggravate ulcerative colitis in some patients.

57. Food intolerance and the irritable bowel syndrome

R. Nanda, et al., *Gut,* 30, 1989, pp. 1099–1104

Fifty per cent of referrals to gastroenterologists are for irritable bowel syndrome, and treatment results are notoriously poor for this condition. This study showed improvement with 48 percent of 200 patients after three weeks of exclusion diet.

58. Positive emotional states and enhancement of the immune system

Kathleen M. Dillon, et al., *International J. Psychiatry in Medicine,* Vol. 15 (1), 1985–86, pp. 13–17

This study showed that the IgA levels in saliva (which is known to have antiviral properties) increased after watching a humorous video but soon returned to normal. Watching a nonhumorous video didn't affect the IgA levels.

59. Glutathione is required for intestinal function

Johannes Mårtensson, et al., *Proc. Natl. Acad. Sci. USA,* Vol. 87, March 1990, pp. 1715–1719

Animal studies show that deficiency of intestinal glutathione leads to severe degeneration of intestinal cells, weight loss, and diarrhea.

60. Intestinal uptake and transmembrane transport systems of intact GSH: characteristics and possible biological role

M. T. Vincenzini, et al., *Biochimica et Biophysica Acta*, 1113, 1992, pp. 13–23

Glutathione in the diet is absorbed intact in the upper small intestine and is put to work protecting the intestine from chemically induced injuries and carcinogens.

61. Glutathione, a first line of defense against cadmium toxicity

Rakesh K. Singhal, et al., *FASEB. J.*, 1, 1987, pp. 220–223

Glutathione has the ability to quickly bind to heavy metals like cadmium until the slower metallothionein enzyme becomes activated.

62. Glutathione and GSH-dependent enzymes in the tumorous and nontumorous mucosa of the human colon and rectum

C. P. Siegers, et al., *J. Cancer Res. Clin. Oncol.*, 107, 1984, pp. 238–241

Glutathione content is higher in mucosal stomach and intestine tissue than in the liver, though glutathione enzyme activity was consistently low in stomach cancer.

63. Selectivity of silymarin on the increase of the glutathione content in different tissues of the rat

Alfonso Valenzuela, et al., *Planta Medica*, 55, 1989, pp. 420–422

The flavonoid silymarin, extracted from the seeds of the herb milk thistle, was found to increase the amount of glutathione in the stomach, intestine, and liver, but not in the kidney, spleen, and lungs. About 80 percent of silymarin in the liver is excreted in the bile as conjugates that are split in the intestine by bacteria so that its effects are increased.

64. Untersuchungen zu pharmakodynamik, angriffspunkt und wirkungsmechanismus von silymarin, dem antihepatotoxischen prinzip aus Silybum mar. (L.) Gaertn. Summary: Studies on pharmacodynamics, site, and mechanism of action of silymarin, the antihepatotoxic principle from Silybum marianum (L.) Gaertn

Von G. Vogel, et al., *Arzneim.-Forsch (Drug Res.)*, 25, No. 2, 1975, pp. 179–188

This study showed that silymarin from the herb Silybum marianum protected the liver from Amanita mushroom poisoning if administered before (not after) the poisoning. The protective effect lasted up to 20 hours after taking silymarin. The effects were on the liver cells, but also, the mast cells made less histamine and the blood cells' membranes were made stronger.

65. Effect of the bioflavonoid silymarin on the in vitro activity and expression of superoxide dismutase (SOD) enzyme

Györgyi Müzes, et al., *Acta Physiologica Hungarica*, Vol. 78 (1), 1991, pp. 3–9

Free radicals produced from alcohol breakdown play a role in liver disease of alcohol consumers. The free radicals reacting with cell membranes cause lipid peroxidation and its toxic end-products, such as malondialdehyde, can affect the rest of the body. This study showed that the use of the bioflavonoid silymarin from the herb milk thistle increased the activity of the enzyme superoxide dismutase (SOD), which decreased the free radical formation of hydrogen peroxide.

66. Enhancement of antioxidant and Phase II enzymes by oral feeding of green tea polyphenols in drinking water to SKH-1 hairless mice: possible role in cancer chemoprevention

Sikandar G. Khan, et al., *Cancer Research*, 52, July 15, 1992, pp. 4050–4052

Feeding green tea extract to mice for 30 days showed increased activity of the Phase 2 conjugation enzymes glutathione peroxidase, catalase, and quinone reductase, in the small intestine, liver, and lungs, and increased glutathione transferase in the small intestine and liver.

67. Diarrhea and colitis associated with antimicrobial therapy in man and animals

W. Lance George, et al., *The American Journal of Clinical Nutrition*, 32, January 1979, pp. 251–257

Antibiotic use can lead to mild diarrhea and colitis. Many cases may be a result of an overgrowth of the bacteria Clostridium difficile or possibly other bacteria.

68. Ulcerative colitis: definition, historical background, aetiology, diagnosis, natural history and local complications

F. T. de Dombal, *Postgrad. Med. J.*, 44, September 1968, pp. 684–692

Emotional factors may play a role in prolonging an existing attack of colitis. Damaging changes in the colonic mucosa can be caused by feelings of anxiety or resentment. Ulcerative colitis that spreads to the entire rectal area increases the risk of large bowel cancer.

69. Faecal bile acids, dysplasia, and carcinoma in ulcerative colitis

M. J. Hill, et al., *The Lancet*, July 25, 1987, pp. 185–186

Patients with extensive ulcerative colitis for 10 years or more are at higher risk of colon cancer. These patients have high concentrations of bile acids that may be the cause of cancer. Since diet affects bile acids in animal studies, it might also affect bile acids in humans.

70. Experimental colorectal cancer: the relationship of diet and faecal bile acid concentration to tumour induction

D. J. Galloway, et al., *Br. J. Surg.*, Vol. 73, No. 3, March 1986, pp. 233–237

Current theories to explain the role of diet in cancer of the large intestine implicate the action of the intestinal flora on the food and bile salts, and these bacterial populations can be altered by dietary changes.

71. Metabolic epidemiology of colorectal cancer

Ernest L. Wynder and Bandaru S. Reddy, *Cancer,* Vol. 34, September 1974 Supplement, pp. 801–806

Colon cancer is rare in Japan but there is a higher incidence of it among Japanese immigrants to the US, indicating the large role of diet. Studies have shown a correlation between the intestinal bacteria, bile acids, and cholesterol, and the risk of colon cancer.

72. Effect of diet on human fecal flora comparison of Japanese and American diets

Sydney M. Finegold, et al., *The American Journal of Clinical Nutrition,* 27, December 1974, pp. 1456–1469

Japanese have a low incidence of bowel cancer unless they move to the US and adopt a Western diet high in fat and animal protein. High fat diets result in high fecal concentration of bile acids which may be converted by the intestinal bacteria Clostridium paraputrificum into carcinogens. Since breast cancer incidence is closely related to that of colon cancer, a similar relationship between diet, bowel flora, and breast cancer may occur.

73. Antibacterial activity of the pancreatic fluid

Ethan Rubinstein, et al., *Gastroenterology,* Vol. 88, No. 4, 1985, pp. 927–932

A small protein that has strong antibacterial activity at alkaline pH was found in pancreatic fluid.

74. Adaptation of the exocrine pancreas to diet

P. M. Brannon, *Annu. Rev. Nutr.,* 10, 1990, pp. 85–105

Ninety to 95 percent of the pancreas makes digestive enzymes and 2 to 3 percent makes hormones. The pancreas normally makes and secretes 10 times more digestive enzymes than needed and cholecystokinin is the mediator of protease secretion. The more protein eaten, the more chymotrypsin is secreted.

75. Further studies on the absorption of chymotrypsin

S. Avakian, *Clinical Pharmacology and Therapeutics,* Vol. 5, No. 6, Part I, 1964, pp. 712–715

This study shows that supplementation with the enzyme chymotrypsin results in it being absorbed into the blood without being broken down by other digestive enzymes.

76. Enteropancreatic circulation of digestive enzymes

Charles Liebow and Stephen S. Rothman, *Science,* Vol. 189, August 8, 1975, pp. 472–474

Intact digestive enzyme molecules are absorbed by the intestine and subsequently resecreted by the pancreas.

77. Transport of large breakdown products of dietary protein through the gut wall

W. A. Hemmings and E. W. Williams, *Gut,* 19, 1978, pp. 715–723

Not all protein is completely digested in the gut, and up to half of the protein eaten may be found lodged in cells throughout the body.

78. Cytochrome P450 enzymes and the mixed function oxidase system

Anderson and Kappas, *Annual Review of Nutrition,* 11, 1991, pp. 141–167

P450 enzymes are found throughout the body but especially in the liver. They help to inactivate chemicals from the diet, hormones, and other internal chemicals. Some products of the P450 enzymes are even more active and need to be neutralized by conjugation enzymes or they can cause even more cellular damage. High-carbohydrate, low-protein diets can reduce the effectiveness of conjugation enzymes. Cruciferous vegetables, especially those high in indole-3-carbinol, enhance P450 enzymes. Some flavonoids can reduce the toxic effects of P450 products made from polycyclic aromatic hydrocarbons.

79. Effects of nutritive factors on metabolic processes involving bioactivation and detoxication of chemicals

F. Peter Guengerich, *Ann. Rev. Nutr.,* 4, 1984, pp. 207–231

Some foods that the body chemically converts into toxins, as well as synthetic chemicals such as industrial chemicals, pesticides, drugs, and pollutants, can cause cancer because the Phase I liver enzymes can, during detoxification, make some things more carcinogenic.

80. Normal bacterial populations of the intestine and their relation to intestinal function

Robert M. Donaldson, Jr., *The New England Journal of Medicine*, Vol. 270, No. 18, April 30, 1964, pp. 938–945

In the late 1800s, Metchnikoff believed that toxins from the intestinal bacteria, when absorbed, were the cause of many of man's afflictions. Scientific reaction against the theory may have impeded further investigations into the significance of the intestinal flora. Recent investigations show that the concept of autointoxication must receive serious reconsideration.

81. The anti-toxic function of the liver

M. Pavlov, *The Lancet*, 2, 1893, page 34

If by means of a ligature placed on the portal vein, the blood is compelled to deviate from the liver, poisonous symptoms appear consisting of fever and nephritis. The conclusion is that when the blood is prevented from passing through the liver, toxemia occurs, which is solely due to the fact that the liver plays a protective role against toxins that are being continually fabricated in the intestinal canal.

82. Intestinal endotoxins as mediators of hepatic injury – an idea whose time has come again

James P. Nolan, *Hepatology*, Vol. 10, No. 5, 1989, pp. 887–891

When gut bacteria die, parts of their outer cell wall become toxic compounds called endotoxins. If the gut barrier is weakened by alcohol or inflammation, endotoxins can flood into the liver via the portal vein where Kupffer cells detoxify them. If the Kupffer cells are unable to handle the endotoxins, hepatocyte membranes can be disrupted, P450 enzymes can be decreased, mitochondrial function can be impaired, and damage can occur from free radicals and leukotrienes.

83. Endotoxin shock: a manifestation of intravascular coagulation

Robert M. Hardaway, et al., *Annals of Surgery*, Vol. 154, No. 5, November 1961, pp. 791–802

Endotoxins in the bloodstream cause decreased blood oxygenation and blood pressure and increased portal vein pressure, vascular clotting, and lactic acid, which contribute to damage to the gastrointestinal system, kidneys, liver, and pancreas.

84. Hypotension (shock) in dogs produced by Escherichia coli endotoxin

Lloyd D. MacLean and Max H. Weil, *Circulation Research*, Vol. 4, September 1956, pp. 546–556

Endotoxin from bacteria was injected into dogs; this resulted in liver failure and increased portal vein pressure, which led to edema of the gallbladder, small intestine, and—to a lesser extent—the large intestine. The greatest damage occurred between the bottom of the stomach and the ileocecal valve.

85. Canine intestinal and liver weight changes induced by E. coli endotoxin

L. D. MacLean, et al., *Proc. Soc. Exp. Biol. & Med.*, Vol. 92, 1956, pp. 602–605

Injection of endotoxin from E. coli bacteria into a dog was followed one to two minutes later by a dramatic increase in weight of the liver, with a lesser increase in weight of the small intestine, probably due to back-pressure from the liver. At the same time, a sudden drop occurred in systemic blood pressure.

86. Portal-systemic encephalopathy: neurological complications of liver disease

Sheila Sherlock, et al., *The Lancet*, September 4, 1954, pp. 453–457

Toxic nitrogenous substances from the portal vein can pass through a damaged liver and/or through portal collateral channels into the systemic circulation. This can cause clouded consciousness, apathy, confusion, grimacing, blinking, a vacant look, bizarre behaviour, nocturnal ramblings, evacuation of bowels and bladder in inappropriate places, flapping tremour, and coma.

87. Hepatic sphincters: brief summary of present-day knowledge

Melvin H. Knisely, et al., *Science*, Vol. 125, Number 3256, May 24, 1957, pp. 1023–1026

The liver and portal vein, as well as the intestinal veins and spleen, can store vast amounts of blood. The "pooling" of blood in the liver and portal vein bed is thought to be a major factor in some types of circulatory shock. The outlet sphincters of the liver provide precise control of the flow of blood out of each and every sinusoid of the liver and thereby control the rate of filling of the heart and thus the cardiac output.

88. A dynamic and static study of hepatic arterioles and hepatic sphincters

Robert S. McCuskey, *American Journal of Anatomy*, 119, pp. 455–478

All species observed were found to have sphincters that regulated blood flow through the liver sinusoids and consisted of afferent (inlet sphincter) and efferent (outlet sphincter) orifices. All sphincters were similar and consisted of contractile endothelial cells, which by bulging were capable of reducing the diameter of the sinusoid vessel to as low as zero and were like "gatekeeper" cells. These sphincters react to local substances or to substances in the blood to cause rapid changes in blood flow through the sinusoids.

89. The liver as an organ

Arthur C. Guyton, *Textbook of Medical Physiology*, Eighth Edition, Chapter 70, pp. 771–776

The millions of spaces of Disse in the liver sinusoids in turn connect with lymphatic vessels. Therefore, excess fluid in these spaces is removed through the lymphatics. Because of the large pores, substances in the plasma move freely into the space of Disse. Even large portions of the plasma proteins diffuse freely into this space.

90. Portals of entry - a review

Lewis W. Mayron, *Annals of Allergy*, Vol. 40, June 1978, pp. 399–405

Allergens are proteins that enter the body unchanged and induce hypersensitivity reactions by the immune system. The three possible entry routes are: 1) absorption through the mouth and esophagus; 2) via the portal vein to the liver with subsequent transfer to the systemic circulation; and 3) via the lymph system from the intestines to the systemic circulation. Studies have shown that proteins can pass through via the second and third routes, although rapid reaction following ingestion is probably via the third portal of entry.

91. Passage of undegraded dietary antigen into the blood of healthy adults

S. Husby, et al., *Scand. J. Immunol*, 22, 1985, pp. 83–92

This study shows that undigested protein is regularly absorbed into the blood in healthy adults.

92. Food allergy - or enterometabolic disorder?

J. O. Hunter, *The Lancet*, Vol. 338, August 24, 1991, pp. 495–496

Exclusion diets have shown to be effective in migraine, irritable bowel syndrome, Crohn's disease, eczema, hyperactivity, and rheumatoid arthritis, yet no evidence of typical allergic reaction can be found in most patients. This may be due to the intestinal flora producing chemicals that the liver enzymes are unable to neutralize; these chemicals pass into the circulation and produce distant symptoms.

93. Effect of diet on faecal and urine urobilinogen excretion and its possible relationship to the pathogenesis of peptic ulceration

S. L. Malhotra, *Gut*, 9, 1968, pp. 183–186

Diets that require a lot of chewing are much less likely to produce peptic ulcers.

94. Diet and diverticulosis - new leads

K. W. Heaton, *Gut*, 26, 1985, pp. 541–543

A Greek study found that patients with diverticulosis eat less brown bread and vegetables and more dairy and meat, especially lamb. The lower fibre could be an important factor, since diverticulosis is less prevalent in vegetarians. The high meat protein may result in the intestinal bacteria making a toxin that may weaken the intestinal walls.

95. Low-residue diets and hiatus hernia

Denis P. Burkitt and Peter A. James, *The Lancet,* July 21, 1973, pp. 128–130

Stools of individuals in the Western world are half the weight and take twice as long to pass as those of African villagers. It's proposed that difficulties in passing stool raises abdominal pressure enough to create hiatal hernia. The refined-carbohydrate diet of the West can also contribute to higher rates of diverticulosis, gallstones, and obesity.

96. Treatment of hepatic encephalopathy by alteration of intestinal flora with Lactobacillus acidophilus

William A. A. G. Macbeth, et al., *The Lancet,* February 20, 1965, pp. 399–403

Lactobacillus acidophilus is effective in treating a liver that's enlarged due to high ammonia levels entering from the intestine via the portal vein.

97. Origin and fate of biliary sludge

Sum P. Lee, et al., *Gastroenterology,* 94, 1988, pp. 170–176

Biliary sludge is a mixture of cholesterol that crystallizes in the gallbladder along with granules of calcium bilirubinate, in a bile thickened with proteins. This study followed 96 patients with biliary sludge over three years. In 17 percent of the patients, the biliary sludge disappeared and didn't return. In 60 percent, it disappeared but later returned. In 8 percent, gallstones developed without any symptoms. In 6 percent, gallstones developed with bile attack symptoms, but another 6 percent with bile sludge experienced the same severe bile attack symptoms without there being any stones present.

98. Gallstone dissolution in man using cholic acid and lecithin

J. Toouli, et al., *The Lancet,* December 6, 1975, pp. 1124–1126

Seven patients with gallstones were treated with soybean lecithin and cholic acid supplements. Bile quality improved in five patients. Stones disappeared in two patients, and were reduced in size in one patient over six months.

99. The action of choline and other substances in the prevention and cure of fatty livers

Charles H. Best and Harold John Channon, *Biochem.*, XXIX, 1935, pp. 2651–2658

Choline and protein help reduce fat infiltration in the liver.

100. Dietary betaine promotes generation of hepatic S-adenosylmethionine and protects the liver from ethanol-induced fatty infiltration

Anthony J. Barak, et al., *Alcoholism: Clinical and Experimental Research*, Vol. 17, No. 3, May/June 1993, pp. 552–555

Dietary betaine supplementation elevated the levels of S-adenosylmethionine (SAM) in the liver by increasing its production from homocysteine via the enzyme betaine homocysteine methyltransferase (BHMT). This helped protect the liver from alcohol-induced fatty infiltration.

101. New insights about an old problem

Keith W. Sehnert, *Townsend Letter for Doctors and Patients*, October 1997, pp. 132–133

This article is a review of the book *The Homocysteine Revolution* by Kilmer S. McCully who has done research on homocysteine for 35 years. McCully's theory is that homocysteine plays a role in arteriosclerosis. When levels of vitamins B_6, B_{12}, and folic acid are too low, homocysteine levels get too high and the stage is set for an increase in calcium deposits and fibrous tissue which contribute to hardening of the arterial walls. As a result, there is a greater risk of blood clots and vascular disease.

Homocysteine is converted to methionine but vitamin B_{12} and folic acid are required for this to take place. Homocysteine is also converted to cystathionine but this process is controlled by vitamin B_6. So low levels of these vitamins mean higher levels of homocysteine. These vitamins are destroyed by food processing and freezing.

102. Food and its service: inadequate nutrition with adequate diets

I. M. Rabinowitch, *The Canadian Hospital*, 1948, pp. 44–46

In diabetes with anemia, restoring stomach acidity and normal duodenal pH will permit iron and vitamins B_1 and C to be absorbed.

103. Gastrointestinal absorption of aluminium from single doses of aluminium containing antacids in man

R. Weberg and A. Berstad, *European Journal of Clinical Investigation*, 16, 1986, pp. 428–432

Antacids that contain aluminum are widely used and the

aluminum is absorbed even at low doses. Absorption is much higher when antacids are taken with citric acid, even in the form of orange juice.

104. Antibacterial activity of garlic and onions: a historical perspective

Karen S. Farbman, et al., *The Pediatric Infectious Disease Journal*, Vol. 12, No. 7, July 1993, pp. 613–614

Ancient civilizations understood the medicinal properties of garlic and onions, which are members of the lily family. Fresh garlic is effective against Gram-positive and Gram-negative bacteria, including those resistant to antibiotics. Allicin is the agent in garlic that's responsible for its antibacterial activity. Boiling reduces the effectiveness of allicin in garlic and since onions have no allicin, they have little antimicrobial effect.

105. Inhibition of growth of Entamoeba histolytica by allicin, the active principle of garlic extract (Allium sativum)

David Mirelman, et al., *The Journal of Infectious Diseases*, Vol. 156, No. 1, July 1987, pp. 243–244

Extracts of garlic and its active component allicin were tested on the protozoan parasite Entamoeba histolytica and the inhibition of the parasite suggested that garlic inactivates the amoeba's sulfhydryl-containing enzymes.

106. Dietary fiber and giardiasis: dietary fiber reduces rate of intestinal infection by Giardia lamblia in the gerbil

G. J. Leitch, et al., *Am. J. Trop. Med. Hyg.*, 41(5), 1989, pp. 512–520 (89–129)

Gerbils on a low-fibre diet were more likely to become infected when inoculated with cysts of Giardia lamblia than were animals on a high-fibre diet.

107. Effect of berberine sulphate on Entamoeba histolytica

T. V. Subbaiah and A. H. Amin, *Nature*, Vol. 215, July 29, 1967, pp. 527–528

In experiments with rabbits, berberine sulphate kills intestinal amoebae and aids in the treatment of dysentery.

108. Liver function in moderate obesity – study in 534 moderately obese subjects among 4,613 male company employees

Fumio Nomura, et al., *International Journal of Obesity*, Vol. 10, 1986, pp. 349–354

This study showed that 24 percent of moderately obese (30 to 50 percent overweight) nondrinking males had high liver enzymes, which are a measure of liver damage.

109. Necropsy studies in myocardial infarction with minimal or no coronary luminal reduction due to atherosclerosis

R. S. Eliot, et al., *Circulation*, Vol. 49, June 1974, pp. 1127–1131

Some patients who died of heart attacks showed no sign of coronary heart disease.

110. Sudden death and acute myocardial infarction - clues to differences in pathophysiology

Robert S. Eliot and Emily A. Salhany, *Postgraduate Medicine*, Vol. 64, No. 4, October 1978, pp. 52–58

Although both sudden death and acute myocardial infarction are almost always associated with long-standing obstructive coronary artery disease, both may originate in the myocardium. Spasm has been suggested as a factor contributing to sudden death. Not all persons dying of acute myocardial infarction have narrowed coronary arteries, nor do all persons with obstructed arteries die of heart disease.

111. Atherosclerotic involvement of the coronary arteries of adolescents and young adults

Doina Velican and C. Velican, *Atherosclerosis*, 36, 1980, pp. 449–460

Hardening of the arteries can be found in many adolescents in Europe and North America, even between 10 to 14 years of age, particularly in cigarette smokers. The same has not been seen in Japanese studies.

112. [Vitamin D levels and the buildup of calcium in fatty plaque]

Circulation, 96, September 1997, pp. 1755–1760

This study found that the lower the level of vitamin D, the greater the chance that calcium will build up in atherosclerotic plaques. The inverse is also true: higher levels of vitamin D means that calcium is less likely to build up in fatty plaques in the coronary arteries.

113. [Calcium and atherosclerosis in middle-aged males]

J. Clin. Epidemiol., 50, 1997, pp. 967–973

In middle-aged males, elevated calcium levels appear to contribute to atherosclerosis.

114. Coronary disease among United States soldiers killed in action in Korea

Major William F. Enos, et al., *JAMA*, Vol. 152, No. 12, July 18, 1953, pp. 1090–1093

Autopsies were performed on 300 US casualties in Korea. The average age was 22.1 years. Over 77 percent showed some gross evidence of hardening of the coronary arteries.

115. Paleolithic nutrition: a consideration of its nature and current implications

S. Boyd Eaton and Melvin Konner, *The New England Journal of Medicine,* Vol. 312, No. 5, January 31, 1985, pp. 283–289

Dietary habits of the last 100 years make Western society more prone to coronary heart disease, hypertension, diabetes, and some cancers. Even young people show the early stages of these diseases. Neanderthals had massive bones, showing high calcium levels, even though no dairy foods were eaten.

116. Nutrition and Physical Degeneration: A Comparison of Primitive and Modern Diets and Their Effects

Weston A. Price, copyright 1945, The Price-Pottenger Nutrition Foundation, Las Mesa, CA

This dentist travelled the world in the 1930s, studying the health of people on traditional as well as modern diets. He found that lower nutrient intake—especially calcium—in modern diets, quickly led to dental cavities and narrowing of the jaw, with associated buckling of the teeth. He found that this was often accompanied by other physical symptoms as well as mental and emotional problems.

117. Diet and overall survival in elderly people

Antonia Trichopoulou, et al., *BMJ,* Vol. 311, December 2, 1995, pp. 1457–1460

The Greek diet is low in saturated fat, high in monounsaturated fat from olive oil, high in legumes, vegetables, whole grain bread, fish, and yogurt, and favourably affects life expectancy in elderly people.

118. Trans-fatty acid patterns in patients with angiographically documented coronary artery disease

Edward N. Siguel and Robert H. Lerman, *The American Journal of Cardiology,* Vol. 71, April 15, 1993, pp. 916–920

Trans fatty acids formed from food processing and cooking behave like saturated fats and increase the risk of coronary heart disease.

119. Effects of high dietary sugar

John Yudkin, et al., *British Medical Journal,* Vol. 281, November 22, 1980, page 1396

Fourteen healthy young men increased their sugar intake from 115 grams per day to 260 grams per day. In three weeks, their HDL cholesterol levels had fallen to levels associated with coronary heart disease. The activity of the enzyme n-acetyl-glucosaminidase increased; this increase is considered to be an early indication of kidney damage.

120. Relationship between impairment of liver function and premature development of arteriosclerosis in diabetes mellitus

I. M. Rabinowitch, *Canad. M. A. J.*, Vol. 58, June 1948, pp. 547–556

Impairment of the detoxifying capacity of the liver may be a factor in the premature development of arteriosclerosis in diabetes mellitus as products of intestinal putrefaction may reach the general circulation and damage the tissues.

121. Effect of oxygen concentration on the metabolic pathway of anisole in rat liver microsomes

M. Hirobe, *Biochemical Pharmacology*, Vol. 35, No. 3, 1986, pp. 541–544

This study showed that the P450 enzymes' function decreased with decreased oxygen levels and the products that the enzymes made were also altered.

122. Malonaldehyde content of food

Raymond J. Shamberger, et al., *Journal of Nutrition*, Vol. 107, 1997, pp. 1404–1409

High levels of malonaldehyde have been found in rancid foods. It is highest in animal fat and rancid meats. Fresh, fresh-frozen, or canned vegetables or fruits have little or no malonaldehyde. Malonaldehyde is a breakdown product of unsaturated fatty acids. It is mutagenic and may also be a carcinogenic initiator.

123. Antioxidant vitamins and low-density-lipoprotein oxidation

Mavis Abbey, et al., *The American Journal of Clinical Nutrition*, 58, 1993, pp. 525–532

Supplementing with alpha tocopherol, beta carotene, and vitamin C increased the blood concentrations of these antioxidants after three months. Malondialdehyde in low-density-lipoprotein (LDL) was the same as in unsupplemented controls, but the onset of oxidation of LDL was delayed.

124. Spontaneously occurring angiotoxic derivatives of cholesterol

C. B. Taylor, et al., *The American Journal of Clinical Nutrition*, 32, January 1979, pp. 40–57

In tests done in 1912, cholesterol fed to rabbits resulted in damage to their arteries resembling atherosclerosis. Likely, the cholesterol used was rancid, as more recent studies using pure cholesterol have not shown the same results. It does, however, prove that rancid cholesterol may cause hardening of the arteries. Fried or hard-boiled eggs raised cholesterol levels by 10 to 14 times. Scrambled or baked eggs raised cholesterol by 6 to 7 times, and soft-boiled eggs by only 3 to 4 times.

125. Cholesterol vehicle in experimental atherosclerosis

D. Kritchevsky and Shirley A. Tepper, *J. Atheroscler. Res.*, 7, 1967, pp. 647–651

When heated, corn oil produces more free fatty acids, which increases atherogenicity and cholesterol. Olive oil is not affected by heating.

126. Effects of cadmium on glutathione peroxidase, superoxide dismutase, and lipid peroxidation in the rat heart: a possible mechanism of cadmium cardiotoxicity

Ijaz S. Jamall and J. Crispin Smith, *Toxicology and Applied Pharmacology*, 80, 1995, pp. 33–42

This study showed that cadmium toxicity resulted in damage to the heart due to lipid peroxidation, without damage to liver or kidneys. The lipid peroxidation was due to the loss of selenium in glutathione peroxidase enzyme and the loss of copper in the superoxide dismutase (SOD) enzyme, due to the high cadmium levels. Supplementing selenium restored some of the activity of glutathione peroxidase enzyme, but high doses of selenium can also damage the heart.

127. Pathogenesis of atherosclerosis

Mohamad Navab, et al., *The American Journal of Cardiology*, Vol. 76, September 28, 1995, pp. 18c–23c

The beginning of atherosclerosis occurs when LDL (low density lipoprotein) cholesterol gets oxidized because the protective antioxidant enzymes of HDL (high density lipoprotein) cholesterol were unable to destroy lipid peroxides in the blood. LDL becomes trapped in the artery wall and is oxidized. This forms a fatty streak in the artery which then stimulates macrophages to attack.

128. The pathogenesis of atherosclerosis: an overview

C. J. Schwartz, et al., *Clin. Cardiol.*, 14, 1991, pp. I-1 to I-16

If LDL (low density lipoprotein) cholesterol becomes oxidized in the intima of an artery, it forms a fatty streak. The oxidized LDL is ingested by macrophages, which can become bloated foam cells. If the foam cells die from this, they can form a toxic fat core that can lead to progression of the problem into plaque. Lymphocytes invade the plaque and by secreting interferon, can develop an autoimmune response. If conditions are improved, it is possible for the macrophages to remove the plaques from the arteries.

129. Serial arteriography in atherosclerosis
G. C. Willis, et al., *Canadian Medical Association Journal*, Vol. 71, December 1954, page 562–568

Men with an average age of 64 who were diagnosed with atherosclerosis were monitored by x-ray of the thigh arteries. Ten were given 500 mg of ascorbic acid three times per day orally for two to six months. X-rays showed decrease in the artery plaque in six of them. All those in the control group became worse or stayed the same.

130. The reversibility of atherosclerosis
G. C. Willis, *Canadian Medical Association Journal*, Vol. 77, July 15, 1957, pp. 106–109

Ascorbic acid therapy may reduce atherosclerosis lesions in some people. Early-stage plaques are reduced more rapidly and this is done by the macrophages.

131. Physiologic levels of ascorbate inhibit the oxidative modification of low density lipoprotein
Ishwarlal Jialal, et al., *Atherosclerosis*, 82, 1990, pp. 185–191

Both vitamin C and vitamin E protect LDL (low density lipoprotein) from oxidation; vitamin C has a greater effect than vitamin E.

132. Tocotrienols modify coronary heart disease risk factors
Randall E. Wilkinson, *Townsend Letter for Doctors and Patients*, December 1997, pp. 96–98

There are eight forms of vitamin E: the four tocopherols (alpha-, beta-, delta-, and gamma-tocopherol) and the four tocotrienols (alpha-, beta-, delta-, and gamma-tocotrienol). Tocotrienols can lower cholesterol by inhibiting HMG-CoA reductase, an enzyme responsible for cholesterol synthesis. Tocotrienols may also inhibit thromboxanes.

133. Randomized controlled trial of vitamin E in patients with coronary diseases
N. G. Stevens, et al., *The Lancet*, 347, 1996, pp. 781–786

Supplementation with alpha-tocopherol (vitamin E) was shown to reduce the rate of deaths from heart attack due to hardening of the arteries.

134. Coronary heart disease in former football players
William C. Pomeroy and Paul D. White, *JAMA*, Vol. 167, No. 6, June 7, 1958, pp. 711–714

A long-range study of ex-football players found that those who exercised the most were less likely to develop coronary heart disease.

135. Regression of atherosclerosis effected by intravenous phospholipid

Walter W. Stafford and Charles E. Day, *Artery*, 1(2), pp. 106–114

"Although numerous agents actively inhibit the formation of atherosclerotic plaques in experimental animals, only one has been shown repeatedly to cause regression of preestablished atherosclerosis. However, the compound is active only if it is administered intravenously. In 1957, Friedman, Byers and Rosenman caused regression of atherosclerosis with intravenous infusions of lecithin."

136. Body weight and mortality

Tim Byers, *The New England Journal of Medicine*, Vol. 333, No. 11, September 14, 1995, pp. 723–724

Weight control usually cannot be maintained without regular physical activity.

137. Drug-related morbidity and mortality: a cost-of-illness model

Jeffrey A. Johnson and J. Lyle Bootman, *PhD, Arch. Intern. Med.*, Vol. 155, October 9, 1995, pp. 1949–1956

Preventable illnesses and deaths related to prescription drugs cost $76.6 billion dollars annually in the US, mostly due to drug-related hospitalizations.

138. Potentiation of effects of weight loss by monounsaturated fatty acids in obese NIDDM patients

Cecelia C. Low, et al., *Diabetes*, Vol. 45, May 1996, pp. 569–575

Weight loss on a high carbohydrate, low-fat diet may be accompanied by irregularities of blood sugar levels, which may be improved by adding in monounsaturated fats.

139. Oat-bran cereal lowers serum total and LDL cholesterol in hypercholesterolemic men

James W. Anderson, et al., *Am. J. Clin. Nutr.*, 52, 1990, pp. 495–499

Consuming 25 grams of oat bran per day for two weeks lowered cholesterol by 5.4 percent, reducing the risk of coronary heart disease by over 10 percent. Similar results have been seen with other soluble fibers such as psyllium, pectin, and guar gum.

140. Meta-analysis of the effects of soy protein intake on serum lipids

James W. Anderson, et al., *The New England Journal of Medicine*, Vol. 333, No. 5, August 3, 1995, pp. 276–282

Consumption of soy protein, rather than animal protein, lowered cholesterol and triglycerides.

141. Hypocholesterolemic effect of sesame lignan in humans
Fumihiko Hirata, et al., *Atherosclerosis,* 122, 1996, pp. 135–136

In this study, sesamin—a lignan found in sesame seeds—was shown to reduce blood cholesterol levels by a number of mechanisms, including inhibition of delta-5 desaturase enzyme.

142. The treatment of bovine xanthine oxidase initiated atherosclerosis by folic acid
Kurt A. Oster, *Clinical Research,* Vol. unknown, page 512A

Homogenization of cow's milk results in the milk enzyme xanthine oxidase, which causes damage to the membrane of the human artery, thus creating atherosclerosis. Supplementation with folic acid (40 to 80 mg/day) prevented the progression of the disease.

143. A factor in yoghurt which lowers cholesteremia in man
George V. Mann, *Atherosclerosis,* 26, 1977, pp. 335–340

Yogurt contains a factor that inhibits the synthesis of cholesterol and can cause low cholesterol even in people who eat large amounts of cholesterol, such as the Masai tribe in Africa.

144. Long-term human studies on the lipid effects of oral calcium
Marvin L. Bierenbaum, et al., Lipids, Vol. 7., No. 3, pp. 202–206

Eight men and two women with high cholesterol showed a 25 percent decrease in cholesterol levels after ingestion of two grams of calcium carbonate per day over a period of one year.

145. Allium sativum (garlic) and atherosclerosis: a review
Benjamin H. S. Lau, et al., *Nutrition Research,* Vol. 3, 1983, pp. 119–128

Regular consumption of garlic may help reduce atherosclerosis and cholesterol.

146. The effect of fried versus raw garlic on fibrinolytic activity in man
S. K. Chutani and Arun Bordia, *Atherosclerosis,* 38, 1981, pp. 417–421

Raw or cooked garlic, or its essential oil, acts quickly to reduce fibrinolytic activity in myocardial patients. Effects are maintained when treatment is continuous.

147. Coffee consumption and myocardial infarction in women
Carlo La Vecchia, et al., *American Journal of Epidemiology,* Vol. 130, No. 3, 1989, pp. 481–485

Women who drink more than three cups of coffee daily may be at risk of acute myocardial infarction.

148. Body weight and mortality among women

JoAnn E. Manson, et al., *The New England Journal of Medicine,*
Vol. 333, No. 11, September 14, 1995, pp. 677–685

In middle-aged women, body weight correlated with death rate.
The lowest rate was for women slightly under the US average, and
those whose weight had been stable since early adulthood.

149. The heart as a target organ in systemic allergic reactions

Norine Capurro and Roberto Levi, *Circulation Research,* Vol. 36,
April 1975, pp. 520–528

Systemic anaphylaxis was induced in guinea pigs made sensitive to
antigen. Exposure to antigen resulted in rapid and sometimes
irregular beating of the heart within 20 seconds. This was followed by
respiratory and blood pressure changes.

150. Physical fitness and immunity to heart-disease in Masai

George V. Mann, et al., *The Lancet,* December 25, 1965, pp. 1308–1310

The Masai of Tanzania have a diet high in milk and meat yet are
free of cardiovascular disease. American men can increase their food
intake without developing cardiovascular disease if they use up the
energy with strenuous exercise.

151. The inverse relation between fish consumption and 20-year mortality from coronary heart disease

Daan Kromhout, et al., *The New England Journal of Medicine,*
Vol. 312, No. 19, May 9, 1985, pp. 1205–1209

Eskimos and Japanese both have low levels of coronary heart
disease, which may be related to their high fish diets. Fish contains
EPA from which prostaglandin I_3 and thromboxane A_3 are made.
These are anticlotting compared to thromboxane A_2, which is made
from arachidonic acid, usually found in red meat.

152. Hypoxia and drug metabolism

Dean P. Jones, *Biochemical Pharmacology,* Vol. 30, No. 10, 1981,
pp. 1019–1023

Half of the deaths in the US are of cardiovascular or respiratory
origin and most involve some degree of hypoxia (low oxygen). The
low oxygen alters the function of enzymes that require oxygen such as
oxidases and oxygenases.

153. Italian multicenter study on the safety and efficacy of coenzyme Q_{10} as adjunctive therapy in heart failure (interim analysis)

E. Baggio, et al., *Clinical Investigator,* 71, 1993, pp. S145–S149

CoQ_{10} may help lower blood pressure and offer protection against
congestive heart failure.

154. Reduction of plasma lipids, lipoproteins, and apoproteins by dietary fish oils in patients with hypertriglyceridemia

Beverley E. Phillipson, et al., *The New England Journal of Medicine,* Vol. 312, No. 19. May 9, 1985, pp. 1210–1216

Fatty fish containing omega-3 fatty acids such as EPA can lower high triglyceride levels better than a low-fat diet.

155. Fish oil and the development of atherosclerosis

Author(s) unknown, *Nutrition Reviews,* Vol. 45, No. 3, March 1987, pp. 90–92

EPA from fish oil reduces atherosclerosis probably by making prostaglandins and thromboxanes of the 3-series, rather than those of the 2-series from arachidonic acid, which stimulate greater platelet aggregation and inflammation.

156. Frozen shoulder and lipids

T. D. Bunker and C. N. A .Esler, *The Journal of Bone and Joint Surgery,* Vol. 77-B, No. 5, September 1995, pp. 684–686

This study showed that people with frozen shoulder had a higher incidence of high cholesterol and triglyceride levels.

157. Effect of citrus pectin on blood lipids and fecal steroid excretion in man

Ruth M. Kay and A. Stewart Truswell, *The American Journal of Clinical Nutrition,* 30, February 1977, pp. 171–175

Wheat fibre helps bowel function but doesn't lower cholesterol or triglyceride levels. Pectin, guar gum, and psyllium lower cholesterol.

158. Syndrome X: 6 years later

G. M. Reaven, *Journal of Internal Medicine,* 236 (Supplement 736), 1994, pp. 13–22

Twenty-five per cent of the population at large have resistance to insulin so they have to make more insulin to maintain normal blood sugar levels. The high insulin can cause high urinary calcium, hypertension, poor fat metabolism, and coronary heart disease; altogether this is called Syndrome X.

159. Hyperinsulinemia or increased sympathetic drive as links for obesity and hypertension

Michaela Modan and Hillel Halkin, *Diabetes Care,* Vol. 14, No. 6, June 1991, pp. 470–487

Chronic overeating and/or low physical activity and/or mental stress can lead to increased sympathetic nervous system drive and high insulin, which can result in insulin resistance. This, in combination with elevated glucose and free fatty acids, can lead to obesity, high blood pressure, and hardening of the arteries.

160. Insulin levels, hunger, and food intake: an example of feedback loops in body weight regulation
Judith Rodin, *Health Psychology*, 4 (1), 1985, pp. 1–24

Elevations in insulin produce increased hunger, heightened pleasantness of sweets, and increased food intake.

161. Insulin resistance and breast cancer risk
Peter F. Bruning, et al., *Int. J. Cancer*, 52, 1992, pp. 511–516

Abdominal fat is related to high levels of triglycerides and available estradiol. High insulin and insulin resistance from overeating and lack of exercise may be a common link between diseases such as hypertension, breast cancer, and non-insulin-dependent diabetes, which are so common in industrialized countries.

162. The metabolic basis for the "apple" and the "pear" body habitus
Author(s) unknown, *Nutrition Reviews*, Vol. 49, No. 3, March 1991, pp. 84–86

People who deposit fat in the abdominal area (apple shape) are more prone to cardiovascular disease, stroke, and diabetes than those who deposit fat in the hips and buttocks (pear shape).

163. Hyperinsulinemia, sex, and risk of atherosclerotic cardiovascular disease
Michaela Modan, et al., *Circulation*, Vol. 84, No. 3, September 1991, pp. 1165–1175

Hyperinsulinemia and insulin resistance may contribute to cardiovascular disease (CVD) in men. CVD is prevalent in industrialized society and is correlated with excessive caloric intake and sedentary lifestyle.

164. Pathophysiology of insulin secretion in non-insulin-dependent diabetes mellitus
W. Kenneth Ward, et al., *Diabetes Care*, Vol. 7, No. 5, Sept.–Oct. 1984, pp. 491–502

Non-insulin-dependent diabetes mellitus (NIDDM) usually has some degree of abnormality of the pancreatic beta cells. As blood sugar levels rise because of impaired insulin levels, eventually the sugar will spill into the urine.

165. Variations in insulin-stimulated glucose uptake in healthy individuals with normal glucose tolerance

Clarie Hollenbeck and Gerald M. Reaven, *Journal of Clinical Endocrinology and Metabolism,* Vol. 64, No. 6, 1987, pp. 1169–1173

Individuals vary widely in the rate at which their bodies take up glucose in response to insulin and these differences may be independent of the blood sugar level. Insulin resistance is associated with high insulin levels in the blood.

166. Insulin resistance and cigarette smoking

Francesco S. Facchini, et al., *The Lancet,* Vol. 339, May 9, 1992, pp. 1128–1130

Chronic cigarette smokers are insulin resistant, have high insulin levels, and have triglyceride and cholesterol problems, which may explain why they are more prone to coronary heart disease.

167. Diet-induced changes in serum transaminase and triglyceride levels in healthy adult men: role of sucrose and excess calories

Katherine P. Porikos and Theodore B. Van Itallie, *The American Journal of Medicine,* Vol. 75, October 1983, pp. 624–630

High sugar intake may damage the livers of healthy males very quickly.

168. Perspectives in diabetes: early environment events as a cause of IDDM

R. David Leslie, et al., *Diabetes,* Vol. 43, July 1994, pp. 843–850

Insulin-dependent diabetes mellitus (IDDM) is caused by destruction of the insulin-secreting beta cells of the pancreas by a destructive immune system process that may take place in early childhood, but a long time may pass before symptoms might appear.

169. Childhood immunisation and diabetes mellitus

J. Barthelow Classen, *New Zealand Medical Journal,* May 24, 1996, page 195

Vaccinations can cause autoimmune diseases like alopecia (hair loss) and diabetes through the stimulation of release of interferon. In New Zealand, hepatitis B vaccinations were followed by a 60 percent increase in diabetes, which was similar to that seen after the Haemophilus influenza B vaccine.

170. Nicotinamide treatment in subjects at high risk of developing IDDM improves insulin secretion

R. Manna, et al., *BJCP,* Vol. 46, No. 3, Autumn 1992, pp. 177–179

The autoimmune process that destroys the pancreatic insulin-producing beta cells is a slow process that includes a pre-diabetic phase. Nicotinamide treatment in the early stage has been shown to reverse beta cell damage and increase insulin secretion, but it does not reverse the autoimmune activity.

171. The coronary artery disease paradox: the role of hyperinsulinemia and insulin resistance and implications for therapy

Henry R. Black, *Journal of Cardiovascular Pharmacology*, Vol. 15 (Suppl. 5), 1990, pp. S26–S38

High insulin levels and insulin resistance are the link between high blood pressure, obesity, and non-insulin-dependent diabetes, all of which can increase the risk of coronary artery disease. Measures that reduce high insulin levels, such as weight loss and exercise, are highly recommended.

172. Why do low-fat high-carbohydrate diets accentuate postprandial lipemia in patients with NIDDM?

Y.D. Ida Chen, et al., *Diabetes Care*, Vol. 18, No. 1, January 1995, pp. 10–16

Patients with non-insulin-dependent diabetes who replace saturated fat with carbohydrate are more at risk of coronary heart disease and might be better advised to replace saturated fat with monounsaturated fat.

173. Duodenal and ileal lipid suppresses postprandial blood glucose and insulin responses in man: possible implications for the dietary management of diabetes mellitus

I. McL. Welch, et al., *Clinical Science*, 72, 1987, pp. 209–216

Adding fat-containing food early in a carbohydrate meal may help reduce blood sugar problems after the meal.

174. Effect of method of administration of psyllium on glycemic response and carbohydrate digestibility

Thomas M. S. Wolever, et al., *Journal of the American College of Nutrition*, Vol. 10, No. 4, 1991, pp. 364–371

Viscous fibres like psyllium help to stabilize blood sugar levels by reducing the digestion rate of carbohydrates, and therefore should be mixed thoroughly with the carbohydrate.

175. Apparent deficiency of vitamin B_6 in typical individuals who commonly serve as normal controls

Junichi Azuma, et al., *Research Communications in Chemical Pathology and Pharmacology*, Vol. 14, No. 2, June 1976, pp. 343–348

The average person's diet does not provide an adequate intake of vitamin B_6.

176. Evidence for synergism between chromium and nicotinic acid in the control of glucose tolerance in elderly humans

Martin Urberg and Michael B. Zemel, *Metabolism*, Vol. 36, No. 9, September 1987, pp. 896–899

GTF (glucose tolerance factor) contains chromium and two molecules of nicotinic acid, and can optimize glucose metabolism.

177. Hypocholesterolemic effects of nicotinic acid and chromium supplementation

Martin Urberg, et al., *The Journal of Family Practice*, Vol. 27, No. 6, 1988, pp. 603–606

When nicotinic acid and chromium were taken together, cholesterol levels were decreased and glucose tolerance levels have also been shown to be improved.

178. Effects of supplemental chromium on patients with symptoms of reactive hypoglycemia

Richard A. Anderson, et al., *Metabolism*, Vol. 36, No. 4, April 1987, pp. 351–355

Hypoglycemic symptoms improved with chromium supplementation. Another study found that not only was the glucose tolerance of subjects with marginally elevated blood glucose improved by supplemental chromium, but chromium also appeared to increase the blood sugar levels of subjects with low blood sugar.

179. Anabolic effects of insulin on bone suggest a role for chromium picolinate in preservation of bone density

M. F. McCarty, *Medical Hypothesis*, 45, 1995, pp. 241–246

Insulin causes the kidneys to eliminate calcium and this can be reduced by the administration of chromium, which, at the same time increases DHEA levels, which could have an "age-retarding" effect.

180. The action of chromium on serum lipids and on atherosclerosis in cholesterol-fed rabbits

Abraham S. Abraham, et al., *Atherosclerosis*, 42, 1982, pp. 185–195

Chromium helps to protect arteries and reduce atherosclerosis in rabbits, even in those with high cholesterol levels.

181. Chromium supplementation of human subjects: effects on glucose, insulin, and lipid variables

Richard A. Anderson, et al., *Metabolism*, Vol. 32, No. 9, September 1983, pp. 894–899

Chromium supplementation didn't change blood insulin levels, but it appeared to make the insulin more effective.

182. Insulin resistance after oral glucose tolerance testing in patients with major depression

Andrew Winokur, et al., *Am. J. Psychiatry*, 145:3, March 1988, pp. 325–330

Depressed patients had normal glucagon hormone response but wider swings in insulin levels, indicating insulin resistance.

183. Relative hypoglycemia as a cause of neuropsychiatric illness

Harry M. Salzer, *Journal of the National Medical Association*, Vol. 58, No. 1, January 1966, pp. 12–17

Relative hypoglycemia occurs as a result of a relative drop in blood sugar level after intake of high-carbohydrate foods and caffeine-containing drinks. It can create any neuropsychiatric disorder including anxiety, depression, schizophrenia, manic depression, psychosis, and alcoholism. Many patients reported being worse after Thanksgiving, Christmas, and Easter, when intake of sweets and other carbohydrates was increased.

184. Depressive symptoms and the glucose tolerance test and insulin tolerance test

George R. Heninger, et al., *The Journal of Nervous and Mental Disease*, Vol. 161, No. 6, 1975, pp. 421–432

Patients with severe depression have shown high insulin levels with reduced rate of glucose utilization and increased fatty acid levels. Decreased glucose utilization is related to emotional withdrawal, blunt affect, and motor retardation, and increased fatty acid levels are related to anxiety.

185. Evidence for abnormal glucose tolerance test among violent offenders

M. Virkkunen and M. O. Huttunen, *Neuropsychobiology*, 8, 1982, pp. 30–34

Fifty-six male violent offenders and 20 male controls from the psychiatric personnel were studied by means of the glucose tolerance test. The results revealed some abnormal findings among those violent offenders who had an antisocial personality. Their blood glucose concentrations, having risen usually to a rather high level, fell to clinically significant hypoglycemia from which the return to the original basal values was slow. This abnormal glucose tolerance in the antisocial personality may have some connection with the etiology and poor prognosis of this disorder. The exact reason for these findings is not clear.

186. Reactive hypoglycemic tendency among habitually violent offenders: a further study by means of the glucose tolerance test

M. Virkkunen, *Neuropsychobiology*, 8, 1982, pp. 35–40

Sixty-eight male, habitually violent offenders had their blood sugar tested and those with an intermittent explosive disorder had much the same abnormal hypoglycemic pattern as the antisocial personality group.

187. Age of alcoholism onset

Laure Buydens-Branchey, et al., *Arch. Gen. Psychiatry*, Vol. 46, March 1989, pp. 231–236

Alcoholics who start abusing alcohol before the age of 20 have more problems with mood and aggression control than patients with a later onset of alcoholism. This is due to low serotonin levels, which may be a result of alcohol stimulating the liver enzyme tryptophan oxygenase. This enzyme breaks down tryptophan, thus lowering the levels of tryptophan, from which serotonin is made.

188. The impact of a low food additive and sucrose diet on academic performance in 803 New York City public schools

Stephen J. Schoenthaler, et al., *Int. J. Biosocial Research*, Vol. (8)2, 1986, pp. 185–195

In children, reducing the daily consumption of artificial food colours and flavours, food preservatives (BHA and BHT), and high-sucrose foods resulted in higher academic performance.

189. Linking school-based diet with behavior disorders

Joseph Jiggetts and Felicia Drury Klement, *PPNF Nutrition Journal*, Vol. 17, Issue No. 3/4, pp. 1–5

The behaviour of emotionally disturbed children was more strongly affected by foods such as chocolate milk, pancakes or waffles with syrup, and sugary canned fruit than was the behaviour of children who were well adjusted.

190. Tryptophan and nutritional status of patients with senile dementia

D. E. Thomas, et al., *Psychological Medicine*, 16, 1986, pp. 297–305

Patients with senile dementia were found to have low levels of tryptophan, vitamin C, and folate.

191. Changes in serum tryptophan, glucose, and related measures in psychotics & neurotics

J. A. Yaryura-Tobias, et al., *Nutrition*, Vol. unknown, #4557, page 1132

Tryptophan levels were lower in the psychotic population than in the normal and neurotic populations.

192. Tryptophanase of fecal flora as a possible factor in the etiology of colon cancer

King-Thom Chung, et al., *Journal of the National Cancer Institute,* Vol. 54, No. 5, May 1975, pp. 1073–1078

Of 23 intestinal anaerobic bacteria studied, four were found to make indole from tryptophan. Indole from tryptophan is suspected of playing a role in colon cancer and possibly bladder cancer and leukemia. The incidence of colon cancer is greater in a population with a high-meat diet than in a population with a low-meat diet.

193. Serum folate values in 423 psychiatric patients

M. W. P. Carney, *British Medical Journal,* 4, December 2, 1967, pp. 512–516

Affective disturbances and organic psychoses are the typical psychiatric manifestations of folate deficiency.

194. On the stimulation by insulin of tryptophan transport across the blood-brain barrier

C. Cangiano, et al., *Biochemistry International,* Vol. 7, No. 5, 1983, pp. 617–627

The amino acids tryptophan, tyrosine, phenylalanine, leucine, isoleucine and valine pass through the blood-brain barrier by a single transport system, thus competing with each other. Insulin causes an increased uptake of tryptophan through the blood-brain barrier.

195. Aggression, suicidality, and serotonin

V. Markku I. Linnoila and Matti Virkkunen, *Journal of Clinical Psychiatry,* 53:10 (Suppl), October 1992, pp. 46–51

Low serotonin in young adults and children has been correlated with aggressive and violent behaviours, including lying, stealing, pet-killing in a rage, impulsive fire-setting, and suicidal behaviour. Low blood sugar has been observed in habitual offenders, and insulin resistance has been reported in depressed and suicidal patients.

196. The mood molecule

Michael D. Lemonick, *Time Magazine,* September 29, 1997, pp. 54–62

Serotonin plays an important role in mood and emotion. It is produced in the raphe nuclei, deep in the brainstem and then travels to all parts of the brain and down into the spinal cord. Serotonin is sent to all parts of the nervous system, whereas other neurotransmitters only work in certain areas. At least 15 different receptors for serotonin have been identified.

197. Blood serotonin and tryptophan in Tourette syndrome
David E. Comings, *American Journal of Medical Genetics,* 36, 1990, pp. 418–430

Serotonin and tryptophan tend to be decreased in individuals with Tourette syndrome. Low brain serotonin has been implicated in sleep disorders, premenstrual tension, migraine headaches, depression, bulimia, alcoholism, attention deficit disorder, and obsessive-compulsive disorders, among others.

198. Low illumination experienced by San Diego adults: association with atypical depressive symptoms
Rachele C. Espiritu, et al., *Biol. Psychiatry,* 35, 1994, pp. 403–407

In San Diego, even with its long hours of sunshine, people who spent little time outdoors reported depressive symptoms similar to those of seasonal affective disorder.

199. Seasonality in panic disorder
Peter F Marriott, et al., *Journal of Affective Disorders,* 31, 1994, pp. 75–80

Seasonal changes have been reported in bulimia, obsessive-compulsive disorder, anxiety, panic attacks, and possibly agoraphobia. Reduction of light intensity is thought to instigate the onset of seasonal affective disorder (SAD), and daylight walks are capable of relieving symptoms.

200. Carbohydrate craving, mood changes, and obesity
Judith J. Wurtman, *J. Clin. Psychiatry,* 49:8 (Suppl.), August 1988, pp. 37–39

A large proportion of obese subjects craved carbohydrates at 4 P.M. or 9 P.M., at which time they would eat more than 800 calories of starches and sweets. Meal intake, however, was more balanced. It is likely that these carbohydrate cravings are used to raise brain serotonin levels.

Patients with seasonal affective disorder craved carbohydrates starting with the shorter days of mid-fall until the longer days of mid-spring, when the cravings disappeared. Associated with the cravings were depression, fatigue, and the desire to sleep.

201. Masked food allergy as a factor in the development and persistence of obesity
Theron G. Randolph, *J. Lab. Clin. Med.,* 32, 1947, page 1547

If an allergenic food is eaten several times daily, a masked or chronic smoldering allergic reaction may develop, which is characterized by an improvement in chronic symptoms occurring immediately after eating a specific food allergen and which persists for approximately two hours, but is then followed by a progressive increase in symptoms.

202. Effect of nutrient intake on premenstrual depression

Judith J. Wurtman, et al., *Am. J. Obstet. Gynecol.*, Vol. 161, No. 5, November 1989, pp. 1228–1234

Low serotonin may play a role in premenstrual syndrome (PMS) because eating a carbohydrate-rich meal in the latter part of the menstrual cycle improved symptoms of depression, tension, anger, confusion, sadness, and fatigue. Low serotonin is known to be improved after carbohydrate intake.

203. Low cerebrospinal fluid 5-hydroxyindoleacetic acid concentration differentiates impulsive from nonimpulsive violent behavior

M. Linnoila, et al., *Life Sciences*, Vol. 33, No. 26, 1983, pp. 2609–2614

Low levels of 5-hydroxyindoleacetic acid (the major metabolite of serotonin) seem to be associated with a tendency toward repeated impulsive, violent behaviour. Depressed patients with low serotonin were more likely to attempt suicide using particularly violent means. Impulsive, violent offenders often had higher levels of insulin after eating sugar; this resulted in prolonged hypoglycemia, which was worsened by alcohol.

204. Serotonin and psychiatric disorders

J. J. López-Ibor, Jr., *International Clinical Psychopharmacology*, Vol. 7, Supplement 2, 1992, pp. 5–11

Serotonin deficiency contributes to self-destructive behaviours, alcoholism, bulimia, depression, impulsivity, aggression, and suicidal behaviour.

205. The role of whole blood serotonin levels in monitoring vitamin B_6 and drug therapy in hyperactive children

M. Coleman, et al., *Agents Actions*, 5, 1975, page 496

The hyperactive syndrome (poor attention span, restlessness, failure of impulse control, and poor peer relationships) shows low levels of blood serotonin. Serotonin levels can be raised by various drugs or by vitamin B_6, with clinical improvement in the symptoms.

206. The influence of phototherapy on serotonin and melatonin in non-seasonal depression

M. L. Rao, et al., *Pharmacopsychiatry*, 23, 1990, pp. 155–158

Light treatment only slightly affected melatonin levels of healthy and depressed patients, but it increased serotonin levels in all.

207. Type A personalities tend to have low platelet monoamine oxidase activity

D. F. Smith, *Acta Psychiatr. Scand.*, 89, 1994, pp. 88–91

Monoamine oxidase (MAO) is an enzyme in the mitochondria that breaks down certain hormones, such as adrenaline. Low levels of MAO correlate with the coronary-prone type A personality, which is characterized by impatience, a heightened pace of living, ambitiousness, dissatisfaction with life, excessive drive, and easily aroused hostility. Type A individuals, under stress, exhibit enhanced sympathetic nervous activity, which may be a result of low levels of MAO.

208. Effect of insulin and glucose infusions on sympathetic nervous system activity in normal man

John W. Rowe, et al., *Diabetes*, Vol. 30, March 1981, pp. 219–225

Fasting or carbohydrate restriction decreases activity of the sympathetic nervous system while glucose increases its activity.

209. Effects of glycyrrhetinic acid and its derivatives on Δ^4–5α- and 5β-reductase in rat liver

Y. Tamura, et al., *Arzneim.-Forsch./Drug Res.*, 29 (I), Nr. 4, 1979, pp. 647–649

Cortisol is mainly deactivated in the liver by the enzyme 5β-reductase, which can be suppressed by extracts of licorice. In Addison's disease, licorice extract can be used with a low dose of cortisol, as they appear to work synergistically.

210. Physical exercise and psychological health

Siegfried Weyerer and Brigitte Kupfer, *Sports Med.*, 17 (2), 1994, pp. 108–116

Physically inactive people are twice as likely to develop coronary heart disease as those who engage in regular physical activity. Some of the benefits may be because exercise also decreases depression and anxiety, and improves self-esteem.

211. Effects of systemic nicotine on serotonin release in rat brain

Eliane B. Ribeiro, et al., *Brain Research*, 621, 1993, pp. 311–318

Nicotine increases serotonin levels in the brain. This may explain the appetite and mood disturbances associated with nicotine withdrawal.

212. Effect of caffeine on the recognition of and responses to hypoglycemia in humans

David Kerr, et al., *Annals of Internal Medicine*, Vol. 119, No. 8, October 15, 1993, pp. 799–804

Caffeine can cause symptoms of hypoglycemia even though blood sugar may not be low.

213. Psychological distress and diet – effects of sucrose and caffeine
Larry Christensen, *Journal of Applied Nutrition*, Vol. 40, No. 1, 1988, pp. 44–50
Mood disturbances may be prevented in some cases by restricting consumption of sucrose or caffeine.

214. Wake up and smell the coffee: caffeine, coffee, and the medical consequences
Tony Chou, *The Western Journal of Medicine*, Vol. 157, No. 5, November 1992, pp. 544–553
Caffeine is the most widely consumed stimulant drug worldwide, with 75 percent of it in the form of coffee. It is broken down by the liver P450 enzymes. Caffeine reinforces nicotine addiction and can cause restlessness, nervousness, anxiety, and insomnia. It has also been reported to aggravate psychiatric disease. Withdrawal symptoms can occur about 18 hours after the last caffeine intake and include headaches, anxiety, fatigue, and nausea.

215. Anxiety or caffeinism: a diagnostic dilemma
John F. Greden, *American Journal of Psychiatry*, 131:10, October 1974, pp. 1089–1092
High doses of caffeine, or "caffeinism," can produce the same symptoms as anxiety. Most forms that are used to assess mental status make no inquiry about the consumption of coffee.

216. Anxiety and depression associated with caffeinism among psychiatric inpatients
John F. Greden, et al., *American Journal of Psychiatry*, 135:8, August 1978, pp. 963–966
Caffeine from coffee, tea, cola drinks, and medications was shown to produce various psychiatric symptoms including anxiety, depression, fatigue, tension, the blues, worrying, feeling like crying, and feeling upset. High caffeine consumers were more likely to use more sedatives, tranquilizers, alcohol, and cigarettes.

217. Caffeinism complicating hypersomnic depressive episodes
John F. Neil, et al., *Comprehensive Psychiatry*, Vol. 19, No. 4 (July/August), 1978, pp. 377–385
Caffeine may be the most popular psychotropic drug in North America. There exists a threshold beyond which the effects on the central nervous system cease to be "therapeutic" and become "toxic."

Chronic caffeine excess can create symptoms of anxiety, restlessness, irritability, sleep disturbance, and rebound depression.

218. Regional cerebral blood flow and cognitive function in patients with chronic liver disease

R. E. O'Carroll, et al., *The Lancet*, Vol. 337, May 25, 1991, pp. 1250–1253

Patients with chronic liver disease may have subtle impaired brain function.

219. Actions of ginsenoside Rb$_1$ on choline uptake in central cholinergic nerve endings

Christina G. Benishin, *Neurochem. Int.*, Vol. 21, No. 1, 1992, pp. 1–5

The herb ginseng has many saponins, one of which was studied to see why it improved memory. The Rb$_1$ fraction was found to increase the uptake of choline.

220. Chronic central nervous system effects of acute organophosphate pesticide intoxication

Linda Rosenstock, et al., *The Lancet*, Vol. 338, July 27, 1991, pp. 223–227

About two years after they had been exposed to organophosphate pesticides, a group of workers was found to still have decreased neuropsychological performance.

221. Synthetic food coloring and behavior: a dose response effect in a double-blind, placebo-controlled, repeated-measures study

Katherine S. Rowe and Kenneth J. Rowe, *Journal of Pediatrics*, Vol. 125, No. 5, Part 1, November 1994, pp. 691–698

Twenty-four children had reactions to a synthetic food colour (tartrazine) at six dosage levels. Test results showed irritability, restlessness, and sleep disturbance in all ages and both sexes, and a dose-related response was observed.

222. The relationship between idiopathic mental retardation and maternal smoking during pregnancy

Carolyn D. Drews, et al., *Pediatrics*, Vol. 97, No. 4, April 1996, pp. 547–553

This study predicts that approximately one-third of idiopathic mental retardation among children of women who smoke can be attributed to the mother smoking during pregnancy.

223. Psychotropic treatment of chronic fatigue syndrome and related disorders

Paul J. Goodnick and Ricardo Sandoval, *J. Clin. Psychiatry*, 54:1, January 1993, pp. 13–20

Chronic fatigue syndrome, fibrositis, fibromyalgia, and depression overlap in many of their symptoms and have similar endocrinologic changes and seasonality of occurrence.

224. A preliminary investigation of chlorinated hydrocarbons and chronic fatigue syndrome

R. Hugh Dunstan, et al., *The Medical Journal of Australia*, Vol. 163, September 18, 1995, pp. 294–297

Patients with chronic fatigue syndrome were found to have higher than normal levels of chlorinated hydrocarbon pesticide residues, even if they had no direct history of exposure.

225. Allergy and the chronic fatigue syndrome

Stephen E. Straus, et al., *J. Allergy Clin. Immunol.*, Vol. 81, No. 5, Part 1, May 1988, pp. 791–795

Chronic fatigue can include a number of symptoms such as easy fatigability, muscle weakness, muscle pain, joint pain, sore throat, tender lymph nodes, feverishness, difficulty concentrating, headaches, sleep difficulties, depression, and allergies. Of 24 patients with chronic fatigue, 21 started with an acute infection and 12 of them now showed a higher than normal incidence of allergies. Other studies hypothesize that chronic fatigue syndrome is a manifestation of recurrent Epstein-Barr virus infection.

226. Persisting illness and fatigue in adults with evidence of Epstein-Barr virus infection

Stephen E. Straus, et al., *Annals of Internal Medicine*, 102, 1985, pp. 7–16

Of 31 patients with chronic illness and fatigue, 23 showed Epstein-Barr virus activity.

227. Evidence for active Epstein-Barr virus infection in patients with persistent, unexplained illnesses: elevated anti-early antigen antibodies

James F. Jones, et al., *Annals of Internal Medicine*, Vol. 102, No. 1, January 1985, pp. 1–6

Forty-four patients with chronic illnesses were tested and 39 showed IgM or IgG antibodies to Epstein-Barr virus.

228. Influenza A virus: a possible precipitating factor in fibromyalgia?

Allen N. Tyler, *Alternative Medicine Review*, Vol. 2., No. 2., 1997, pp. 82–86

"Ten fibromyalgia patients were selected at random for blood testing to determine if viral infections could play a part in development of fibromyalgia. Screening volunteers for antibodies to influenza A viral antigen yielded positive results in nine of 10 patients. In the fibromyalgia cases tested, the patients related a history of upper respiratory infection, along with associated neurological symptoms prior to the onset of fibromyalgia symptoms."

229. Effect of high doses of essential fatty acids on the postviral fatigue syndrome

P. O. Behan, et al., *Acta Neurol. Scand.*, 82, 1990, pp. 209–216

Post-viral fatigue syndrome is characterized by severe fatigue, usually with muscle pain and often with depression, anxiety, and difficulty with concentration. Epstein-Barr and Coxsackie viruses may be involved and enlargement of mitochondria is seen. Omega-6 fatty acids high in GLA and omega-3 fatty acids high in EPA and DHA, taken over three months, gave improvement in 85 percent of the patients involved.

230. Effective treatment of severe chronic fatigue: a report of a series of 64 patients

Jacob Teitelbaum and Barbara Bird, *Journal of Musculoskeletal Pain*, Vol. 3(4), 1995, pp. 91–110

Patients with chronic fatigue improve when treated for fungal overgrowth, adrenal dysfunction, sleep disorders, fibromyalgia, hypothyroidism, and bowel parasites. Adding new life goals, vitamins, and magnesium, and deleting excess sugar, caffeine, and alcohol also helps in treatment.

231. Management of fibromyalgia: rationale for the use of magnesium and malic acid

Guy E. Abraham and Jorge D. Flechas, *Journal of Nutritional Medicine*, 3, 1992, pp. 49–59

Fibromyalgia is a common syndrome of muscle pain often associated with irritable bowel, tension headaches, menstrual cramping, mitral valve prolapse, and chronic fatigue syndrome. It is seen nine times more often in women between the ages of 30 and 50 years than in men.

Fibromyalgia patients have normal blood flow in muscle at rest, but decreased blood flow under aerobic conditions. They also have low oxygen pressures in the muscles, especially in the most tender points. Biopsies showed swollen mitochondria and low levels of ATP at tender points.

Magnesium and malate have been shown to strengthen mitochondrial membranes and have oxygen-sparing effects.

232. The role of red blood cell morphology in the pathogenesis of M.E./CFIDS

Maryann Spurgin, *The CFIDS Chronicle,* Summer 1995, pp. 55–58

Capillaries are the most important part of the circulation system as this is where red blood cells do their work delivering oxygen. Capillaries are often narrower than the red blood cells so the red blood cells have to "squeeze" through them. Capillary size varies throughout the body and from person to person, but women generally have smaller capillaries. Malformed red blood cells can't squeeze through the capillaries as well, and can result in a 45 percent decrease in oxygen uptake and 23 percent decline in oxygen release rate.

Stress and free radicals are possible causes of misshapen red blood cells, which may result in poor detoxification. Vitamin B_{12}, omega-3 fatty acids, and antioxidants such as glutathione have been shown to improve red blood cell shape.

233. International tables of glycemic index

Kaye Foster-Powell and Janette Brand Miller, *Am. J. Clin. Nutr.,* 62, 1995, pp. 8715–8935

"The glycemic index (GI) is a ranking of carbohydrate foods based on the postprandial blood glucose response compared with a reference food. Despite early controversy, most studies have found the GI concept to be reproducible, predictable within the context of mixed meals, and clinically useful in the dietary management of diabetes and hyperlipidemia.

The particle size of food has a marked effect: as particle size decreases, the GI increases. Furthermore, the greater the degree of gelatinization of the starch granules, the higher the GI. Differences in particle size and gelatinization help to explain the wide differences in the GIs of pasta and bread.

Low-GI foods eaten before prolonged strenuous exercise were found to increase endurance time, and provided higher concentrations of plasma fuels toward the end of the exercise. In contrast, high-GI foods led to faster replenishment of muscle glycogen after exercise. In other studies, low-GI foods were found to produce greater satiety than did foods with high glycemic and insulin responses."

234. Glycemic index of foods in individual subjects

Thomas M. S. Wolever, et al., *Diabetes Care,* Vol. 13, No. 2, February 1990, pp. 126–132

People's reaction to sugars released from carbohydrates are quite similar and therefore, the glycemic index can be used to predict responses of mixed meals.

235. Glycemic index of foods: a physiological basis for carbohydrate exchange

David J. A. Jenkins, et al., *The American Journal of Clinical Nutrition*, 34, March 1981, pp. 362–366

Studies show that carbohydrates raise blood glucose levels at widely different rates that are not strictly related to their fibre content.

236. Food processing and the glycemic index

Janette C. Brand, et al., *The American Journal of Clinical Nutrition*, 42, December 1985, pp. 1192–1196

"Differences in the glycemic response to carbohydrate meals can be brought about by the cook. A much greater blood glucose response occurs after the consumption of cooked compared with raw starch, and pureed compared with whole foods. Many foods eaten in Western countries today are prepared under factory-processing conditions very different from conventional cooking methods. The food industry has developed a wide range of convenient and novel snack products that are ready-to-eat or that minimize preparation in the home and have increased storage life. New processes such as extrusion cooking, explosion puffing, and instantization make use of extreme temperature and pressure or repeated wetting and drying. Since such extremes may affect the digestibility of the starch, the aim of this study was to compare the rate of digestion and postprandial glucose response in a range of conventionally-cooked and factory-processed rice, corn, and potato products."

Results support the view that the more processed a food is, the higher the glycemic response it will produce.

237. Application of glycemic index to mixed meals

Irene Chew, et al., *Am. J. Clin. Nutr.*, 47, 1988, pp. 53–56

"During the last few years it has been found that the same weight of carbohydrate in different foods can produce widely different blood glucose responses (glycemic index). Tables are now available that compare the glycemic index of many different foods.

This study shows that there are significant differences in the glycemic and insulin responses of healthy individuals to different mixed meals. Moreover, the glycemic indices of the mixed meals could be predicted from the glycemic indices of the component carbohydrate foods. Rank orders coincided for measured and predicted values almost completely. The incorporation of low-glycemic index carbohydrate foods such as legumes into the diet has been shown to reduce the glucose profile in individuals with diabetes. Unfortunately legumes are not a major component of Western diets and the required change in diet pattern may be difficult to achieve."

238. Low glycemic index carbohydrate foods in the management of hyperlipidemia

David J. A. Jenkins, et al., *The American Journal of Clinical Nutrition,* 42, October 1985, pp. 604–617

Diets that contain low glycemic index carbohydrates resulted in a reduction in cholesterol and triglyceride levels in hyperlipidemic patients. Pumpernickel bread, barley, and spaghetti were used instead of white and wholemeal bread and potatoes because of their lower glycemic index.

239. Carbohydrate ingestion before exercise: comparison of glucose, fructose, and sweet placebo

Veikko A. Koivisto, et al., *J. Appl. Physiol.: Respirat. Environ. Exercise Physiol.,* 51 (4), 1981, pp. 783–787

"This study suggests that glucose ingestion prior to exercise results in hypoglycemia during vigorous exercise. This rapid fall in plasma glucose is mediated, at least in part, by hyperinsulinemia. Fructose ingestion is associated with a modest rise in plasma insulin and does not result in hypoglycemia during exercise."

240. Fructose and glucose ingestion and muscle glycogen use during submaximal exercise

L. Levine, et al., *J. Appl. Physiol.: Respirat. Environ. Exercise Physiol.,* 55 (6), 1983, pp. 1767–1771

"These data suggest that fructose ingested before 30 minutes of submaximal exercise maintains stable blood glucose and insulin concentrations, which may lead to the observed sparing of muscle glycogen."

241. Effects of carbohydrate restriction on glucose tolerance of normal men and reactive hypoglycemic patients

James W. Anderson and Robert H. Herman, *The American Journal of Clinical Nutrition,* 28, July 1975, pp. 748–755

Normal men can maintain a normal glucose tolerance on a low carbohydrate diet unless the fat content of the diet exceeds 43 percent. For patients with reactive hypoglycemia, a diet that contains about 45 percent of calories from carbohydrates that are slowly absorbed is usually recommended.

242. Plasma glucose, insulin and lipid responses to high-carbohydrate low-fat diets in normal humans

Ann M. Coulston, et al., *Metabolism,* Vol. 32, No. 1, January, 1983, pp. 52–56

Lowering fats and increasing carbohydrates in the diet to prevent hardening of the arteries could cause the opposite effect, unless the carbohydrates have a low glycemic index (such as legumes) instead of a high glycemic index (such as sucrose).

243. A high-monounsaturated-fat/low-carbohydrate diet improves peripheral insulin sensitivity in non-insulin-dependent diabetic patients

M. Parillo, et al., *Metabolism,* Vol. 41, No. 12, December 1992, pp. 1373–1378

Replacing some of the carbohydrates in the diet with monounsaturated fats helps improve blood sugar control and insulin sensitivity in non-insulin-dependent diabetic patients.

244. Fish oil prevents insulin resistance induced by high-fat feeding in rats

Leonard H. Storlien, et al., *Science,* Vol. 237, August 21, 1987, pp. 885–888

Diets high in omega-6 fats, such as linoleic acid (from vegetable oils) and saturated fat (from meat) lead to insulin resistance. Omega-3 fish oils prevented the development of insulin resistance, especially in the liver and skeletal muscle.

245. Traditional diet and food preferences of Australian aboriginal hunter-gatherers

Kerin O'Dea, *Phil. Trans. R. Soc. Lond.* B, 1991), 334, pp. 233–241

Traditional Australian Aborigines consumed a diet low in saturated fat and sugar and high in fibre and minerals. It protected them against obesity, diabetes, and cardiovascular disease.

246. Marked improvement in carbohydrate and lipid metabolism in diabetic Australian Aborigines after temporary reversion to traditional lifestyle

Kerin O'Dea, *Diabetes,* Vol. 33, June 1984, pp. 596–603

Urbanized Australian Aborigines who reverted to their traditional diet and lifestyle for three to 12 weeks, experienced weight loss, improved glucose tolerance, reduced insulin, and lower triglycerides. Diabetic Aborigines who reverted to a traditional hunter-gatherer lifestyle for seven weeks also showed these improvements.

247. Effect of fenugreek seeds on endocrine pancreatic secretions in dogs

Gerard Ribes, et al., *Ann. Nutr. Metab.,* 28, 1984, pp. 37–43

The dietary fibres of fenugreek seeds help reduce both mild and severe diabetes.

248. Effect of insulin and glucose on feeding behavior

Judith Rodin, et al., *Metabolism*, Vol. 34, No 9, September 1985, pp. 826–831

"Four experimental groups of human subjects, in whom plasma glucose and insulin were independently raised or lowered, were tested for perceptions of hunger, taste, bodily state, and food intake. The data showed that hyperinsulinemia, unrelated to change in plasma glucose concentration, resulted in increased hunger, heightened palatability of sucrose or sweetness, and greater food intake."

249. Role of cholecystokinin and opioid peptides in control of food intake

Clifton A. Baile, et al., *Physiological Reviews*, Vol. 66, No. 1, January 1986, pp. 172–234

Cholecystokinin (CCK) hormone is found in both the brain and the gastrointestinal tract and levels vary with feeding. Opioid hormone and CCK levels play a role in stimulating and ending feeding, respectively, and may work together to regulate energy balance.

250. Modulation of memory processing by cholecystokinin: dependence on the vagus nerve

James F. Flood, et al., *Science*, Vol. 236, May 15, 1987, pp. 832–834

The gastrointestinal hormone cholecystokinin (CCK) enhances memory by activating vagal nerve fibres. The memory helps to recall what was successful in acquiring food.

251. Cholecystokinin in the brains of obese and nonobese mice

Eugene Straus and Rosalyn S. Yalow, *Science,* Vol. 203, January 5, 1979, pp. 68–69

Mice that tend to overeat have lower brain levels of the hormone cholecystokinin.

252. Gastrin and cholecystokinin in central and peripheral neurons

J. F. Rehfeld, *Federation Proceedings*, Vol. 38, No. 9, August 1979, pp. 2325–2329

Many gut proteins have been found to also have an effect on the brain. The largest amount of gut protein in the brain is cholecystokinin.

253. Regional distribution of cholecystokinin-like immunoreactivity in the human brain

Flor L. Geola, et al., *Journal of Clinical Endocrinology and Metabolism,* Vol. 53, No. 2, 1984, pp. 270–275

The peptide cholecystokinin (CCK) stimulates the gallbladder and pancreatic enzyme secretions, and may regulate the neurons in the brain that control appetite. Gastrin is another digestive hormone that is found in all regions of the brain, except the cerebellum.

254. Melatonin: a mammalian pineal hormone

Daniel P. Cardinali, *Endocrine Reviews*, Vol. 2, No. 3, 1981, pp. 327–346

The pineal gland takes up the amino acid tryptophan and converts it to serotonin which, under the influence of light changes, it converts to melatonin. Melatonin affects the function of a variety of endocrine glands.

255. The contribution of extrapineal sites of melatonin synthesis to circulating melatonin levels in higher vertebrates

G. Huether, *Experientia*, 49, 1993, pp. 665–670

The intestinal tract is the largest source of melatonin and after tryptophan administration, the intestine produces melatonin, which can raise blood levels of melatonin. Pineal gland production of melatonin, however, is increased as light levels get lower.

256. Role of the pineal gland in immunity: melatonin antagonizes the immunosuppressive effect of acute stress via an opiatergic mechanism

G. J. M., Maestroni, et al., *Immunology*, 63, 1988, pp. 465–469

Acute stress reduces the thymus gland and its immune response but melatonin in the evening counteracts this.

257. Melatonin as a free radical scavenger: implications for aging and age-related diseases

Russel J. Reiter, et al., *Annals New York Academy of Sciences*, Vol. unknown, pp. 1–12

Every cell of every species of animal uses melatonin as a free radical scavenger, especially against the hydroxyl radical, which is considered to be the most damaging of the free radicals. In vertebrates, melatonin is also produced in the pineal gland with the highest level present at night, and it has the ability to pass through cell membranes and membranes of subcellular compartments. In mammals, ageing reduces the production of pineal melatonin and ageing itself may be a consequence of free radical oxidative damage to cells.

258. A study of the mechanisms involved in the immunostimulatory action of the pineal hormone in cancer patients

P. Lissoni, et al., *Oncology*, 50, 1993, pp. 399–402

Melatonin made by the pineal gland at night has been shown to stimulate immune functions, including antitumour defenses.

259. A randomized study with the pineal hormone melatonin versus supportive care alone in patients with brain metastases due to solid neoplasms
Paolo Lissoni, et al., *Cancer*, Vol. 73, No. 3, February 1, 1994, pp. 699–701

This study concludes that the pineal hormone melatonin may be able to improve the survival time and the quality of life in patients with brain metastases due to solid tumours.

260. Food restriction retards aging of the pineal gland
Karl-Arne Stokkan, et al., *Brain Research*, 545, 1991, pp. 66–72

The pineal gland's production of melatonin is 10 to 20 times higher at night and it decreases with age, except if food intake is restricted with increased age. Food restriction and melatonin supplementation both resulted in improved health and prolonged life in mice.

The results of the present study indicate that extrapineal production of melatonin may be of importance in old animals where pineal function, and therefore melatonin levels, are normally low. In a separate study, when food restriction was continued for the whole life span, it was reported that old rats had preserved a "youthful pineal."

261. Effects of human growth hormone in men over 60 years old
Daniel Rudman, et al., *The New England Journal of Medicine*, Vol. 323, No. 1, July 5, 1990, pp. 1–6

In old age, the decrease of growth hormone is responsible in part for decrease in muscle mass, increase of fat, and thinning of the skin.

262. Effect of growth hormone on human sleep energy
Christina Aström and Werner Trojaborg, *Clinical Endocrinology*, 36, 1992, pp. 241–245

Growth hormone disturbance results in sleep disturbances.

263. Effects of vitamin B$_{12}$ on plasma melatonin rhythm in humans: increased light sensitivity phase-advances the circadian clock?
K. Honma, et al., *Experientia*, 48, 1992, pp. 716–720

"It is concluded that vitamin B$_{12}$ phase-advances the circadian rhythm of plasma melatonin, and increases the sensitivity of plasma melatonin to bright light. The phase-advance shift of plasma melatonin rhythm by vitamin B$_{12}$ may be mediated by an increased sensitivity of the circadian clock to light."

264. Schizophrenia: an evolutionary defense against severe stress
Abram Hoffer, *Townsend Letter for Doctors and Patients*, Feb./Mar. 1996, pp. 52–59

A deficiency of NAD can lead to an increase in the amount of the breakdown products of adrenalin, such as adrenochrome. Adrenochrome and its derivatives can cause psychotic ideas in some people.

265. Depressed nocturnal plasma melatonin levels in drug-free paranoid schizophrenics

Palmiero Monteleone, et al., *Schizophrenia Research*, 7, 1992, pp. 77–84

The cortisol levels of paranoid schizophrenics were slightly higher than normal, but the circadian rhythm of melatonin was absent.

266. The immuno-reconstituting effect of melatonin or pineal grafting and its relation to zinc pool in aging mice

Eugenio Mocchegiani, et al., *Journal of Neuroimmunology*, 53, 1994, pp. 189–201

The pineal gland hormone melatonin affects the regulation of the immune system by improving zinc retention. Zinc deficiency causes thymic atrophy and reduced immune response. Melatonin also suppresses the zinc-depleting efforts of the glucocorticoids.

267. Scleroderma autoantigens are uniquely fragmented by metal-catalyzed oxidation reactions: implications for pathogenesis

Livia Casciola-Rosen, et al., *J. Exp. Med.*, Vol. 185, No. 1, January 6, 1997, pp. 71–79

The autoimmune disease scleroderma involves antibodies developed to attack proteins that appear to have been fragmented from the person's own cells by free radical activity. This free radical self-destruction requires metals such as iron or copper, but may be inhibited by zinc, and it involves dysfunction of small arteries and arterioles of the extremities and the internal organs.

268. What if multiple sclerosis isn't an immunological or a viral disease? The case for a circulating toxin

Frederick Wolfgram, *Neurochemical Research*, 4, 1979, pp. 1–14

MS is believed to be a viral and/or immunological disease, but a circulating toxin, due to a disorder of the liver, should not be ruled out.

269. Chronic methanol poisoning with the clinical and pathologic-anatomical features of multiple sclerosis

H. Henzi, *Medical Hypotheses*, 13, 1984, pp. 63–75

This theory is that fermentation of sugars in the gut leads to formaldehyde production, which can result in damage to the nerves in MS.

270. Multiple sclerosis: prevention of serious illness – vision of a desired future for newly ascertained patients

R. U. Schwyzer, *Medical Hypotheses,* 37, 1992, pp. 115–118

It is proposed that MS first appeared when sugar became more predominant in the diet in the early 1800s. Fructose in large amounts can overwhelm the liver's ability to convert it, and can lead to methanol, aldehyde, and formaldehyde, which can react with myelin, making it subject to attack from the immune system.

271. Nutrition, latitude, and multiple sclerosis mortality: an ecologic study

M. Luisa Esparza, et al., *American Journal of Epidemiology,* Vol. 142, No. 7, 1995, pp. 733–737

Multiple sclerosis, usually found in higher latitudes, is less prevalent in coastal, fish-eating populations.

272. Vitamin B_{12} metabolism in multiple sclerosis

E. H. Reynolds, et al., *Arch. Neurol.,* Vol. 49, June 1992, pp. 649–652

There is a significant association between vitamin B_{12} deficiency and MS.

273. Vitamin B_{12} and its relationship to age of onset of multiple sclerosis

Reuven Sandyk and Gavin I. Awerbuch, *Intern. J. Neuroscience,* Vol. 71, 1993, pp. 93–99

This study shows that patients with early onset of MS had significantly lower levels of vitamin B_{12}, which has been shown to play an important role in immune function. Vitamin B_{12} is necessary for the production of methionine and its product SAM, which is required for the synthesis of myelin and melatonin.

274. Xenobiotic metabolism in motorneuron disease

G. Steventon, et al., *The Lancet,* September 17, 1988, pp. 644–647

Patients with motorneuron disease were studied and shown to have normal P450 enzyme function but deficient liver sulphur conjugation enzyme function. This study suggests that an internal or external sulphur compound, over a long period of time, may be the toxin that causes the brain damage.

275. Xenobiotic metabolism in Alzheimer's disease

G. B. Steventon, et al., *Neurology,* 40, July 1990, pp. 1095–1098

Patients with Alzheimer's, Parkinson's, and motor neuron disease show reduced ability to conjugate toxins containing sulphur. A long-term inability to neutralize toxins can lead to eventual nerve damage.

276. Parkinson's disease and brain levels of organochlorine pesticides

Lora Fleming, et al., *Annals of Neurology*, Vol. 36, No. 1, July 1994, pp. 100–103

Studies done on postmortem brains from Parkinson's disease, Alzheimer's disease, and nonneurological cases showed higher levels of DDT in Alzheimer brains and higher levels of the mitochondrial-damaging pesticide dieldrin in some of the Parkinson's brains.

277. Dietary factors in the management of Parkinson's disease

P. A. Kempster and M. L. Wahlqvist, *Nutrition Reviews*, Vol. 52, No. 2, February 1994, pp. 51–58

Parkinson's disease is caused by degeneration in the brainstem neurons, which can lead to a deficiency of dopamine. *Vicia faba* (broad beans), especially the pods, have been found to be a rich source of L-dopa. Some cases of Parkinson's disease may respond better to *vicia faba* than to conventional L-dopa medication.

278. Methylation of inorganic mercury in experimental jejunal blind-loop

M. Abdulla, et al., *Scand. J. Gastroent.*, 8, 1973, pp. 565–567

Inorganic mercury is relatively nontoxic but bacteria in the intestine, especially in the presence of methylcobalamin, a vitamin B_{12} analogue, can methylate the mercury, making it highly toxic to the nervous system.

279. Specific adaptation

Theron G. Randolph, *Annals of Allergy*, Vol. 40, May 1978, pp. 333–345

In the last half-century, a number of hazardous stressors have slowly put pressure on people's ability to adapt. They include coffee, tea, chocolate, colas, cigarettes, alcohol, sugars, drugs, air pollutants, and food and water contaminants. The ability of people to adapt to these will vary widely.

280. The role of activated T lymphocytes in gastrointestinal disease

T. T. MacDonald, *Clinical and Experimental Allergy*, Vol. 20, 1990, pp. 247–252

T cells are present in the Peyer's patches, between the cells of the lamina propria, and within the absorptive epithelium. The main stimulus for the induction of mucosal T cells is antigenic stimulation by food antigens and bacteria at birth. Inflammatory diseases of the

human gut are usually associated with increased numbers of l
propria and epithelial T cells. Epithelial integrity prevents exce
antigen entry. IgA binds antigen in the lumen.

281. Adverse reactions to food

A. E. Bender and Diana R. Matthews, *Br. J. Nutr.*, Vol. 46, 1981,
pp. 403–404

In London, of 560 people queried, 26 percent of males and 39
percent of females avoided specific foods because they experienced
unpleasant symptoms after consuming them. The commonest
symptoms were nausea, vomiting, headaches, skin reactions,
indigestion, diarrhea, and tremor. Of the 67 foods that were
specifically mentioned as a cause of adverse reaction, the most
common aggravants were alcohol, vegetables, meat, dairy, sugar,
chocolate, and fish.

282. Food intolerance: a community survey

M. L. Burr and T. G. Merrett, *Br. J. Nutr.*, Vol. 49, 1983, pp. 217–218

In Wales, of 475 people queried, 19 percent of men and 26 percent
of women reported adverse affects after eating certain foods.
Symptoms included indigestion, vomiting, diarrhea, headache, skin
symptoms, mouth ulcer, and sore throat. Offending foods were fruit,
onions, cheese, fats and fried food, vegetables, meat, chocolate, and
shellfish. Those with food intolerances were found to have *lower* IgE
levels than those with fewer intolerances, suggesting that allergy may
not be a common cause of food intolerance.

283. Hair element content in learning disabled children

R. O. Pihl and M. Parkes, *Science,* Vol. 19, October 1977, pp. 204–206

Learning disabled children were found to have higher levels of
lead, cadmium, and other elements that appeared to also affect their
behaviour.

284. Food allergy in its relation to gastrointestinal disorders

Julius Friedenwald and Samuel Morrison, *American Journal of
Digestive Diseases and Nutrition,* 5;1, 1934, pp. 100–103

Allergy may be related to problems with calcium metabolism.
Substances that pass through the intestine and the liver can intoxicate
the organism and affect the endocrine glands and the nervous system,
which can amplify the symptoms. The most frequent gastrointestinal
allergy symptoms are fullness, distention, eructations, acidity,
constipation, nausea, vomiting, cramping, fatigue, malaise, and
cankers.

...ations of food allergy

...l *Journal and Record,* September 2, 1925,

...ids can cause spasm varying from
...iy pain and the areas of greatest
...ocecal region, transverse colon, pelvic
...uncter. Symptoms may persist after surgery.

...ergy elimination diet as the most effective gallbladder diet

J. C. Breneman, *Annals of Allergy,* Vol. 26, February 1968, pp. 83–87

Standard gallbladder diets don't allow for the individuality of food intolerances.

287. Food allergies and migraine

Ellen C. G. Grant, *The Lancet,* May 5, 1979, pp. 966–969

Migraine can be caused by birth control pills, ergotamine, smoking, alcohol, stress, hunger, and food allergies. Sixty patients showed adverse reactions to certain foods, ranging from one to 30 foods per person, with an average of ten foods each. Seventy-eight percent had reactions to wheat, 65 percent to oranges, 45 percent to eggs, 40 percent to tea and coffee, 37 percent to chocolate and milk, 35 percent to beef, 33 percent to corn, cane sugar, and yeast, 30 percent to mushrooms, and 28 percent to peas.

Diet therapy resulted in no migraines in 51 individuals and fewer migraines in the other nine, and little medication was needed (an average of 115 tablets used per month before the dietary change went down to one-half tablet per month). Fifteen of the patients had reductions in blood pressure that previously had been high.

288. Amelioration of severe migraine by fish oil fatty acids

T. McCarren, et al., *Am. J. Clin. Nutr.,* 41, 1985, page 874

Chronic migraine sufferers were treated with either omega-3 fish oils or omega-6 vegetable oils, and results were much better with fish oils.

289. Effect of diet treatment on enuresis in children with migraine or hyperkinetic behavior

J. Egger, et al., *Clinical Pediatrics,* May 1992, pp. 302–307

Children with migraines and/or hyperactivity often also experience bedwetting, headaches, stomach aches, limb pains, and epileptic seizure. Of 21 children on food-restricted diets, 12 showed complete remission of bedwetting, along with improvement of other symptoms.

290. Controlled trial of oligoantigenic treatment in the hyperkinetic syndrome

J. Egger, et al., *The Lancet*, March 9, 1985, pp. 540–545

Of 76 overactive children treated with a low allergy diet, 62 improved and of these, 21 achieved a normal range of behaviour. Forty-eight foods were found to provoke symptoms and the most common were artificial colours and preservatives.

291. Artificial food additive intolerance in patients with angio-oedema and urticaria

G. Supramaniam and J. O. Warner, *The Lancet*, October 18, 1986, pp. 907–909

Forty to 50 percent of children with urticaria and/or angio-oedema don't show allergies on standard tests and 75 percent of them respond to a diet free of azo-dye and benzoate preservatives.

292. Omega-3 fatty acids in boys with behavior, learning, and health problems

Laura J. Stevens, et al., *Physiology & Behavior*, Vol. 59, Nos. 4/5, 1966, pp. 915–920

This study of 100 boys aged 6 to 12 measured the levels of omega-3 fatty acids (found mainly in the brain) and omega-6 fatty acids (found throughout the body), and compared the levels of these fatty acids with the health and behaviour of the boys. Boys with lower levels of omega-3 fatty acids had increased frequency of behavior problems (hyperactivity, impulsivity, conduct, anxiety, temper tantrums, and sleep problems). Boys with lower levels of omega-6 fatty acids had more problems with dry skin and hair, increased thirst, and more colds.

293. Salicylates, oligoantigenic diets, and behaviour

Anne Swain, et al., *The Lancet*, July 6, 1985, pp. 41–42

In this study, 86 children with urticaria (skin inflammation) who responded to a diet free from antigens were later challenged with a diet containing salicylates. Three out of four of them reacted to food preservatives like benzoates and nitrates, food colourings, amines, and MSG.

294. Treatment of Crohn's disease with an unrefined-carbohydrate, fibre-rich diet

K. W. Heaton, et al., *British Medical Journal*, September 29, 1979, pp. 764–766

An unrefined-carbohydrate diet improves Crohn's disease if the fibre intake is increased slowly and food is chewed thoroughly.

295. Effect of an enteric-coated fish-oil preparation on relapses in Crohn's disease

Andrea Beluzzi, et al., *The New England Journal of Medicine*, Vol. 334, No. 24, June 13, 1996, pp. 1557–1560

In this study of Crohn's disease patients in remission, 69 percent of the control group had the Crohn's disease return. Only 28 percent of those people on fish-oil relapsed, which may be due to decreased production of leukotriene B_4 and thromboxane A_2.

296. n-3 fatty acids decrease colonic epithelial cell proliferation in high-risk bowel mucosa

Yun-Ching Huang, et al., *Lipids*, Vol. 31, Supplement 1996, pp. S313–S317

Patients at high risk for bowel cancer due to abnormal proliferation of the intestinal cells showed improvement on fish oil supplementation.

297. Effects of fish oil on fecal bacterial enzymes and steroid excretion in healthy volunteers: implications for colon cancer prevention

Hans-Peter Bartram, et al., *Nutrition and Cancer*, Vol. 25, No. 1, 1996, pp. 71–78

Saturated and polyunsaturated omega-6 fatty acids have been shown to increase colon cancer risk and growth, while omega-3 fish oils have been shown to be protective. This study showed that excretion of a putative colon carcinogen was lower during fish oil supplementation than during corn oil supplementation.

298. Children with allergic rhinitis and/or bronchial asthma treated with elimination diet

Kim A. Ogle and Joseph D. Bullock, *Annals of Allergy*, Vol. 39, July 1977, pp. 8–11

Low IgA levels in infants may allow large proteins to penetrate the gastrointestinal mucosa, which can lead to food allergies and later in life, to respiratory allergies.

299. Symptoms of respiratory allergies are worse in subjects with coexisting food sensitization

G. Fiorini, et al., *Clinical and Experimental Allergy*, Vol. 20, 1990, pp. 689–692

Food allergies that occur early in life may contribute to respiratory allergies later in life.

300. Perennial nasal allergy due to food sensitization

Albert H. Rowe and Albert Rowe, Jr., *The Journal of Asthma Research*, Vol. 3, No. 2, December 1965, pp. 141–154

Food allergy is commonly the underlying factor in chronic nasal allergy, although it can also have an inhalant allergy component. Sneezing and itching are less than in inhalant allergies but symptoms can include tickling, picking, or pushing of the nose; loss of smell and taste; sniffling; mouth-breathing; noisy breathing; and snoring. Nasal polyps are usually due to food allergy and correcting the allergies often prevents reoccurrence. Accompanying symptoms could include digestive symptoms, restlessness, insomnia, fatigue, depression, asthma, headaches, and achiness. These symptoms can often be managed with diet.

301. Some developmental and behavioral problems associated with bilateral otitis media with effusion

Phil A. Silva, et al., *Journal of Learning Disabilities*, Vol. 15, No. 7, Aug./Sept. 1982, pp. 417–421

Chronic dysfunction of the eustachian tube can result in middle ear inflammation, which can lead to hearing loss, impaired intelligence, and problems with reading, speech, language, and behaviour.

302. Food allergy – its role in emphysema and chronic bronchitis

Albert H. Rowe and Albert Rowe, Jr., *Diseases of the Chest*, Vol. 48, No. 6, December 1965, pp. 609–612

Food allergy is the sole cause of asthma in 25 to 40 percent of cases, regardless of age. Chronic bronchitis and even emphysema can be related to food allergies. Chronic bronchitis is worsened in fall and winter. The most common foods that cause an allergic response are cereals, milk, eggs, chocolate, and others.

303. Increased consumption of polyunsaturated oils may be a cause of increased prevalence of childhood asthma

L. Hodge, et al., *Aust. NZ. J. Med.*, 24, 1994, page 727

Worldwide increase in childhood asthma in affluent countries is likely due to dietary changes than to air pollution or allergens. Increased use of omega-6 vegetable oils increases inflammatory eicosanoids. In Australia, New Zealand, the US, and the UK, the increased prevalence of childhood asthma coincides with the increased use of polyunsaturated oils.

"On the other hand, the prevalence of asthma is low in some Mediterranean and Scandinavian countries where consumption of olive oil, which is low in omega-6 fatty acids, or oily fish, which is rich in omega-3 fatty acids, is high."

304. Chronic respiratory effects of indoor formaldehyde exposure

Michal Krzyzanowski, et al., *Environmental Research*, 52, 1990, pp. 117–125

Increased rates of childhood asthma and chronic bronchitis were seen in children living in houses with high levels of formaldehyde, especially in those who were exposed to tobacco smoke.

305. Pertussis vaccination and asthma: is there a link?

Michel R. Odent, et al., *JAMA*, Vol. 272, No. 8, August 24/31, 1994, pp. 592–593

In children immunized with pertussis vaccination, 10.69 percent were later found to have developed asthma while only 1.97 percent of unvaccinated children had developed asthma.

306. A randomized, controlled trial of vitamin A in children with severe measles

Gregory D. Hussey and Max Klein, *New England Journal of Medicine*, July 19, 1990, pp. 160–164

This study showed remarkable protective effects of vitamin A (total dose, 400,000 IU) in severe cases of measles. Recovery was much faster than in the control group, and of the 12 that died, 10 were on placebo.

307. The capillary syndrome in hemorrhagic cystitis: therapeutic evaluation of bio-flavonoids

Clarence C. Saelhof, *Amer. Jour. Dig. Dis.*, 22, 1955, pp. 204–206

Bioflavonoids have been shown to reduce capillary fragility, and they act as antiinflammatory agents in viral and bacterial infections.

308. Asthma with sulfite intolerance in children: a blocking study with cyanocobalamin

Belén Añíbarro, et al., *J. Allergy Clin. Immunol.*, Vol. 90, No. 1, July 1992, pp. 103–109

Some people with asthma experience bronchospasm on exposure to sulfites but in pretreatment with 1.5 mg oral cyanocobalamin (vitamin B_{12}), four of five child asthmatics did not develop reactions.

309. Children with allergic rhinitis and/or bronchial asthma treated with elimination diet: a five-year follow-up

Kim A. Ogle and Joseph D. Bullock, *Annals of Allergy*, Vol. 44, May 1980, pp. 273–278

Most children with respiratory allergy showed significant improvement of symptoms when placed on a hypoallergenic diet, and gradually lost their allergies to those foods over three to eighteen months. The younger the child, the shorter the time period.

310. B-cell memory is short-lived in the absence of antigen

David Gray and Helena Skarvall, *Nature*, Vol. 336, November 3, 1988, pp. 70–73

This study shows that in the complete absence of antigen, memory B-cells are gone after 10 to 12 weeks.

311. Allergy of the nervous system: a review

Kay Hall, *Annals of Allergy,* Vol. 36, January 1976, pp. 49–64

Eighty-five percent of patients with headaches also had nasal symptoms; 70 percent also had throat or bronchial symptoms, and 36 percent had asthma. Chronic indigestion and constipation have been reported as other complaints in headache patients.

The frontal headache was the most common type of recurring headache by 10 times, and was related to pressure and pain in the sinuses. Allergic headaches are more often related to food allergies than inhalant allergies. Behavioural reactions commonly occur with allergic headache, gastrointestinal disorders, and nasal symptoms.

Ninety percent of schizophrenics and 70 percent of neurotics had food allergies that could provoke delusions, hallucinations, catonia, depression, mania, and tics. Central nervous system allergies are often caused by chemicals such as food preservatives, colourings, fertilizers, insecticides, plastics, stove and heater hydrocarbons, car exhaust, and aerosols. People with allergies may have deficiencies in vitamins A, B, C, and D, calcium and/or salt.

312. Identical intestinal permeability changes in children with different clinical manifestations of cow's milk allergy

Taina Jalonen, *J. Allergy Clin. Immunol.,* Vol. 88, No. 5, November 1991, pp. 737–741

Reduced mucosal barrier function and overstimulation of the immune system by excess antigens may cause cow's milk allergy (CMA). Patients with gastrointestinal allergy and those with CMA presenting as skin symptoms show high intestinal permeability.

313. Regulation and deregulation of human IgE synthesis

Sergio Romagnani, *Immunology Today,* Vol. 11, No. 9, 1990, pp. 316–321

Immediate hypersensitivity to environmental allergens is from overproduction of IgE from normal plasma cells, due to helper T cells either making too much interleukin-4 or too little gamma interferon, which have opposite effects on IgE production. This pattern is particularly seen in persons with parasites.

314. Thymomodulin: biological properties and clinical applications

N. M. Kouttab, et al., *Med. Oncol. & Tumor Pharmacother.,* Vol. 6, No. 1, 1989, pp. 5–9

Thymomodulin, a calf thymus extract, has low toxicity and remains active when administered orally. It stimulates T cells, which regulate B cell antibody production thereby increasing IgA and IgG, but reducing IgE, giving improvement in allergic symptoms. When given to cancer patients undergoing radiation, starting one week prior, blood tests showed less damage to their white blood cell levels.

315. Effect of an orally administered thymic derivative, thymomodulin, in chronic type B hepatitis in children

F. Bortolotti, et al., *Current Therapeutic Research,* Vol. 43, No. 1, January 1988, pp. 67–72

This study found that in children with chronic hepatitis B treated with thymus hormone, 45 percent had remission, while only 18 percent of controls had remission.

316. Food allergy in children: an attempt to improve the effects of the elimination diet with an immunomodulating agent (thymomodulin). A double-blind clinical trial

G. Cavagni, et al., *Immunopharmacology and Immunotoxicology,* 11(1), 1989, pp. 131–142

The main food allergy symptoms in children are gastrointestinal, respiratory, and dermatological, and most commonly, reactions are to cow's milk proteins, eggs, and vegetables. This study showed that children with atopic dermatitis who were placed on food avoidance diets achieved improvement in symptoms. Those who were given thymus hormone—in addition to the avoidance diet—had lowered IgE levels after three months, apparently due to increased activity of T helper cells. After three months, both groups were rechallenged with the food allergens and the children on thymus hormone had far less reaction than those only on dietary avoidance.

317. Cow's milk exposure and type 1 diabetes mellitus

Hertzel C. Gerstein, *Diabetes Care,* Vol. 17, No. 1, January 1994, pp. 13–19

Damage to the insulin-producing beta cells of the pancreas (Type 1 diabetes mellitus) is an autoimmune disease that may be triggered by exposure to a protein in cow's milk in the first few months of life.

318. Antibiotics in milk

Author unknown, *British Medical Journal,* Saturday, June 8, 1963, pp. 5344–5345

The amount of penicillin found in milk varies by season and by region.

319. Casein: a milk protein with diverse biologic consequences

Mark J. S. Miller, et al., Journal unknown (Copyright 1990 by the Society for Experimental Biology and Medicine), pp. 143–159

The proteins in milk can be divided into two main groups: casein and whey. Caseins are proteins found only in milk. Casein proteins curdle in the presence of the cow stomach enzyme rennin. Whey consists of a number of proteins—such as beta-lactoglobulin, alpha-lactalbumin, peptones, serumalbumins and immunoglobulins—that are similar to proteins found in blood and other vital secretions.

While cow's milk whey and human milk whey are similar, their caseins are quite different in structure. Human milk protein is less than 25 percent casein while cow's milk protein is greater than 80 percent casein. Cow's milk and cow's milk-based formulas can greatly reduce stomach function in infants, and may contribute to inflammatory bowel disease and other disease in adults. Casein stimulates phospholipase A_2 and lipoxygenase enzymes, as well as neutrophils and neighbouring cells.

320. Uptake and transport of macromolecules by the intestine

W. Allan Walker and Kurt J. Isselbacher, *Gastroenterology*, 67, 1974, pp. 531–550

Bacteria and their toxins entering the body through the mucus membranes and portal vein can damage the liver, and, particularly if the person is low in IgA, can lead to connective tissue disease and cancer.

321. Gastrointestinal candidiasis: fact or fiction?

Timothy C. Birdsall, *Alternative Medicine Review*, Vol. 2, No. 5, 1997, pp. 346–354

Gastrointestinal candidiasis can cause systemic symptoms even in people with normal immune systems. It's capable of passing from the intestinal system to the internal organs through the bloodstream. It also produces gliotoxins which can weaken the immune system and disrupt glutathione metabolism.

322. A short review of the relationship between intestinal permeability and inflammatory joint disease

P. J. Rooney, et al., *Clinical and Experimental Rheumatology*, 8, 1990, pp. 75–83

Inflammatory arthritis is directly related to the passage of pathogens across the gut mucosa into the circulation system.

323. Small intestinal bacterial overgrowth in patients with rheumatoid arthritis

A. E. K. Henriksson, et al., *Annals of Rheumatic Diseases*, 52, 1993, 503–510

This study showed that a high percentage of patients with rheumatoid arthritis had bacterial overgrowth in the upper small intestine and the greater the bacterial overgrowth, the worse the arthritis was. Fifty percent of the patients who had low stomach acid had bacterial overgrowth, while 35 percent of those with normal stomach acid had bacterial overgrowth. The overgrowth was more frequent in those with O blood type.

324. Association between villous atrophy in rheumatoid arthritis and a rheumatoid factor and gliadin-specific IgG

Cliona O'Farrelly, et al., *The Lancet*, October 8, 1988, pp. 819–822

The immune system can interact with antigens, such as gluten from wheat, in the small intestine and create immune complexes that can cause celiac disease. Lupus, myasthenia gravis, and other autoimmune diseases often exhibit an antigen that is common in celiac disease.

325. Antibodies to Proteus in rheumatoid arthritis

Alan Ebringer, et al., *The Lancet*, August 10, 1985, pp. 305–308

Rheumatoid arthritis and ankylosing spondylitis patients have high antibodies to Proteus and Klebsiella bacteria, respectively.

326. Klebsiella antibodies in ankylosing spondylitis and Proteus antibodies in rheumatoid arthritis

A. Ebringer, et al., *British Journal of Rheumatology*, 27, (Suppl. II), 1988, pp. 72–85

Ankylosing spondylitis(AS) and rheumatoid arthritis (RA) are probably immune reactions in which antibodies to intestinal bacteria (Klebsiella in AS, Proteus in RA) cross-react to antigens in the joints.

327. Do antioxidant micronutrients protect against the development and progression of knee osteoarthritis?

Timothy E. McAlindon, et al., *Arthritis and Rheumatism*, Vol. 39, No. 4, April 1966, pp. 648–656

The progression of osteoarthritis of the knee and associated knee pain appears to be inhibited by high intake of antioxidants such as vitamin C, beta carotene, and vitamin E.

328. Infective arthritis due to Blastocystis hominis

M. G. Lee, et al., *Annals of the Rheumatic Diseases*, 49, 1990, pp. 192–193

The protozoan Blastocystis hominis in the intestinal tract may cause recurrent diarrhea and arthritis.

329. Intestinal Clostridium perfringens in rheumatoid arthritis and other connective tissue disorders

Ingmar Månsson and Börje Olhagen, *Acta Rheum. Scand.*, 12, 1966, pp. 167–174

Clostridium perfringens flora exotoxin is present in many patients with rheumatoid arthritis, lupus, and psoriatic arthritis.

330. Arthritis in pigs induced by dietary factors

I. Månsson, et al., *Clin. Exp. Immunol.*, 9, 1971, pp. 677–693

Pigs fed a high protein diet developed arthritis within weeks. They showed an increase in the intestinal bacteria Clostridium perfringens. It is hypothesized that antigens formed against the Clostridium perfringens leaked into the system, affecting kidneys, joints, and heart. Symptoms could be quickly reduced by the addition of zinc, which possibly decreased the leakage of antigens from the gut. Similar conditions may exist in humans with rheumatoid arthritis, psoriatic arthritis, ankylosing spondylitis, entero-arthritis, and systemic lupus erythematosus.

331. The naeglerial causation of rheumatoid disease and many human cancers. A new concept in medicine.

R. Wyburn-Mason, *Medical Hypotheses*, 5, 1979, pp. 1237–1249

Rheumatoid arthritis, systemic lupus erythematosus, scleroderma, dermatomyositis, and polyarteritis nodosa are closely related diseases of the collagen that is damaged by the person's immune system. These are linked to many other immune diseases such as Hashimoto's thyroiditis, Raynaud's disease, and lymphoma. Underlying the immune reactions in some of these cases may be amoebae of the genus Naegleria.

332. Intestinal flora bacteria and arthritis: why the joint?

M. P. Hazenberg, *Scand. J. Rheumatol.*, 24 (Suppl 101), 1995, pp. 207–211

Patients with inflammatory bowel disease suffer joint inflammation that may parallel the problems in the bowel. Bacterial overgrowth is related to increased rheumatoid arthritis. It is proposed that immune complexes from the gut get into the blood and become trapped in the joints where T cells that had been primed to gut antigens recognize and attack the joint.

333. Review of dietary therapy for rheumatoid arthritis

L. G. Darlington and N. W. Ramsey, *British Journal of Rheumatology,* 32, 1993, pp. 507–514

Bacteria like Proteus or Clostridium perfringens may create substances which pass through gaps in an irritated intestinal epithelium or through its M cells, that eventually trigger inflammation in the joints, called rheumatoid arthritis. Foods such corn, wheat, pork, oranges, milk, oats, rye, eggs, beef, coffee, malt, cheese, grapefruit, tomato, peanuts, sugar, butter, lamb, lemon, and soy have been shown to aggravate rheumatoid arthritis.

334. Platelet serotonin release in rheumatoid arthritis: a study in food-intolerant patients

Colin H. Little, et al., *The Lancet,* August 6, 1983, pp. 297–299

Patients with rheumatoid arthritis may have IgG antibodies attached to food antigens that trigger the release of serotonin from platelets. The serotonin may cause the immune complexes to bind to the synovial membranes of joints, contributing to the inflammatory response.

335. Tryptophan and rheumatic diseases

Alan D. Broadhurst, *British Medical Journal,* August 13, 1977, page 456

Using tryptophan as an antidepressant resulted in amelioration of rheumatoid symptoms in some patients.

336. Changes of faecal flora in rheumatoid arthritis during fasting and one-year vegetarian diet

R. Peltonen, et al., *British Journal of Rheumatology,* 33, 1994, pp. 638–643

Disease activity in rheumatoid arthritis patients changes with alterations in intestinal flora, which can be affected by dietary changes.

337. Dietary fat aggravates active rheumatoid arthritis

Charles P. Lucas and Lawrence Power, *Clinical Research,* Vol. 29, No. 4, 1981, page 754A

Dietary fats in the American diet aggravate rheumatoid arthritis.

338. A new dietary regimen for arthritis

Charles A. Brusch and Edward T. Johnson, *Journal of the National Medical Association,* Vol. 51, No. 4, July 1959, pp. 266–270

Cod liver oil can give improvement in arthritis after four to five months, probably due to its vitamin D content.

339. Bromelains therapy in rheumatoid arthritis

Abraham Cohen and Joel Goldman, *The Pennsylvania Medical Journal,* 67, June 1964, pp. 27–30

In rheumatoid arthritis, swelling of the joint capsule leads to stiffness and soreness on moving the joint, and it is not necessarily improved by long-term steroid therapy. In this study, 72 percent of those tested showed good improvement using bromelain enzymes (from pineapple). It is believed that fibrin is deposited during inflammation to block fluid flow and that the enzymes break up the fibrin, restoring drainage.

340. n-3 polyunsaturated fatty acids: update 1995

S. Endres, et al., *European Journal of Clinical Investigation,* 25, 1995, pp. 629–638

Omega-3 fish oils have been shown to have positive effects on rheumatoid arthritis and hypertension, but not on psoriasis or lupus nephritis.

341. Effects of fish oil supplementation in rheumatoid arthritis

Hille van der Tempel, et al., *Annals of the Rheumatic Diseases,* 49, 1990, pp. 76–80

This study showed that fish oil supplementation reduces the symptoms of rheumatoid arthritis, possibly due to effects on prostaglandins and leukotrienes.

342. The effect of diet in rheumatoid arthritis

J. A. Hicklin, et al., *Clinical Allergy,* Vol. 10, 1980, pp. 463–467

Of 22 rheumatoid arthritis patients tested for food allergies and put on an exclusion diet, 20 noted an improvement in symptoms. Food sensitivities included grains, milk, nuts, beef, cheese, eggs, chicken, fish, potatoes, onion, and liver.

343. Dietary fish oil and olive oil supplementation in patients with rheumatoid arthritis

Joel M Kremer, *Arthritis and Rheumatism,* Vol. 33, No. 6, June 1990, pp. 810–820

The ingestion of olive oil and fish oil reduces inflammation and bolsters the immune system. Fish oil contains EPA, which competitively inhibits the utilization of arachidonic acid, resulting in a decrease of leukotriene B_4. Fish oil may also help asthmatic patients.

344. Treatment of rheumatoid arthritis with gammalinolenic acid

Lawrence J. Leventhal, et al., *Annals of Internal Medicine,* Vol. 119, No. 9, November 1, 1993, pp. 867–873

Borage seed oil contains gammalinolenic acid (GLA). Patients who were given 1.4 grams of GLA per day for 12 weeks showed improvement of 28 to 45 percent, while controls showed no improvement.

345. Treatment of rheumatoid arthritis with blackcurrant seed oil

L. J. Leventhal, et al., *British Journal of Rheumatology*, 33, 1994, pp. 847–852

Black currant seed oil contains gammalinolenic acid (GLA) which is rapidly converted to dihomogammalinolenic acid (DGLA), which can be converted to prostaglandin E_1 (PGE$_1$). PGE$_1$ decreases the production of the inflammatory PGE$_2$ and leukotriene B_4. Treatment of rheumatoid arthritis with 10.5 grams of black currant seed oil per day resulted in modest reduction in overall pain and joint tenderness.

346. Cetyl myristoleate - a unique natural compound valuable in arthritis conditions

Charles Cochran and Raymond Dent, *Townsend Letter for Doctors and Patients*, July 1997, pp. 70–74

Mice are immune to arthritis due to an oil called cetyl myristoleate that circulates in their blood. This oil can be manufactured from fish oils, whale oils, dairy butter, and kombo butter. It appears that cetyl myristoleate stimulates the production of series 1 and series 3 prostaglandins, thereby reducing pain and inflammation. It is taken in a dose of 13 grams over one month. Glucosamine sulfate taken during the same period, at a dose of 500 mg three times a day, seems to improve the effectiveness of cetyl myristoleate.

347. The effect of *cis*-9-cetyl myristoleate (CMO) and adjunctive therapy on arthritis and auto-immune disease: a randomized trial

H. Siemandi, *Townsend Letter for Doctors and Patients*, August/September 1997, pp. 58–63

This study of patients with arthritis showed that treatment with *cis*-9-myristoleate (CMO) plus other natural remedies, such as glucosamine sulphate, gave an 88.2 percent improvement over a four-week period. Treatment with CMO alone gave a 59.2 percent improvement and the placebo group reported a 16.1 percent improvement.

348. Adjuvant treatment of recent onset rheumatoid arthritis by selenium supplementation: preliminary observations

A. Peretz, et al., *British Journal of Rheumatology*, 31,1992, pp. 281–282

Women with recent onset rheumatoid arthritis were given 200

micrograms of yeast-based selenium for three months and six of eight showed reduction in pain and joint involvement, while those on placebo showed no improvement.

349. The effect of niacinamide on osteoarthritis: a pilot study

W. B. Jonas, et al., *Inflamm. Res.*, 45, 1996, pp. 330–334

Patients with osteoarthritis were given 500 mg of niacinamide six times per day for 12 weeks, and showed 29 percent improvement, while the control group worsened by 10 percent.

350. Cherry diet control for gout and arthritis

Ludwig W. Blau, Source unknown, 1950, pp. 309–311

In 12 cases of gout, the uric acid was brought to normal and arthritis was prevented by eating one-half pound of fresh or canned cherries per day. Juice appeared to be equally effective, and dark, yellow, or sour cherries appeared to be effective.

351. Ginger (zingiber officinale) in rheumatism and musculoskeletal disorders

K. C. Svivastava and T. Mustafa, *Medical Hypotheses*, 39, 1992, pp. 342–348

Improvement of arthritis by use of ginger indicates that the benefit may be due to ginger inhibiting cyclooxygenase (COX) and lipoxygenase (LOX) enzymes, thus reducing prostaglandins and leukotrienes from arachidonic acid.

352. Dual activities of tannins from Hamamelis virginiana and related polyphenols on 5-lipoxygenase and lyso-PAF:acetyl CoA transferase

C. Hartisch, et al., *Planta Medica*, 63, 1997, pp. 106–110

Proanthocyanidins were shown to inhibit lipoxygenase (LOX) enzymes.

353. Vitamin B_{12} in acute subdeltoid bursitis

I. S. Klemes, *Industrial Medicine and Surgery*, June 1957

Many neurological symptoms like neuropathies, trigeminal neuralgias, and nervous degeneration diseases have been treated with vitamin B_{12}. This study showed that bursitis with calcification would respond quickly to B_{12} and as the neurological symptoms improved, the absorption of calcium deposits would follow.

354. The carpal tunnel syndrome as a probable primary deficiency of vitamin B_6 rather than a deficiency of a dependency state

Satoshi Shizukuishi, et al., *Biochemical and Biophysical Research Communications*, Vol. 95, No. 3, 1980, pp. 1126–1130

Ten patients with severe carpal tunnel syndrome were found to be deficient in vitamin B_6 and all achieved great clinical improvement on treatment with B_6 supplementation.

355. Type 1 allergic reactions to plant-derived foods: a consequence of primary sensitization to pollen allergens

Rudolf Valenta and Dietrich Kraft, *J. Allergy Clin. Immunol.*, Vol. 97, No. 4, April 1996, pp. 893–895

This study hypothesizes that allergies to pollen can overlap into allergies to foods that contain similar proteins. For example, IgE allergic reactions to a mugwort protein, could lead to cross-reaction allergies to celery, apples, peanuts, and kiwi fruit. Allergic reactions to birch pollen proteins can cause cross-reaction allergies to hazelnuts or apples.

356. Identification of a simple chemical compound (chlorogenic acid) as an allergen in plant materials causing human atopic disease

Samuel O. Freedman, et al., *The American Journal of the Medical Sciences*, November 1962, pp. 548–555

People who develop asthma, rhinitis, or dermatitis from coffee beans, castor beans, or oranges were all found to be allergic to the phenol chlorogenic acid.

357. Allergy and chronic simple glaucoma

Louis F. Raymond, *Annals of Allergy*, Vol. 22, March 1964, pp. 146–150

Chronic simple glaucoma appears to be a systemic immunological disease that causes vasospasm of the fine blood vessels with subsequent congestion and edema of the eye.

358. High frequency of thyroid dysfunction in patients with vitiligo

Lazlo Hegedus, et al., *Acta Derm. Venereol. (Stockholm)*, Vol. 74, 1994, pp. 120–123

This study showed that 43 percent of patients with vitiligo had problems with their thyroid, indicating that vitiligo may be an autoimmune disease.

359. Decreased tuftsin concentrations in patients who have undergone splenectomy

Zvi Spirer, et al., *British Medical Journal*, December 17, 1977, pp. 1574–1576

Tuftsin is a protein made by the spleen that stimulates the immune system, especially against bacteria. In patients with Hodgkin's disease, tuftsin levels are similar to those of individuals who have had their spleens removed.

360. Immunrestitutive wirkung eines hydrolysates bzw. ultrafiltrates aus rindermilz (Immunorestitution by a bovine spleen hydrolysate and ultrafiltrate)

H. D. Volk, et al., *Arzneim-Forsch../Drug Res.*, 41 (II), Nr.12, 1991, pp. 1281–1285

Bovine spleen extracts improved immune function in radiated mice in 6 to 8 weeks, while the control group took 10 weeks or longer.

361. Neuroendocrine-immune aging: an integrative view on the role of zinc

Nicola Fabris, *Annals New York Academy of Sciences*, Vol. unknown, pp. 353–368

Zinc is an important trace element in ensuring correct total body growth and function throughout life. It is essential for regulating the thymus, spleen, lymph nodes, and Peyer's patches. Zinc is a component of enzymes that destroy free radicals. Many hormones, including growth hormone, thyroid hormone, and melatonin, may increase zinc turnover, and through this effect, they may increment thymic function.

362. Relative contributions of host and microbial factors in bacterial translocation

Carol L. Wells, et al., *Arch. Surg.*, Vol. 126, February 1991, pp. 247–252

Intestinal bacteria can translocate out of the intestine where they can cause complications. Anaerobic species don't translocate as well as aerobic or facultative bacteria, even though they are much more numerous. Antibiotic therapy coupled with intestinal bacterial overgrowth can increase the incidence of bacterial translocation.

363. Partial sleep deprivation reduces natural killer cell activity in humans

Michael Irwin, et al., *Psychosomatic Medicine*, 56, 1994, pp. 493–498

Sleep loss due to depression or bacterial or yeast infection can reduce natural killer cell function, thereby weakening immunity to viral infections.

364. St. John's Wort clinical monograph

Donald J. Brown, *Townsend Letter for Doctors and Patients*, October 1997, pp. 150–151

St. John's Wort contains hypercin, pseudohypericin, x and flavonoids. It acts as an antidepressant possibly by i interleukin-6, a cytokine that may contribute to the incre cortisone production that occurs in major depression. H〉 pseudohypericin have been shown to be responsible for the antiviral properties of St. John's Wort; they exhibit strong antiviral activity against Epstein-Barr virus, influenza A and B, and Herpes simplex virus I and II.

365. A specific type of organism cultivated from malignancy: bacteriology and proposed classification

Virginia Wuerthele-Caspe Livingston and Eleanor Alexander-Jackson, *Annals New York Academy of Sciences,* 174: art. 2, 1970, pp. 636–654

Even healthy people can carry a microorganism that is capable of changing from a virus-like body to a mycroplasma-like L-form and even to bacterial shapes. These are consistently found in malignant tissue.

366. Allergy of the lower urinary tract

Norborne B. Powell, et al., *The Journal of Urology,* Vol. 107, April 1972, pp. 631–634

Patients with recurrent urinary symptoms improved with treatment for allergies.

367. Allergies of the genito-urinary tract

Norborne B. Powell, *Annals of Allergy,* Vol. 19, September 1961, pp. 1019–1025

Urinary tract allergies are usually caused by foods and drugs. Symptoms can be the same as those of an infection, except no organism is involved but the edema could make the bladder and urethra more susceptible to infection.

The reaction usually peaks four to six hours after the food is eaten. Ninety-five percent of patients can usually overcome allergies to a specific food eventually, and the worst aggravators are citrus, tomatoes, condiments, chocolates, and nuts. The worst times of the year for flareups are Thanksgiving to New Year's and again at Easter, during hayfever season, and when strawberries, tomatoes, and summer fruits are in season.

368. Nonreaginic food allergy in the management of essential hypertension

L. P. Gay, *Journal of Applied Nutrition,* 12, 1959, pp. 71–74

Allergic edema within the capsule of the kidneys can create renal blood and oxygen loss and can result in high blood pressure. Removal of food allergens resulted in reduction of the blood pressure to normal. Reintroduction of allergens caused an increase in blood ressure and pulse rate.

369. Elevation of the pressure in the abdominal inferior vena cava as a cause of a hepatorenal syndrome in cirrhosis

John F. Mullane and Marvin L. Gliedman, *Surgery*, Vol. 59, No. 6, June 1966, pp. 1135–1146

In advanced liver disease, a thickened caudate lobe compresses the inferior vena cava, interfering with kidney function.

370. Hepatic swelling and inferior vena cava constriction

Marvin L. Gliedman, *Annals of Surgery*, March 1965, pp. 344–349

Acute or chronic liver congestion led to liver enlargement that consistently constricted the inferior vena cava. Inferior vena caval constriction has been shown to increase renin output by the kidney.

371. Studies on experimental hypertension. I. The production of persistent elevation of systolic blood pressure by means of renal ischemia

Harry Goldblatt, et al., *J. Exp. Med.*, 59, 1934, pp. 347–379

Constriction of the main renal arteries of both kidneys in dogs is sufficient to elevate systolic blood pressure.

372. Interaction of signals influencing renin release

G. H. Gibbons, et al. *Ann. Rev. Physiol.*, 46, 1984, pp. 291–308

Inferior vena cava constriction can lower arterial pressure, which can interfere with kidney function and lead to increased renin activity, which in turn can result in hypertension.

373. Arterial pressure regulation

Arthur C. Guyton, et al., *The American Journal of Medicine*, Vol. 52, May 1972, pp. 584–594

In a person with essential hypertension, while the output of water and salt may be normal, the function of the kidneys is not normal because the high pressure is necessary to achieve this normal output.

374. Parathyroid hypertensive factor and intracellular calcium regulation

Peter K. T. Pang, et al., *Journal of Hypertension*, 14, 1996, pp. 1053–1060

Low calcium levels can stimulate the parathyroid gland to make parathyroid hypertensive factor (PHF), which makes the smooth muscles of blood vessels more reactive to vasoconstricting hormones. This can result in high blood pressure, which is often seen in people with low renin and salt sensitivity. Similar events may be taking place in type II diabetes and colon and breast cancer. Increasing calcium levels may correct this type of high blood pressure.

375. Inhibited breathing decreases renal sodium excretion

D. E. Anderson, et al., *Psychosomatic Medicine*, 57, 1995, pp. 373–380

Increased sympathetic (adrenal) activity has been shown to raise blood pressure by increasing sodium retention. This study showed that the same result can be observed with inhibited breathing (high normal end tidal CO_2). Inhibited breathing elicited renal sodium and fluid retention, and resulted in increased blood pressure.

376. The rate of increase in blood pressure in children 5 years of age is related to changes in aerobic fitness and body mass index

Steven Shea, et al., *Pediatrics*, Vol. 94, No. 4, October 1994, pp. 465–470

Young children who increase their aerobic fitness or decrease their body mass index reduce their risk of high blood pressure.

377. Effects of cessation of caffeinated-coffee consumption on ambulatory and resting blood pressure in men

H. Robert Superko, et al., *The American Journal of Cardiology*, Vol. 73, April 15, 1994, pp. 780–784

Decreases in ambulatory blood pressure were seen when coffee was discontinued.

378. Does supplementation of diet with 'fish oil' reduce blood pressure?

Lawrence J. Appel, et al., *Arch. Intern. Med.*, Vol. 153, June 28, 1993, pp. 1429–1438

The beneficial effects of omega-3 fish oils include reductions in triglyceride levels, coronary artery disease, and platelet aggravation, as well as a reduction in blood pressure.

379. Does fish oil lower blood pressure?

Martha Clare Morris, et al., *Circulation*, Vol. 88, No 2, August 1993, pp. 523–533

Patients with high cholesterol and cardiovascular disease showed the greatest lowering of blood pressure on omega-3 fish oil, probably due to its effects on inhibiting thromboxane and stimulating prostacyclin.

380. The dose-dependent reduction in blood pressure through administration of magnesium

L. Widman, et al., *American Journal of Hypertension*, Vol. 6, No. 1, January 1993, pp. 41–45

The use of magnesium in the treatment of high blood pressure resulted in a dose-dependent decrease in blood pressure.

381. Reduction of blood pressure with oral magnesium supplementation in women with mild to moderate hypertension

Jacqueline C. M. Witteman, et al., *Am. J. Clin. Nutr.,* 60, 1994, pp. 129–135

The findings suggest that oral supplementation with magnesium aspartate-HCl may lower blood pressure in subjects with mild to moderate hypertension.

382. Effect of coenzyme Q_{10} on essential arterial hypertension

V. Digiesi, et al., *Current Therapeutic Research,* Vol. 47, No. 5, May 1990, pp. 841–845

CoQ_{10} supplementation was shown to reduce high blood pressure in three to four weeks at 100 mg/day.

383. Calcium supplementation prevents pregnancy-induced hypertension by increasing the production of vascular nitric oxide

P. Lopez-Jaramillo, et al., *Medical Hypotheses,* 45, 1995, pp. 68–72

Nitric acid is crucial for maintaining dilation of blood vessels during pregnancy. Low blood levels of ionized calcium can lead to reduced nitric oxide, which can cause hypertension in pregnancy.

384. Calcium diet supplementation increases urinary sodium excretion in essential hypertension

A. N. Lasardis and A. B. Sofos, *Nephron,* 45, 1987, page 250

Oral calcium supplementation has been shown to lower blood pressure and may be due to its stimulating the kidneys to release sodium in the urine.

385. Chinese kidney tonics and osteoporosis

Paul Bergner, *Medical Herbalism,* Vol. 6, No. 2, Summer 1994, pp. 1 & 14

In Traditional Chinese Medicine, there is an intimate relationship between the kidney and the health of the bones. Fifty-eight women with osteoporosis were treated with herbal formulas tailored to their syndromes, and were later shown to have an increase in bone density.

386. Differences in proximal femur bone density over two centuries

Belinda Lees, et al., *The Lancet,* Vol. 341, March 13, 1993, pp. 673–675

X-ray evaluations of bones from an English churchyard showed that women two hundred years ago had much stronger bones, both pre- and post-menopausally. Factors that may influence bone density include exercise, diet, smoking, and alcohol consumption.

387. Acute effects of dietary caffeine and sucrose on urinary mineral excretion of healthy adolescents

Linda K. Massey and Patsy W. Hollingbery, *Nutrition Research,* Vol. 8, 1988, pp. 1005–1012

In this study, 18 teenagers were given morning soft drinks that contained caffeine, sucrose, or both. The ingestion of caffeine increased the loss of calcium in the urine, particularly when combined with sucrose. Use of soft drinks in place of milk may lead to long-term calcium deficiency problems.

388. Are stone-formers maladapted to refined carbohydrates?

P. N. Rao, et al., *British Journal of Urology,* 54, 1982, pp. 575–577

Kidney stones are more common in developed countries and may be related to diet, particularly those rich in refined carbohydrates. Insulin may be responsible for the renal leak of calcium.

389. Anabolic effects of insulin on bone suggest a role for chromium picolinate in preservation of bone density

M. F. McCarty, *Medical Hypotheses,* 45, 1995, pp. 241–246

Efficient insulin activity may have a building effect on bone; this may explain why Type I diabetics tend to have reduced bone density. Chromium (which is necessary to make insulin effective) has been found to reduce urinary loss of calcium in postmenopausal women.

390. Boron an overlooked element of potential nutritional importance

Forrest H. Nielsen, *Nutrition Today,* Jan./Feb. 1988, pp. 4–7

Boron improves calcium and magnesium absorption, particularly if vitamin D is low, which indicates it may play a role in the activation of vitamin D. Rich sources of boron are fruits, vegetables, and nuts; poor sources are meat and fish.

391. Boron enhances and mimics some effects of estrogen therapy in postmenopausal women

Forrest H. Nielsen, et al., *The Journal of Trace Elements in Experimental Medicine,* 5, 1992, pp. 237–246

Lack of boron in the diet can induce problems with estrogen and calcium metabolism. Boron is found mainly in vegetables and fruits.

392. Hip fractures and fluoridation in Utah's elderly population

Christa Danielson, et al., *JAMA,* Vol. 268, No. 6, August 12, 1992, pp. 746–748

Fluoridation of the water supply to 1 ppm was associated with an increase in the rate of hip fracture in men and women.

393. Spinal bone loss and ovulatory disturbances

Jerilynn C. Prior, et al., *The New England Journal of Medicine*, Vol. 323, No. 18, November 1, 1990, pp. 1221–1227

Inadequate production of progesterone is associated with accelerated bone loss, even if estradiol levels and menstrual cycles are normal. The rate of spinal bone loss of 4 percent per year could result in significant bone loss even before menopause.

394. Estrogen promotes apoptosis of murine osteoblast mediated by TGF-beta

D. E. Hughes, *Nat. Med.*, 2, 1996, pp. 1132–1136

Estrogen was found to increase apoptosis by two to three times in osetoclasts, the cells that break down bone. Transforming growth factor beta (TGF-beta), a regulatory protein made by osteoblasts (bone-building cells), also increased apoptosis in osteoclasts. Estrogen may slow down postmenopausal bone loss by inducing apoptosis of osteoclasts.

395. Is natural progesterone the missing link in osteoporosis prevention and treatment?

J. R. Lee, *Medical Hypotheses*, 35, 1991, pp. 316–318

Estrogen supplements have been shown to delay bone loss but do not reverse it. Lifestyle factors can contribute to osteoporosis. In a study of 100 postmenopausal women, progesterone cream was effective in reversing osteoporosis, with no side effects.

396. [Progesterone protects against heart disease]

Nature Medicine, 1997, page 3

Progesterone protects against heart disease by directly inhibiting DNA synthesis in smooth muscle cells. This inhibits the proliferation of arterial smooth muscle cells, which is a major factor in the development of atherosclerotic plaques.

397. Effects of extracts from Cimicifuga racemosa on gonadotropin release in menopausal women and ovariectomized rats

Eva-Maria Düker, et al., *Planta Med.*, 57, 1991, pp. 420–424

Menopausal symptoms occur as decreased estrogen production fails to inhibit pituitary gland production of lutenizing hormone (LH) which then creates hot flushes and depression. This study showed that an alcohol extract of Cimicifuga racemosa (black cohosh), taken for two months, was able to reduce these symptoms due to its estrogen-like properties. Earlier studies showed that Cimicifuga racemosa also reduced vaginal problems due to menopause.

398. Intestinal calcium absorption and serum vitamin D metabolites in normal subjects and osteoporotic patients

J. C. Gallagher, et al., *J. Clin. Invest.,* Vol. 64, September 1979, pp. 729–736

This study showed that osteoporotic patients as well as normal elderly people have normal levels of 25-hydroxyvitamin D (made by the liver), but levels of 1,25-dihydroxyvitamin D are significantly decreased. The 1,25-dihydroxyvitamin D is the much more active version of vitamin D that is made by the kidneys and it stimulates calcium absorption in the intestine.

399. Do tumor promoters affect DNA after all?

Jean L. Marx, *Science,* Vol. 219, January 14, 1983, pp. 158–159

Chemicals that promote cancer may do so by stimulating certain white blood cells, such as neutrophils, to produce a burst of superoxide radicals about 40 seconds after exposure. This appears to activate the formation of arachidonic acid from membrane fats and thus the formation of prostaglandins, thromboxanes, and leukotrienes. The arachidonic acid cascade may be the transmitter of the DNA damage started by the chemical.

400. Evidence that Serenoa repens extract displays an antiestrogenic activity in prostatic tissue of benign prostatic hypertrophy patients

F. Di Silverio, et al., *Eur. Urol.,* 21, 1992, pp. 309–314

In benign prostatic hyperplasia patients, Serenoa repens extract is effective in inhibiting the growth of prostatic tissue by inhibiting estrogen receptors and 5α-reductase enzyme.

401. Benign prostatic hyperplasia – treatment with an extract from the fruit of Sabal serrulata. A drug monitoring study involving 1,334 patients

Von W. Vahlensieck, Jr., et al., *Fortschr. Med.,* 111. Jg, Nr. 18, 1993, pp. 323–326

In this study, 1,334 patients with benign prostatic hyperplasia were treated for 12 weeks with Sabal serrulata (saw palmetto berry) extract and there was a significant reduction in irritative symptoms.

402. Geographic patterns of prostate cancer mortality: evidence for a protective effect of ultraviolet radiation

Carol L. Hanchette and Gary G. Schwartz, *Cancer,* Vol. 70. No. 12, December 15, 1992, pp. 2861–2869

On autopsy, older men are commonly found to have "latent" prostate cancer, regardless of country or race. Black American men have the highest prostate cancer mortality in the world, while black

African men have much lower rates. Japanese men have very low prostate cancer mortality unless they move to the US.

This study indicates an inverse relationship between prostate cancer mortality and ultraviolet light exposure. This is possibly because higher exposure to UV light creates higher levels of vitamin D, which has been shown to have a tumour-inhibiting effect.

403. [The role of ultraviolet light/vitamin D in increased blood pressure]

Hypertension, 30, 1997, pp. 150–156

Lack of exposure to ultraviolet light may contribute to increased blood pressure in higher latitudes. Twenty to 30 percent of ultraviolet B (UVB) radiation is transmitted through white skin, whereas only 5 percent is transmitted through deeply pigmented skin. People with greater amounts of skin pigment require greater amounts of UVB light to produce the same amount of vitamin D found in people with lighter skin.

404. Do diets and androgens alter prostate cancer risk via a common etiologic pathway?

Ronald K. Ross and Brian E. Henderson, *Journal of the National Cancer Institute*, Vol. 86, No. 4, February 16, 1994, pp. 252–254

Prostate cancer is, of all cancers, most closely related to ageing, but race also plays a role. Young adult African-American men have at least 10 percent more testosterone than young adult white men, which may explain the 60 to 70 percent higher prostate cancer rates in older African-American men. Native Chinese and Japanese men have lower 5α-reductase activity than young white and African-American men and have up to 30 times lower incidence of prostate cancer.

The conversion of testosterone to its active form, dihydrotestosterone, is controlled by the enzyme 5α-reductase, which may be manipulated by diet, and red meat may have a negative effect.

High levels of the active form of vitamin D, 1,25-dihydroxyvitamin D, seem to have a strong effect in inhibiting prostate cancer, and levels appear largely unrelated to sunlight exposure and diet.

405. Occupation-related risks for colorectal cancer

Donna Spiegleman and David H. Wegman, *JNCI*, Vol. 75, No. 5, November 1985, pp. 813–821

Colon cancer risk in males increases with exposure to solvents, abrasives, and fuel oil and in those with high-stress jobs. In women, the risk increases with exposure to dyes, solvents, and grinding-wheel dust.

406. Chlorination of drinking water and cancer incidence in Norway

Trond Peder Flaten, *International Journal of Epidemiology,* Vol. 21, No. 1, pp. 6–15

Chlorine is added to drinking water to kill bacteria, but it also reacts with organic molecules to form small amounts of chloroform and chlorinated phenols. Most US studies have shown an association between chlorinated drinking water and cancers of the bladder and the colorectum. This study in Norway showed an increased incidence of cancer of the colon and the rectum.

407. Dietary vitamin D and calcium and risk of colorectal cancer: a 19-year prospective study in men

Cedric Garland, et al., *The Lancet,* February 9, 1985, pp. 307–309

People in northern latitudes and major cities get the least exposure to sunlight and have the highest colon cancer rates. Calcium is believed to have anticancer properties and 1,25-dihydroxyvitamin D inhibits growth of melanoma. Vitamin D and calcium may reduce the risk of colorectal cancer.

408. Oral calcium suppresses increased rectal epithelial proliferation of persons at risk of colorectal cancer

P. Rozen, et al., *Gut,* 30, 1989, pp. 650–655

Patients who have cancer of their bowel often show abnormal proliferation of intestinal cells. Three months of oral calcium carbonate supplementation suppressed much of this abnormal proliferation.

409. [Dietary calcium and colon cancer]

Cancer, 80 (5), 1997, pp. 858–864

Increased levels of dietary calcium appear to be linked to a lower risk of colon cancer.

410. Serum 25-hydroxyvitamin D and colon cancer: eight-year prospective study

Cedric F. Garland, et al., *The Lancet,* November 18, 1989, pp. 1176–1178

These findings suggest that vitamin D metabolites, possibly working in conjunction with calcium, reduce colon cancer risk.

411. Effects of fish oil on rectal cell proliferation, mucosal fatty acids, and prostaglandin E_2 release in healthy subjects

Hans-Peter Bartram, et al., *Gastroenterology,* 105, 1993, pp. 1317–1322

This study showed that dietary fish oil protected against colon cancer, probably by reduction of prostaglandin E_2.

412. Familial clustering of breast and prostate cancers and risk of postmenopausal breast cancer

Thomas A. Sellers, et al., *Journal of the National Cancer Institute*, Vol. 86, No. 24, December 21, 1994, page 1860

Women from families with a history of breast and/or prostate cancer are at increased risk of breast cancer.

413. Enhancing effects of diallyl sulfide on hepatocarcinogenesis and inhibitory actions of the related diallyl disulfide on colon and renal carcinogenesis in rats

Satoru Takahashi, et al., *Carcinogenesis*, Vol. 13, No. 9, 1992, pp. 1513–1518

Diallyl sulfide from garlic was shown to stimulate liver cancer while diallyl disulfide was shown to inhibit colon and kidney cancer.

414. Multistage carcinogenesis in mouse skin

John DiGiovanni, *Pharmac. Ther.*, Vol. 54, 1992, pp. 63–128

In the development of cancer of the skin in mice, three stages were observed. The *initiation* stage involves damage to genes by initiators such as prolonged exposure to polycyclic aromatic hydrocarbons, perhaps epoxides produced by P450 enzymes. This is followed by "locking in" the mutation during DNA replication.

The *promotion* stage consists of a premalignant period of clone hyperplasia and expansion of clone cells to form papillomas. The *progression* stage involves the conversion of papillomas to malignant tumours, though most of the papillomas may spontaneously disappear without becoming malignancies.

Eicosanoids from arachidonic acid may play a major role in the promotion of cancer, and things that inhibit cyclooxygenase enzymes, lipoxygenase enzymes, and phospholipase A_2 enzymes thus counteract cancer promotion. One is quercetin, a bioflavonoid. Other inhibitors are antioxidants, such as vitamins E and C, and the mineral selenium. Agents that stimulate glutathione and superoxide dismutase enzymes also block cancer promotion. Low polyunsaturated fat diets and low caloric diets also inhibit cancer.

415. The induction of ornithine decarboxylase as an early, possibly obligatory, event in mouse skin carcinogenesis

T. G. O'Brien, *Cancer Research*, Vol. 36, July 1976, pp. 2644–2653

Treatment of mouse skin with carcinogenic hydrocarbons resulted in a large increase in the activity of ornithine decarboxylase enzyme and production of putrescine, spermidine, and spermine, which appear to be essential features in preneoplasia. Repeated exposure to carcinogenic hydrocarbons may result in a permanently high level of enzyme activity and an accumulation of putrescine, spermadine, and spermine. Skin tumours showed high levels of ornithine decarboxylase, with malignant tumours having higher levels than benign tumours.

416. Posttranslational regulation of p53 tumor suppressor protein function

Steve A. Maxwell and Jack A. Roth, *Critical Reviews in Oncogenesis*, 5 (1), 1994, pp. 23–57

The p53 protein restricts cell growth but alteration of its shape can shift its function so that it can become a growth promoter instead of a suppressor. Alteration of p53 is the most common denominator seen in human cancers.

417. Flavonoids activate wild-type p53

B. Plaumann, et al., *Oncogene,* 13, 1996, pp. 1605–1614

Certain flavonoids activate p53 protein. This protein causes cells to pause after DNA duplication. These flavonoids also induce apoptosis.

418. Inhibition of neutrophil apoptosis by antioxidants in culture medium

K. Oishi and K. Machida, *Scand. J. Immunol.*, 45, 1997, pp. 21–27

In this study, neutrophils were incubated with superoxide dismutase (the enzyme that converts superoxide radical to hydrogen peroxide and water) and catalase (the enzyme that breaks down hydrogen peroxide). Spontaneous apoptosis of the neutrophils was delayed, suggesting that superoxide radical may be needed for apoptosis.

419. Augmented intracellular glutathione inhibits Fas-triggered apoptosis of activated human neutrophils

R. W. Watson, et al., *Blood,* 89, 1997, pp. 4175–4181

Neutrophils have a receptor protein called Fas that can trigger apoptosis when it binds certain proteins. This study found that added glutathione or N-acetyl cysteine blocked Fas-triggered apoptosis.

420. Peroxynitrite-induced apoptosis in T84 and RAW 264.7 cells: attenuation by L-ascorbic acid

M. Sandoval, et al., *Free Radic. Biol. Med.*, 22, 1997, pp. 489–495

Peroxynitrite is a potent oxidizing agent and generator of free radicals. It is produced during inflammation, as a result of excessive nitric oxide and superoxide. This study showed that when cells were treated with ascorbic acid (vitamin C), peroxynitrite-induced damage and apoptosis was reduced.

421. Taurine modulates platelet aggregation in cats and humans
K. C. Hayes, et al., *Am. J. Clin. Nutr.*, 49, 1989, pp. 1211–1216
Decreased platelet aggregation was associated with decreased thromboxane release on aggregation and with increased platelet taurine. Taurine appears to affect platelet aggregation by increasing the concentration of glutathione.

422. Initiation of chemical carcinogenesis requires cell proliferation
Edmundo Cayama, et al., *Nature*, Vol. 275, September 7, 1978, pp. 60–62
Cancer, whether caused by chemicals, x-rays, or viruses, begins with damage, such as to DNA. This damage must then be "fixed" into the cell by at least one round of cell replication before cancer can develop.

423. Histamine as an autocrine growth factor in experimental mammary carcinomas
G. P. Cricco, et al., *Agents Actions*, 43, 1994, pp. 17–20
Histamine is critical for cell proliferation in experimental breast cancer.

424. The Israeli breast-cancer anomaly
Jerome B. Westin and Elihu Richter, *Annals New York Academy of Sciences*, Vol. unknown, pp. 269–279
Israel is a country with a high incidence of breast cancer but, unlike the rest of the world, breast cancer mortality rates *dropped* by nearly 8 percent between 1976 and 1986. It is believed that this drop was a result of decreasing the use of pesticides that had been contaminating the food chain, especially dairy products. It's likely that lindane, BHC, and DDT had been made carcinogenic by the P450 enzymes.

425. Diet and breast cancer in causation and therapy
Ernst L. Wynder, et al., *Cancer*, 58, October 15 Supplement, 1986, pp. 1804–1813
Postmenopausal breast cancer patients had higher estradiol levels as did the prostatic fluid of prostate cancer patients, which indicates that similar diet-related hormonal dysfunctions underlie both breast and prostate cancer.

426. Cytidine methylation of regulatory sequences near the π-class glutathione S-transferase gene accompanies human prostatic carcinogenesis
Wen-Hsiang Lee, et al., *Proc. Natl. Acad. Sci. USA*, Vol. 91, November 1994, pp. 11733–11737
This study found that prostate cancer patients showed damage to a

gene of the enzyme glutathione transferase, which is important for intracellular detoxification.

427. Inhibition of spontaneous metastasis in a rat prostate cancer model by oral administration of modified citrus pectin

K. J. Pienta, et al., *J. Natl. Cancer Inst.*, 87, 1995, pp. 348–353

Prostate cancer is considered incurable once it has spread (metastasized). Citrus pectin, when its pH is modified, is shown to inhibit rat prostate cancer from spreading.

428. Intake of carotenoids and retinol in relation to risk of prostate cancer

E. Giovannucci et al., *J. Natl. Cancer Inst.*, December 6, 1995, pp. 1767–1776

This study indicated that the risk of prostate cancer was 45 percent lower among those men who consumed at least 10 servings per week of tomato-based foods. Lycopene, a carotenoid in tomatoes, may provide the protective effect.

429. Inhibition of polycyclic aromatic hydrocarbon-DNA adduct formation in epidermis and lungs of SENCAR mice by naturally occurring plant phenols

Mukul Das, et al., *Cancer Research*, 47, February 1, 1987, pp. 767–773

P450 enzymes are capable of converting polycyclic aromatic hydrocarbons into epoxides that can be much more cancer-causing than the original substance. When these epoxides bind to the DNA of lung, skin, or other cells, they can be cancer-causing. P450 enzymes can make four versions of an epoxide, and one of these might be 60 times more cancer-causing than the other three. The plant phenols shown to inhibit this process are tannic acid, quercetin, myricetin, and anthraflavic acid. Ellagic acid has previously been shown to inhibit the binding of epoxides to DNA.

430. Interaction of epicatechins derived from green tea with rat hepatic cytochrome P-450

Zhi Y. Wang, et al., *Drug Metabolism and Disposition*, Vol. 16, No. 1, 1987, pp. 98–103

The phenols of green tea inhibit cancer probably because they inhibit the formation of epoxides by the P450 enzymes. Approximately 25 percent of green tea is flavonoids, which include quercetin, myricetin, and rutin. The most active anticancer component of the flavonoids was epigallocatechin-3-gallate (EGCG).

431. Bacterial vaginosis in pregnancy treated with yoghurt

Alexander Neri, et al., *Acta Obstet. Gynecol. Scand.*, 72, 1993, pp. 17–19

In pregnant women, commercial yogurt applied vaginally helped to restore normal vaginal acidity and flora without side effects.

432. A controlled trial of intravaginal estriol in postmenopausal women with recurrent urinary tract infections

Raul Raz, et al., *The New England Journal of Medicine,* Vol. 329, No. 11, September 9, 1993, pp. 753–756

Vaginal lactobacillus bacteria are stimulated by estrogen to make lactic acid from glycogen, which lowers the vaginal pH enough to inhibit many harmful bacteria. After menopause, the lower estrogen levels lead to a reduction of lactobacillus, higher pH, and an increase in E. Coli bacteria, which are part of the reason for increased postmenopausal urinary tract infections. Application of a vaginal estriol cream showed prevention of urinary tract infections.

433. Menstrual pain in Danish women correlated with low n-3 polyunsaturated fatty acid intake

B. Deutch, *European Journal of Clinical Nutrition,* 49, 1995, pp. 508–516

Women with menstrual cramping are found to have elevated prostaglandins of the 2 series, which are made from omega-6 fatty acids. Increasing the intake of omega-3 fatty acids from fish or whale meat creates more prostaglandins of the 3 series, which result in milder menstrual symptoms.

434. Supplementation with omega-3 polyunsaturated fatty acids in the management of dysmenorrhea in adolescents

Zeev Harel, et al., *Am. J. Obstet. Gynecol.,* Vol. 174, No. 4, April 1996, pp. 1335–1338

This study showed that omega-3 fish oil supplementation reduced the symptoms of dysmenorrhea in adolescents, probably due to decreased production of prostaglandin E_2 and leukotriene A_4.

435. Estrogen replacement therapy and fatal ovarian cancer

Carmen Rodriguez, et al., *American Journal of Epidemiology,* Vol. 141, No. 9, 1995, pp. 828–835

In peri- and postmenopausal women, the prolonged use of estrogen replacement therapy may increase the risk of ovarian cancer.

436. The risk of breast cancer after estrogen and estrogen-progestin replacement

Leif Bergkvist, et al., *The New England Journal of Medicine,* Vol. 321, No 5, August 3, 1989, pp. 293–297

The use of estrogens for menopausal symptoms was associated

with greater risk of breast cancer, which increased to as high as 70 percent with increasing duration of treatment. The stronger estrogens such as estradiol increased the risk while estriol showed no increased risk. Progestin offered no protection against breast cancer development.

437. Biliary excretion and intestinal metabolism of progesterone and estrogens in man

H. Adlercreutz and F. Martin, *Journal of Steroid Biochemistry*, Vol. 13, 1980, pp. 231–244

Estrogens and progesterone are altered by the liver and secreted via the bile into the intestine, where the intestinal flora and digestive enzymes can make them stronger or weaker; some of them are then reabsorbed. This is called enterohepatic circulation of steroid hormones, and liver function can profoundly influence it.

438. In vitro metabolism of estrogens by isolated intestinal micro-organisms and by human faecal microflora

Paula Järvenpää, et al., *Journal of Steroid Biochemistry*, Vol. 13, 1980, pp. 345–349

Antibiotics alter the metabolism of steroid hormones by affecting the intestinal flora's ability to convert hormones. Some strains of bacteria can convert estrone to 16α-hydroxyestrone in the gut.

439. Breast cancer incidence in women with a history of progesterone deficiency

Linda D. Cowan, et al., *American Journal of Epidemiology*, Vol. 114, No. 2, 1981, pp. 209–217

It has been suggested that "in the absence of sufficient cyclic progesterone production, the breast is exposed to a continuous, unopposed estrogen stimulus and that under conditions of altered ovarian function, the breast may also be subjected to the products of disordered secretion of numerous ovarian and pituitary hormones."

In this study, women with a history of low progesterone production had a fivefold increased risk of premenopausal breast cancer, compared to women without such history.

440. Estradiol/progesterone interaction in normal and pathologic breast cells

Pierre Mauvais-Jarvis, et al., *Annals New York Academy of Sciences*, Vol. unknown, pp. 152–167

Estradiol increases breast cell multiplication while progesterone has the opposite effect. Low progesterone, over a period of time, may allow unopposed estradiol to promote breast cancer.

441. The war on cancer: failure of therapy and research

N. J. Temple and D. P. Burkitt, *The Royal Society of Medicine,* Vol. 84, February 1991, pp. 95–98

Therapeutic medicine has had little impact on the toll taken by the major cancers. In fact, medicine has a poor ability to cure virtually any of the Western diseases. The majority of cancer is related to lifestyle factors, and this dictates that the main goal should be prevention.

442. Diet and breast cancer: the possible connection with sugar consumption

Stephen Seely and David F. Horrobin, *Hypotheses,* 11, 1983, pp. 319–327

When women adopt the diet of a country they move to, they acquire the risk of breast cancer of that country. Animal fats and sugar are suspected of influencing carcinogens. Sugar may be linked to breast cancer because insulin secretion rises with increased blood sugar; insulin has effects similar to estrogen and prolactin, and stimulates proliferation of breast tissue.

443. Dietary fat and cancer trends - a critique

Mary G. Enig, et al., *Federation Proceedings,* Vol. 37, No. 9, July 1978, pp. 2215–2220

Cancer may be caused by eating trans fatty acids found in partially hydrogenated vegetable fats, including margarine, refined oils, and vegetable shortening. Trans fatty acids affect cell function and repress mitochondrial enzyme function.

444. Dietary ω-3 polyunsaturated fats and breast cancer

William T. Cave, Jr., *Nutrition,* Vol. 12, No. 1, 1996 Supplement, pp. S39–S42

Dietary increases in omega-6 oils, like corn or sunflower oil, increases the growth rate of many tumours, including breast, whereas equivalent increases in omega-3 fish oils slows the development of tumours. These differences are probably due to the alteration in the production of eicosanoids, especially leukotrienes.

445. Diet and ovarian cancer

David A. Snowdon, *JAMA,* Vol. 254, No. 3, July 19, 1985, pp. 356–357

This study followed the diets of over 16,000 white California Seventh-Day Adventist women to see if diet correlated with death from ovarian cancer. Of 50 women who died of ovarian cancer over a span of 20 years, it was determined that those who frequently ate fried foods, especially fried eggs, had the greatest risk of ovarian cancer.

446. Apparent partial remission of breast cancer in 'high risk' patients supplemented with nutritional antioxidants, essential fatty acids, and coenzyme Q_{10}

K. Lockwood, *Molec. Aspects Med.*, Vol. 15 (Supplement), 1994, pp. S231–S240

Impaired biosynthesis of CoQ_{10} may be a factor in the cause of many immune disorders as it was found that supplementing with CoQ_{10} increased IgG levels. Thirty-two women with breast cancer that had spread to the lymph nodes, and, in some, to the bone, were treated with antioxidants, essential fatty acids, and CoQ_{10} for 18 months. Six of them experienced partial remission and the remaining 26 patients showed improvement in clinical condition. The recommendation is to use 300 mg of CoQ_{10} per day.

447. Cosupplementation with coenzyme Q prevents the prooxidant effect of α-tocopherol and increases the resistance of LDL to transition metal-dependent oxidation initiation

Shane R. Thomas, et al., *Arteriosclerosis, Thrombosis, and Vascular Biology,* Vol. 16, No. 5, May 1996, pp. 687–696

Supplementation with vitamin E *increased* the lipid peroxidation of LDL but supplementation with vitamin E *and* CoQ_{10} improved the LDL's resistance to oxidation.

448. Supplementation with ubiquinone-10 causes cellular damage during intense exercise

C. Malm, et al., *Acta Physiologica Scandanavica*, 157, 1996, pp. 511–512

Two groups of healthy males between the ages of 20 and 34 carried out vigorous exercise. The group supplemented with CoQ_{10} (60 mg, 2 times daily for 20 days) showed increased creatine kinase levels. This study suggests that under conditions of CoQ_{10} supplementation and high intensity anaerobic exercise, there is increased cell damage, possibly due to increased free radical production. High intensity anaerobic exercise can increase the proton concentration in the intramembrane component of the mitochondria, and promote free radical formation at the site of CoQ_{10}.

449. Estriol, the forgotten estrogen?

Alvin H. Follingstad, *JAMA*, Vol. 239, No. 1, January 2, 1978, pp. 29–30

The three active estrogens are estrone (E_1), estradiol (E_2), the main ovarian estrogen, and estriol (E_3), the mildest estrogen. E_3 is mainly converted from E_1 and E_2 and it is made in large quantities by the placenta during pregnancy.

Estrone may be more cancer-causing than estradiol but most estradiol, including the commercial ones, is converted into estrone in the woman's small intestine. Diethylstilbestrol, used in the treatment of breast cancer, is not a steroid but is as cancer-causing as estrone. Estriol, when given orally, remains estriol and may even be anticancerous.

450. Estriol in the management of the menopause
Vassilios A. Tzingounis, et al., *JAMA*, Vol. 239, No. 16, April 21, 1978, pp. 1638–1641

In postmenopausal women, the mild hormone estriol (E_3) relieves symptoms without detrimental side effects.

451. Effects of dietary fish oil on human mammary carcinoma and on lipid-metabolizing enzymes
Charlotte E. Borgeson, et al., *Lipids*, Vol. 24, No. 4, 1989, pp. 290–295

A diet high in polyunsaturated fats increases the risk of breast cancer, possibly by increasing prostaglandin production, while fish oils in the diet may reduce tumours.

452. [Intake of trans fatty acids and breast cancer]
Cancer Epidemiology, Biomarkers, and Prevention, 6, 1997, pp. 705–710

Women who have a higher intake of trans fatty acids may have a greater risk of breast cancer. Trans fatty acids are a type of fat found in items such as margarine, solid vegetable shortening, and fried foods.

453. Consumption of olive oil and specific food groups in relation to breast cancer risk in Greece
Antonia Trichopoulou, *Journal of the National Cancer Institute*, Vol. 87, No. 2, January 18, 1995, pp. 110–116

Greek women have 42 percent of their energy intake from fat while US women have around 35 percent, yet Greek women have substantially lower mortality from breast cancer. This may be because the fat in the Greek diet comes from monounsaturated oils such as olive oil, while the fat in the North American diet comes from margarine and meat.

454. Differential induction of mixed-function oxidase (MFO) activity in rat liver and intestine by diets containing processed cabbage: correlation with cabbage levels of glucosinolates and glucosinolate hydrolysis products
R. McDanell, et al., *Fd. Chem. Toxic.*, Vol. 25, No. 5, 1987, pp. 363–368

Chemicals entering the body can be dealt with in the intestine and liver by the mixed-function oxidase system that consists of Phase 1 and Phase 2 enzymes. The activity of these enzymes can be induced by Brassica (cruciferous) vegetables. The two most active ingredients of cabbage were found to be indole-3-carbinol, which especially stimulates the liver enzymes, and ascorbigen, which has greater effect in the intestine. Brassicas stimulate both Phase 1 and Phase 2 enzymes but the active ingredients can be reduced by long cooking, especially boiling. Savoy cabbage has twice the active ingredients as white cabbage and they are reduced 44 percent by boiling, while the active ingredients in white cabbage are reduced 34 percent. Chopping and then fermenting the cabbage maintained the levels of active ingredients.

455. Plasma concentrations of phyto-oestrogens in Japanese men

Herman Adlercreutz, et al., *The Lancet*, Vol. 342, November 13, 1993, pp. 1209–1210

Seventh Day Adventist men have a lower incidence of prostate cancer, and Japanese men have a low mortality rate from prostate cancer, as it grows very little. Both groups have high quantities of isoflavonoids in their diets, especially from legumes. Isoflavonoids may inhibit the growth of cancer. Genistein from soy may be the most active of these isoflavonoids.

456. Alterations in estradiol metabolism in MCF-7 cells induced by treatment with indole-3-carbinol and related compounds

Toshifuma Niwa, et al., *Steroids*, Vol. 59, September 1994, pp. 523–527

Steroid hormones are broken down in two ways: via the C-2 or the C-16α pathways. The C-16α pathway is somewhat difficult to alter. The C-2 pathway can be enhanced by indole-3-carbinol from cruciferous vegetables. Oral intake is most effective probably because stomach juices enhance the activity of indole-3-carbinol.

457. EcoCancers: do environmental factors underlie a breast cancer epidemic?

Janet Raloff, *Science News*, Vol. 144, July 3, 1993, pp. 10–13

Breast cancer rates are on the rise worldwide, possibly due to exposure to pesticides and other chemicals in the diet that affect estrogen receptors, increasing a person's exposure to estrogen stimulation. Plant estrogens may have the opposite effect.

Alcohol, human papillomavirus, benzo[a]pyrene, and some drugs depress the C-2 hormone breakdown pathway while vigorous exercise, smoking, dioxins, and indole-3-carbinol from cruciferous vegetables stimulate the C-2 pathway to make mild estrogen. Alcohol consumption and electromagnetic waves can inhibit melatonin, and melatonin may inhibit estrogen production at night.

458. Long-term responses of women to indole-3-carbinol or a high fiber diet

H. Leon Bradlow, et al., *Cancer Epidemiology, Biomarkers & Prevention,* Vol. 3, Oct./Nov. 1994, pp. 591–595

Estrogens are broken down by the C-2 or C-16α pathways, the latter of which is suspected to be cancer-inducing, yet difficult to alter. A previous study showed that the C-2 pathway was enhanced within six days of indole-3-carbinol stimulation of P450 enzymes, with few side effects. This three-month study showed a sustained increase in the C-2 pathway in most of the subjects tested.

459. Inhibition of polycyclic aromatic hydrocarbon-induced neoplasia by naturally occurring indoles

Lee W. Wattenberg and William D. Loub, *Cancer Research,* Vol. 38, May 1978, pp. 1410–1413

Indole-3-carbinol (and other indoles from cruciferous vegetables) inhibited breast and stomach tumours in mice.

460. Effects of dietary broccoli on human *in vivo* drug metabolizing enzymes: evaluation of caffeine, oestrone, and chlorzoxazone metabolism

Morten A. Kall, et al., *Carcinogenesis,* Vol. 17, No. 4, 1996, pp. 793–799

Broccoli increases the activity of the Phase 1 liver detoxification enzyme P450 1A2 and the activity of Phase 2 conjugation enzymes involving glutathione and glucuronosyl, thus increasing the C-2 pathway of estrogen breakdown.

461. Effects of dietary indole-3-carbinol on estradiol metabolism and spontaneous mammary tumors in mice

H. Leon Bradlow, et al., Journal unknown, pp. 1571–1574

Cruciferous vegetables contain substances like indole-3-carbinol (I3C) that have anticancer properties due to their ability to stimulate P450 enzymes to break down chemicals and hormones. The P450 enzymes can break steroid hormones at the C-2 or the C-16α positions. The C-16α pathway increases the risk of breast cancer while the C-2 pathway decreases risk. In this study, I3C increased P450 enzyme activity and the C-2 pathway in mice.

462. Role of chemopreventers in human diet

Bozidar Stavric, *Clinical Biochemistry,* Vol. 27, No. 5, 1994, pp. 319–332

Vegetables grown in their optimum growing season have the greatest anticancer effect. Leafy greens from the Brassica family and spinach reduced the cancer-causing effect of some chemicals. Indole-3-carbinol from cruciferous vegetables inhibits the start of cancer.

Lignans have antitumour and antiviral effects. Flavonoids from vegetables, tea, and fruit may reduce heart disease and cancer risk. Curcumin from turmeric is a strong antioxidant that can protect the liver, stimulate glutathione detoxification, and inhibit cancer. Antioxidants in rosemary, sesame, oregano, and ginger can be stronger than α-tocopherol. Isoflavones and phytoestrogens from soybeans appear to lower cancer incidence. Genistein from soy protein can inhibit blood vessels from growing, thus inhibiting tumour growth. Garlic may inhibit stomach cancer and can reduce blood pressure, cholesterol, and triglycerides.

Green tea is anticancerous, and grapes, strawberries, raspberries, citrus, and licorice also have medicinal properties.

463. Caffeic and ferulic acid as blockers of nitrosamine formation
W. Kuenzig, et al., *Carcinogenesis*, Vol. 5, No. 3, 1984, pp. 309–313

Soybeans, oats, and other cereals are high in caffeic acid and ferulic acid, which block nitrosation and reduce the cancer-inducing effect of polycyclic hydrocarbons.

464. High-performance liquid chromatographic determination of glucosinolates in Brassica vegetables
J. M. Betz and W. D. Fox, *American Chemical Society, Symposium Series*, No. 546, 1993, pp. 181–196

Sea cabbage, a small wild plant of Western Europe, is the source of many of the varieties of the Brassica (cruciferae) genus eaten today. They have been used for gout, diarrhea, stomach trouble, deafness, headache, wound-healing, and mushroom poisoning.

There are over 100 sulphur-containing glucosinolates, a few of which may be found in a specific species. In rats, cabbage and cauliflower have been shown to reduce liver and breast tumours. Phase 1 enzymes may detoxify foreign compounds but they can also make inert substances more active, which can be cancer-causing, while Phase 2 enzymes may protect against dietary cancer.

Cabbage increased Phase 1 enzyme activity in the small intestine, while brussels sprouts increased Phase 1 enzyme activity in the intestines and liver, and Phase 2 enzyme activity in the liver. Sulforaphane from broccoli was found to stimulate Phase 2 quinone reductase enzyme. Stir frying for five minutes was the least destructive of the cooking methods. Raw, freeze-dried, and frozen broccoli showed the highest levels of glucosinolates.

465. [Broccoli sprouts provide cancer protection]
Proceedings of the National Academy of Sciences, 94, 1997, pp. 10367–10372

Small amounts of three-day-old broccoli sprouts have been found to contain as much cancer protection as larger amounts of full-grown broccoli. Sulforaphane is the active ingredient that provides cancer protection.

466. Inhibitory effects of the natural products indole-3 carbinol and sinigrin during initiation and promotion phases of 4-nitroquinoline 1-oxide-induced rat-tongue carcinogenesis
Takuji Tanaka, et al., *Jpn. J. Cancer Res.,* 83, August 1992, pp. 835–842

Indole-3 carbinol (found in cruciferous vegetables) was shown to inhibit cancer of the tongue in rats, possibly by activating the enzyme glutathione transferase.

467. Inhibition of the tobacco-specific nitrosamine-induced lung tumorigenesis by compounds derived from cruciferous vegetables and green tea
F. -L. Chung, et al., *Annals New York Academy of Sciences,* Vol. unknown, pp. 186–202

Cruciferous vegetables and green tea may inhibit the formation of cancerous lung tumours by reducing the production of free radicals.

468. Pulmonary carcinogenesis and its prevention by dietary polyphenolic compounds
Andre Castonguay, *Annals New York Academy of Sciences,* Vol. unknown, pp. 177–185

This study shows that ellagic acid inhibits the development of lung cancer, probably by inhibiting Phase 1 detoxification enzymes, and/or stimulating the Phase 2 enzyme glutathione transferase, and/or protecting membranes from free radicals. Ellagic acid is a polyphenol found in grapes, strawberries, raspberries, and pomegranates.

469. Inhibition of chemical carcinogens by minor dietary components
Lee W. Wattenberg, *Molecular Interrelations of Nutrition and Cancer,* 1982, pp. 43–56

Studies show that a diet high in vegetables, especially cabbage, brussels sprouts, cauliflower, mustard greens, kale, lettuce, celery, and tomatoes, inhibits cancer.

470. Altered estrogen metabolism and excretion in humans following consumption of indole-3-carbinol

Jon J. Michnovicz and H. Leon Bradlow, *Nutrition and Cancer,* Vol. 16, No. 1, 1991, pp. 59–64

Diets high in cruciferous vegetables are associated with decreased colon, lung, and other cancers. Indole-3-carbinol (I3C) from cruciferous vegetables has been shown to inhibit breast cancer in rats and mice. Oral administration of I3C stimulates Phase 1 P450 enzymes and Phase 2 detoxification enzymes to break down estradiol through the C-2 pathway, rather than the C-16α pathway, and this results in less active hormones. Low body fat, increased aerobic exercise, and low fat diets have also been shown to increase the C-2 pathway. In this study, both men and women showed increased breakdown of estradiol via the C-2 pathway within seven days on five to seven mg/kg/day of I3C.

471. Phytoestrogens: epidemiology and a possible role in cancer protection

Herman Adlercreutz, *Environmental Health Perspectives,* Vol. 103, Suppl. 7, October 1995, pp. 103–108

The Western diet is one of the main causes of breast, prostate, and colon cancer and coronary heart disease, primarily due to the diet's effect on hormone metabolism. Two plant estrogen groups (phytoestrogens) have been found to reduce these diseases: lignans and isoflavonoids.

Lignans are found bound to the fibre of grains, seeds, berries, and nuts, and are lost with modern milling. The strongest isoflavonoid is genistein, found in soy protein. Lignans and isoflavonoids are converted by the gut bacteria into many active forms that can be blocked by antibiotics. The active forms are anticarcinogenic, antiviral, bactericidic, and fungistatic. Both lignans and genistein stimulate the liver to manufacture sex hormone-binding globulin (SHBG), which reduces the effect of testosterone and estradiol.

Breast cancer patients have low levels of SHBG. Genistein inhibits breast tumour development. Men who eat tofu, dark rye bread, and legumes have less incidence of prostate cancer.

472. Genistein and biochanin A inhibit the growth of human prostate cancer cells but not epidermal growth factor receptor tyrosine autophosphorylation

Greg Peterson and Stephen Barnes, *The Prostate,* 22, 1993, pp. 335–345

Asians get less prostate cancer than Americans, unless they move to the USA and adopt the American diet. A study of the Asian diet shows that soybeans have anticancer properties. Genistein and biochanin A from soy don't affect estrogen receptors and don't completely stop the activation of cancer, but they do appear to inhibit the growth of prostate cancer.

473. Soy metabolite in Asian diet stimulates cancer suppressor gene
Norman Bauman, *Urology Times of Canada*, October 1997, page 6

Genistein, found in soy, inhibits prostate cancer by increasing the transcription of the p21WAF1 gene. This gene is responsible for inducing cell cycle arrest and apoptosis. Genistein also inhibits the 5α-reductase enzyme.

474. Mechanism of antimutagenicity of wheat sprout extracts
Bogumila Peryt, et al., *Mutation Research,* 269, 1992, pp. 201–215

The anticancer effects of wheat sprouts are due to its flavonoids decreasing the activity of P4501A1 and P4502B1.

475. Resting human female breast tissue produces iodinated proteins
Judy M. Strum, et al., *Journal of Ultrastructure Research,* 84, 1983, pp. 130–139

Epithelial cells in the terminal parts of the breast secrete protein bound to iodine when stimulated by hormones.

476. Etiology of mammary gland pathophysiology induced by iodine deficiency
Bernard A. Eskin, et al., *In Medeiros-Neto C. Caitan Eiedsi: Frontiers in Thyroidology.* Proceedings of the Ninth International Congress. 1985. Sao Paolo. Brazil. Vol. 2 Plenum. New York, 1986, pp. 1027–1031

In women, iodine is necessary for normal breast growth, protects against breast cysts, and can reduce the risk of breast cancer.

477. Iodine replacement in fibrocystic disease of the breast
William R. Ghent, et al., *CJS,* Vol. 36, No. 5, October 1993, pp. 453–460

Fifty to 80 percent of North American women experience fibrocystic breast disease, with a buildup of cystic fluid that is high in potassium. Iodine, but not iodide salt, helps the breast neutralize estrogen stimulation, thus protecting against cysts and malignancy.

478. Tamoxifen and quercetin interact with type-II estrogen binding sites and inhibit the growth of human melanoma cells
Mauro Piantelli, et al., *The Journal of Investigative Dermatology,* Vol. 105, No. 2, August 1995, pp. 248–253

Flavonoids, especially quercetin, can bind to some estrogen binding sites in breast, ovarian, colorectal, meningeal, and leukemic tumour cells, thereby inhibiting melanoma cell growth. Tamoxifen acts in a similar way as quercitin.

479. Processed meats and risk of childhood leukemia (California, USA)

John M. Peters, et al., *Cancer Causes and Control* , Vol. 5, 1994, pp. 195–202

A study was done in Los Angeles to explore possible contributing factors of childhood leukemia. Factors that were studied included environmental chemcals, electric and magnetic fields, and parents' and child's medical history and diet, including beverages. The only positive correlations were the number of hot dogs eaten by the child and the father. No protection was apparently provided by fruit intake. Hot dogs are thought to contain precursors (e.g., nitrite) of N-nitroso compounds, which may be associated with leukemia risk.

480. Diabetes produced in mice by smoked/cured mutton

T. Helgason, et al., *The Lancet*, November 6, 1982, pp. 1017–1021

Icelandic children, especially males, that were conceived in January and born in October, have a higher incidence of diabetes. This correlates with the increased consumption of nitrate-cured mutton by Icelanders, from Christmas through New Year's. In this study, mice were fed a diet high in smoked mutton cured with nitrates to see if there might be a connection between nitrate consumption and diabetes in offspring. Sixteen percent of male offspring and 4 percent of female offspring developed diabetes and showed death of the pancreatic cells, while their parents showed no blood sugar problems.

481. Reduced risk of esophageal cancer associated with green tea consumption

Yu Tang Gao, et al. *Journal of the National Cancer Institute*, Vol. 86, No. 11, June 1, 1994, pp. 855–858

Green tea reduced the risk of esophageal cancer 20 percent among men and 50 percent among women; this effect may be due to green tea's strong antioxidant properties. Nonsmokers and those who don't drink alcohol showed even greater risk reductions.

482. Inhibition of 4-nitroquinoline-1-oxide-induced rat tongue carcinogenesis by the naturally occurring plant phenolics caffeic, ellagic, chlorogenic and ferulic acids

Takuji Tanaka, et al. *Carcinogenesis*, Vol. 14, No. 7, 1993, pp. 1321–1325

Four plant phenolics, especially caffeic acid and ellagic acid, found in vegetables, fruits, and nuts, are excellent inhibitors of tongue carcinogenesis when given during the initiation phase of carcinogenesis.

483. Dietary phyto-oestrogens and the menopause in Japan
Herman Aldercreutz, et al., *The Lancet*, Vol. 339, May 16, 1992, page 1233

Japanese women have fewer hot flushes than Canadian women, which may relate to their higher levels of isoflavonoids from soy. Isoflavonoids are phytoestrogens that may reduce menopausal symptoms.

484. Enhancement of tissue glutathione for antioxidant and immune functions in malnutrition
Tammy M. Bray and Carla G. Taylor, *Biochemical Pharmacology*, Vol. 47, No. 12, 1994, pp. 2113–2123

Glutathione concentrations play a critical role in antioxidant and immune functions, help regulate leukotriene and prostaglandin metabolism, and control cell proliferation. Low levels of glutathione can lead to increased toxicity and disease.

485. [Glutathione and T cell funcion]
Leonard A. Herzenberg, *Proceedings of the National Academy of Sciences*, 94, March 1997, pp. 1967–1972

When T cells are depleted of glutathione, T cell function and viability are impaired.

486. Stimulatory effect of Silibinin on the DNA synthesis in partially hepatectomized rat livers: non-response in hepatoma and other malign cell lines
Author(s) unknown, *Biochemical Pharmacology*, Vol. 35, No. 3, 1986, pp. 538–541

The flavonoid lignan Silibinin from the milk thistle plant stimulates liver RNA synthesis activity by 20 percent, which increases the liver's production of protein. No effect on the DNA of normal cells or malignant cells was seen, indicating that Silibinin is unlikely to be a cancer promoter.

487. Endogenous hormones as a major factor in human cancer
Brian E. Henderson, et al., *Cancer Research*, Vol. 42, August 1982, pp. 3232–3239

Failure of the testes to descend in the third trimester may be due to excessive free estrogen in the first trimester of pregnancy. This can result in a twelvefold increased risk of testis cancer in the affected testis and a threefold increased risk in the unaffected testis.

488. Are oestrogens involved in falling sperm counts and disorders of the male reproductive tract?

Richard M. Sharpe and Niels E. Skakkebaek, *The Lancet*, Vol. 341, May 29, 1993, pp. 1392–1395

Male reproductive tract disorders, such as testicular cancer and lower sperm counts, have increased over the last 30 to 50 years in many countries and may have a common cause. Synthetic estrogens like birth control pills, plant estrogens, dairy estrogens, and estrogenic chemicals may create changes during development of the fetus that leads to these problems.

489. Medical hypothesis: xenoestrogens as preventable causes of breast cancer

Devra Lee Davis, et al., *Environmental Health Perspectives*, Vol. 101, No. 5, October 1993, pp. 372–377

Steady increases in breast and testicular cancers and reduced sperm counts may be related to chlorinated chemicals and drugs that alter the breakdown of steroid hormones.

Pathway 1 results in mild hormones and is stimulated by indole-3-carbinol, low-caloric high-fibre diets, and exercise. Pathway 1 is inhibited by cimetidine, an antacid drug. Pathway 2 produces 16α-hormones that increase the risk of cancer. It is stimulated by alcohol and linoleic and arachidonic acids. Chemicals could alter cancer risk by their effects on P450 enzymes.

490. High sperm density among members of organic farmers' association

Annette Abell, et al., *The Lancet*, Vol. 343, June 11, 1994, page 1498

In a study of Danish greenhouse workers, an unexpectedly high sperm density was found in members of an association of organic farmers who used no pesticides or chemical fertilizer.

491. Ascorbic acid protects against endogenous oxidative DNA damage in human sperm

Cesar G. Fraga, et al., *Proc. Natl. Acad. Sci. USA*, Vol. 88 , December 1991, pp. 11003–11006

There are about 20 types of oxidative DNA damage that can occur to sperm cells and these could lead to birth defects, genetic diseases, and cancer. Sperm taken from healthy 20 to 50-year-old males showed approximately 25,000 adducts per sperm cell. Increasing vitamin C from 5 mg/per day doubled the vitamin C in the seminal fluid within four weeks, and reduced sperm adducts by 36 percent.

492. Effect of cadmium and cigarette smoking on human semen quality

S. E. Chia, et al., *Int. J. Fertil.*, 39(5), 1994, pp. 292–298

Human sperm quality has decreased dramatically over the last few decades and pesticides, lead, and radiation are a few of the environmental toxins that might be involved. Cigarette smoke contains several hundred substances. This study shows that cigarette smoking affects sperm density and cadmium could be one of the agents in cigarette smoke that lowers sperm count.

493. Effect of zinc administration on seminal zinc and fertility of oligospermic males

Manorama Tikkiwal, et al., *Ind. J. Physiol. Pharmac.*, Vol. 31, No. 1, January–March 1987, pp. 30–34

Fourteen infertile males between the ages of 24 and 45 were given oral zinc supplement for four months. Blood levels of zinc remained the same but seminal fluid zinc levels rose significantly. Sperm count as well as motility increased and the wives of three patients conceived.

494. One cancer warrants closer look

Richard Stone, *Science*, Vol. 265, July 15, 1994, page 310

Testicular cancer has increased worldwide by a factor of two to four in the last 50 years, mainly in men 20 to 40 years of age. Environmental estrogens may be the missing link.

495. Hypothesis: dietary management may improve survival from nutritionally linked cancers based on analysis of representative cases

James P. Carter, et al., *Journal of the American College of Nutrition*, Vol. 12, No. 3, 1993, pp. 209–226

Reducing the consumption of meat and dairy products and increasing the intake of cereal grains, legumes, and vegetables, especially of the dark green and yellow variety, helps the body fight against nutritionally linked cancer and hormonal imbalance. Monounsaturated olive oil, omega-3 polyunsaturated fish oils, and medium-chain triglycerides may also be beneficial in fighting cancer. This study shows that in pancreatic cancer patients, the one-year survival rate was higher among those who improved their diets. Dietary changes, involving a high-fibre, vegetable, and low-fat diet, may be associated with increased survival in primary pancreatic cancer, prostate cancer, and possibly other cancers.

ʒar, fat, and the risk of colorectal cancer

Bristol, et al., *British Medical Journal*, Vol. 291, November 23, 1985, pp. 1467–1470

Patients with colon cancer were found to consume more energy than control subjects, mainly in the form of carbohydrate and fat. The mortality rate from colorectal cancer is greater among overweight subjects. This study suggests that a high intake of sugars depleted in fibre, especially if they are eaten with fat (as in cakes, cookies, etc.,) predisposes to the development of colon cancer.

497. Diet and carcinogenesis

Adrianne E. Rogers, et al., *Carcinogenesis*, Vol. 14, No. 11, 1993, pp. 2205–2217

The following are found to inhibit some cancers: vitamin A and other retinoids, natural product diets, diets high in whole grains, fruit, fibre and vegetables (especially cruciferous), selenium and other minerals, and free phytic acid.

498. Inhibitory effects of α-carotene on proliferation of the human neuroblastoma cell line GOTO

Michiaki Murakoshi, et al., *Journal of the National Cancer Institute*, Vol. 81, No. 21, November 1, 1989, pp. 1649–1652

Carotene in palm oil consists of 30 percent α-carotene, 60 percent β-carotene, and 10 percent other carotenoids, which is about the same as those in carrots. This study showed that α-carotene from palm oil was 10 times more inhibitory to neuroblastoma cancer development than β-carotene.

499. Potent preventive action of α-carotene against carcinogenesis: spontaneous liver carcinogenesis and promoting stage of lung and skin carcinogenesis in mice are suppressed more effectively by α-carotene than β-carotene

Michiaki Murakoshi, et al., *Cancer Research*, 52, December 1, 1992, pp. 6583–6587

This study showed that α-carotene inhibited cancer of the liver, lungs, and skin far more than β-carotene.

500. Lycopene as the most efficient biological carotenoid singlet oxygen quencher

Paolo Di Mascio, et al., *Archives of Biochemistry and Biophysics*, Vol. 274, No. 2, November 1, 1989, pp. 532–538

Lycopene has a singlet oxygen-quenching rate more than 100 times greater than α-tocopherol and β-carotene has a rate 50 times greater. Bilirubin also has a greater quenching ability than α-tocopherol.

501. Intake of carotenoids and retinol in relation to risk of prostate cancer

Edward Giovannucci, et al., *Journal of the National Cancer Institute,* Vol. 87, No. 23, December 6, 1995, pp. 1767–1776

Lycopene from tomatoes may reduce the risk of prostate cancer while other carotenoids are unrelated to risk.

502. Tomatoes and risk of digestive-tract cancers

Silvia Franceschi, et al., *Int. J. Cancer,* 59, 1994, pp. 181–184

This study of Northern Italians showed that a high intake of tomatoes provided protection against cancer of the mouth, throat, esophagus, stomach, colon, and rectum.

503. Lycopene is a more potent inhibitor of human cancer cell proliferation than either α-carotene or β-carotene

Joseph Levy, et al., *Nutrition and Cancer,* Vol. 24, No. 3, 1995, pp. 257–266

The novel finding in this report is that lycopene is much more potent than α- and β-carotene in inhibiting human endometrial, mammary, and lung cancer cell growth.

504. Skin lycopene is destroyed preferentially over β-carotene during ultraviolet irradiation in humans

Judy D. Ribaya-Mercado, et al., *J. Nutr.,* 125, 1995, pp. 1854–1859

When skin is exposed to UV light, the free radical stress is dealt with in the body cells by lycopene rather than β-carotene, indicating it is a much greater protector of free radical damage.

505. Marked differences in the skin tumor-initiating activities of the optical enantiomers of the diastereomeric benzo[*a*]pyrene 7,8-diol-9,10-epoxides

T. J. Slaga, et al., *Cancer Research* 39, January 1979, pp. 67–71

Polycyclic aromatic hydrocarbons that are chemically unreactive become cancer-causing when metabolized into epoxides that can bind to and damage DNA. The (+)-BP-diol-epoxide 2 is the ultimate carcinogenic form of benzo[*a*]pyrene epoxide.

506. Tumorigenicity of the optical enantiomers of the diastereomeric benzo[*a*]pyrene 7,8-diol-9,10-epoxides in newborn mice: exceptional activity of (+)-7,8-dihydroxy-9,10-epoxy-7,8,9,10-tetrahydrobenzo[*a*]pyrene

M. K. Buening, et al., *Proc. Natl. Acad. Sci. USA,* Vol. 75, No. 11, November 1978, pp. 5358–5361

When benzo[*a*]pyrene is activated into epoxides by liver enzymes, some epoxides can generate up to 40 times more cancers than others.

This appears to be related to the position of the oxygen added by the liver enzymes.

507. Repair of DNA damage induced by benzo[a]pyrene diol-epoxides I and II in human alveolar tumor cells

Peter A. Cerutti, et al., *Cancer Research*, 38, July 1978, pp. 2118–2124

Approximately 1,300 tons of the polycyclic aromatic hydrocarbon benzo[a]pyrene are released into the air in the USA each year. When activated into epoxides that bind to DNA, they can cause DNA damage that can lead to cancer. This DNA damage can be repaired to a degree.

508. Formation and disappearance of benzo[a]pyrene DNA-adducts in mouse epidermis

John DiGiovanni, et al., *Carcinogenesis*, Vol. 6., No. 5, 1985, pp. 741–747

Polycyclic aromatic hydrocarbons have been implicated in cancer of the lung and skin. When they are metabolically activated to epoxides, they can create problems by binding to DNA, where they can become mutagenic and/or carcinogenic. This study with mice found that DNA binding peaked at 24 hours after application of the hydrocarbon. Between 24 to 48 hours after application, the hydrocarbon bound to DNA decreased rapidly as repair began. Hydrocarbons bound to adenine were removed faster than those bound to guanine.

509. Inactivation of DNA-binding metabolites of benzo[a]pyrene and benzo[a]pyrene-7,8-dihydrodiol by glutathione and glutathione S-transferases

S. Hesse, et al., *Carcinogeneis*, Vol. 3, No. 7, 1982, pp. 757–760

Binding of benzo[a]pyrene epoxides to DNA was inhibited slightly by glutathione, and to a greater extent by glutathione transferase enzymes.

510. Regression of aflatoxin B_1-induced hepatocellular carcinomas by reduced glutathione

Anna M. Novi, *Science*, Vol. 212, May 1, 1981, pp. 541–542

Glutathione was administered to rats with aflatoxin-induced liver cancer, and 81 percent were still alive four months after the controls had died. Autopsies suggested a reversion of malignancy was occurring.

511. Effect of ellagic and caffeic acids on covalent binding of benzo[a]pyrene to epidermal DNA of mouse skin in organ culture

Lee Shugart and John Kao, *Int. J. Biochem.*, Vol. 16, No. 5, 1984, pp. 571–573

Ellagic acid, from plant tannins, was shown to inhibit damage to DNA from benzo[a]pyrene epoxides by binding to the epoxide. Caffeic acid, a similar plant phenol, showed no inhibitory effect.

512. Chemoprevention of mouse urinary bladder carcinogenesis by the naturally occurring carotenoid astaxanthin

Takuji Tanaka, et al., *Carcinogenesis*, Vol. 15, No. 1, 1994, pp. 15–19

Approximately 600 carotenoids are found in vegetables, fish, and sea algae. About 10 percent of them are precursors of vitamin A. Lycopene, lutein, astaxanthin, canthaxanthin, and fucoxanthin are not vitamin A precursors. This study was done to see if astaxanthin and canthaxanthin had any anticancer properties. The results showed that astaxanthin inhibited cancer in mice but canthaxanthin was much weaker.

513. Effects of selenium supplementation for cancer prevention in patients with carcinoma of the skin: a randomized controlled trial

Larry C. Clark, et al., *JAMA*, Vol. 276, No. 24, December 25, 1996, pp. 1957–1963

This study used 200 micrograms of selenium per day to see if it would help prevent skin cancer in those with a history of it. While no improvement was seen in skin cancer, there was a significant reduction in incidences of lung, colon, and prostate cancer. No toxicity was observed on 200 micrograms per day, even though it is above the daily recommended dose.

514. Synergistic effect of vitamin E and selenium in the chemoprevention of mammary carcinogenesis in rats

Paula M. Horvath and Clement Ip, *Cancer Research*, 43, November 1983, pp. 5335–5341

Although vitamin E is a stronger antioxidant than selenium, its ability to suppress lipid peroxidation isn't adequate to inhibit tumour formation. However, when used with selenium, it potentiates selenium's ability to inhibit the development of breast tumours in rats fed a diet high in corn oil and subjected to polycyclic aromatic hydrocarbons.

515. The effectiveness of a mixture of β-carotene, α-tocopherol, glutathione, and ascorbic acid for cancer prevention

Gerald Shklar, et al., *Nutrition and Cancer*, Vol. 20, No. 2, 1993, pp. 145–151

Six groups of rats were exposed to a chemical to induce cancer. One group received no supplementation; another group received equal parts of β-carotene, vitamin E, glutathione, and vitamin C. The other four groups received only one of the four supplements. The tumour burden of each group was obtained, a value based on the total number of tumours and mean tumour volume. The group without supplementation had a tumour burden of 11.9 per cubic millimeter, while the group with all four supplements had a tumour burden of only 1 per cubic millimeter. The two groups that received only β-carotene or only glutathione each had a value of 3.5. The vitamin E group had 6.27 and the group that only received vitamin C showed a value of 13.51, which was *greater* than the unsupplemented group. This shows that vitamin C, when used alone, could worsen the growth of cancer, but if used together with other antioxidants, would work synergistically to inhibit cancer growth.

516. Chemopreventive effects of β-carotene, α-tocopherol, and five naturally occurring antioxidants on initiation of hepatocarcinogenesis by 2-amino-3-methylimidazo[4,5-*f*]quinoline in the rat

Hiroyuki Tsuda, et al., *Jpn. J. Cancer Res.*, 85, December 1994, pp. 1214–1219

This study tested a number of antioxidants to see if they could inhibit the initiation of liver cancer in rats exposed to carcinogens. The ones that successfully inhibited the cancer were α-tocopherol (vitamin E), glutathione, vanillin, quercetin, β-carotene, and diallyl sulphide. The reasons for their success could be that they inhibit P450 enzymes (P450 enzymes increase the toxicity of the chemical used), that they neutralize the free radicals produced by the P450 enzymes, and/or that they stimulate Phase 2 conjugation enzymes, which then neutralize the chemical so that it can't bind to DNA. The one antioxidant not successful at inhibiting the initiation of liver cancer was ellagic acid.

517. Inhibition of epidermal xenobiotic metabolism in SENCAR mice by naturally occurring plant phenols

Mukul Das, et al., *Cancer Research,* 47, February 1, 1987, pp. 760–766

The plant phenol, ellagic acid, has been shown to inhibit P450 enzymes, thereby reducing the binding of polycyclic aromatic hydrocarbons with DNA, and therefore reducing the formation of tumours. This study showed that the plant phenols tannic acid, quercetin, and myricetin showed similar results at inhibiting P450 enzyme-produced epoxides.

518. Glutathione-ascorbic acid antioxidant system in animals

Alton Meister, *The Journal of Biological Chemistry,* Vol. 269, No. 13, April 1, 1994, pp. 9397–9400

When glutathione production is inhibited in young animals, damage occurs in the liver, kidney, lung, and brain, and cataracts form in the eyes. Damage mainly involves the mitochondria. Some of these symptoms can be lessened by the use of ascorbate (vitamin C). Symptoms of scurvy (vitamin C deficiency) can be delayed by the administration of glutathione. Ascorbate and glutathione can both react with hydrogen peroxide and oxygen free radicals and reduce their toxicity.

519. Flavonoids inhibit the oxidative modification of low density lipoproteins by macrophages

Catherine V. de Whalley, et al., *Biochemical Pharmacology*, Vol. 39, No. 11, 1990, pp. 1743–1750

Previous studies have shown that flavonoids can scavenge free radicals, can prevent lipid peroxidation, are antiinflammatory, and can inhibit COX and LOX enzymes as well as phospholipase A_2. This study shows that flavonoids also inhibit oxidation of LDL, probably by conserving the vitamin E content of LDL.

520. Inhibition by dietary curcumin of azoxymethane-induced ornithine decarboxylase, tyrosine protein kinase, arachidonic acid metabolism, and aberrant crypt foci formation in the rat colon

Chinthalapally V. Rao, et al., *Carcinogenesis*, Vol. 14, No. 11, 1993, pp. 2219–2225

Curcumin, a phenol from turmeric, has antioxidant and antiinflammatory properties. This study showed that curcumin inhibited precancerous lesions in the colon by reducing the formation of prostaglandins and thromboxanes made from arachidonic acid. Curcumin may also inhibit a variety of enzymes including P4502EI.

521. Case-control study of malignant melanoma in Washington State

Constance S. Kirkpatrick, et al., *American Journal of Epidemiology*, Vol. 139, No. 9, 1994, pp. 869–880

Among 16 nutrients from food and among four nutrients from food and supplements that were studied, only vitamin E from food and zinc from food and supplements were associated with a decreased risk of melanoma.

522. Carnitine supplementation in human idiopathic asthenospermia: clinical results

G. Vitali, et al., *Drugs Exptl. Clin. Res.*, XXI (4), 1995, pp. 157–159

L-carnitine transports fatty acids across the inner membrane of the mitochondria. L-carnitine helps protect against heart and muscle disease, and it increases sperm count and sperm motility.

523. The role of free oxygen radicals and sperm function

R. J. Aitken, *International Journal of Andrology,* 12, 1989, pp. 95–97

The membrane of a sperm is high in polyunsaturated fats that have a large number of double bonds to give the sperm fluidity. A sperm is able to generate superoxide radicals, which can create hydrogen peroxide and hydroxyl radicals. This can make sperm highly susceptible to lipid peroxidation, especially in the presence of metals like iron. Free radicals from neutrophils or macrophages can further aggravate lipid peroxidation, which can activate phospholipase A_2 whose products can have a severe perturbing effect on the sperm motility and viability. Defective sperm function is the largest defined cause of human infertility.

524. Wheat germ oil and reproduction: a review

W. Richard Dukelow, *Acta Endocrinologica,* Supplementum 181, pp. 5–15

Wheat germ oil contains other factors besides vitamin E that show benefits for reproduction.

525. Oxidants, antioxidants, and the degenerative diseases of aging

Bruce N. Ames, et al., *Proc. Natl. Acad. Sci. USA,* Vol. 90, September 1993, pp. 7915–7922

The DNA of each cell is exposed to approximately 10,000 free radicals per day, and the DNA of its mitochondria is exposed to 10 times more. DNA-repair enzymes are constantly working to repair this damage and mitochondria are constantly being replaced, but DNA lesions gradually accumulate with age. The degenerative diseases associated with ageing include cancer, cardiovascular disease, immune system disease, brain dysfunction, and cataracts. Sperm DNA lesions increase 250 percent with inadequate vitamin C.

526. Effects of antioxidant nutrient deficiency on the retina and retinal pigment epithelium of albino rats: a light and electron microscopic study

Martin L. Katz, et al., *Exp. Eye Res.,* 34, 1982, pp. 339–369

Rats were raised in two groups, each with antioxidant deficiency diets. The group deficient in vitamin E and selenium showed a loss of photoreceptor cells in the eye and a buildup of lipofuscin "age" pigment. The group deficient in vitamin E, selenium, chromium, and sulphur amino acids had the same damage, but more severe.

527. Serum antioxidant vitamins and risk of cataract

Paul Knekt, et al., *British Medical Journal,* Vol. 305, December 5, 1992, pp. 1392–1394

Low levels of β-carotene and α-tocopherol antioxidants were shown to increase the risk of cataract of the eye with ageing, while selenium and vitamin A showed no association.

528. Evidence for protection against age-related macular degeneration by carotenoids and antioxidant vitamins

D. Max Snodderly, *American Journal of Clinical Nutrition*, 62 (Suppl), 1995, pp. 1448S–1461S

The retina of the eye doesn't contain β-carotene but does contain lutein and zeaxanthin, which accumulate as the macular pigment. Low levels of these carotenoids, especially in smokers, may cause macular degeneration. High doses of β-carotene may reduce the levels of lutein and zeaxanthin. Lutein and zeaxanthin are found in leafy greens such as collard greens and spinach.

529. Aging, energy, and oxidative stress in neurodegenerative diseases

M. Flint Beal, *Annals of Neurology*, Vol. 38, No. 3, September 1995, pp. 357–366

Neurodegenerative diseases such as Alzheimer's, Huntington's, Parkinson's, and amyotrophic-related sclerosis are mysterious diseases that involve the death of neurons. Damage to the nerves may be caused by free radicals originating in the mitochondrial respiratory chain, of which the two main sources might be ubiquinone (CoQ_{10}) and NADH, which originates from nicotinamide.

530. Prostaglandin biosynthesis can be triggered by lipid peroxides

Martin E. Hemler, et al., *Archives of Biochemistry and Biophysics*, Vol. 193, No. 2, April 1, 1979, pp. 340–345

Any substance that generates peroxides may activate cyclooxygenase (COX) enzyme to make prostaglandins. Things that inhibit or remove peroxides counter this effect, especially glutathione peroxidase enzyme.

531. The nature of oxidants and antioxidant systems in the inhibition of mutation and cancer

Paul Hochstein and Ahmed S. Atallah, *Mutation Research*, 202, 1988, pp. 363–375

Superoxide anion is of low toxicity and is quickly converted by superoxide dismutase enzyme into oxygen and hydrogen peroxide. This is the main way that peroxide is formed from electrons leaking from the mitochondrial electron transport chain. Other enzymes within cells can also form peroxide directly from oxygen. White blood cells like macrophages and neutrophils have enzymes in their cell membranes that can make peroxide from oxygen for secretion outside.

These enzymes can be activated by chemicals and inflammation products.

The toxicity of hydrogen peroxide appears to be related mainly to its ability to generate hydroxyl radicals, though it can also react with chlorine to form hypochlorous acid (a technique generated by neutrophils) and with iodine (including that in thyroid hormone) to form lipid peroxides.

The hydroxyl radical is among the most reactive of free radicals and its release from hydrogen peroxide by metals leads to lipid peroxidation, which can tie in with the arachidonic cascade in the initiation and promotion of cancer. Selenium-containing glutathione peroxidase enzyme is the main detoxifier of hydrogen peroxide. Damage to DNA is inhibited by removal of oxygen or by the presence of either superoxide dismutase enzymes or EDTA. Free radical scavengers and detoxifiers inhibit tumour promotion.

532. Uric acid provides an antioxidant defense in humans against oxidant- and radical-caused aging and cancer: a hypothesis

Bruce N. Ames, et al., *Proc. Natl. Acad. Sci. USA,* Vol. 78, No. 11, November 1981, pp. 6858–6862

Uric acid levels in the blood are much higher than ascorbate (vitamin C) levels. Uric acid is a good scavenger of free radicals and a powerful antioxidant. It protects DNA and red blood cells from lipid peroxidation. Its evolution appears to have increased lifespan and decreased cancer rates.

533. Flavonoids, a class of natural products of high pharmacological potency

B. Havsteen, *Biochemical Pharmacology,* Vol. 32, No. 7, 1983, pp. 1141–1148

Plants have developed over 500 types of flavonoids and these are found mainly in the areas of photosynthesis. When the photosynthesizing cells die, the flavonoids are released into the plant juice and resin. Bees gather these fluids and make Propolis, with which they seal their hive and help keep it sterile.

Flavonoids inhibit cyclooxygenase and lipoxygenase enzymes, thus reducing prostaglandin inflammation without the side effects of aspirin and glucocorticoids.

Flavonoids stimulate the enzyme proline hydroxylase which makes connective tissue stronger and they can also inhibit microbleeding such as is found in diabetes. Flavonoids reduce histamine and serotonin, thereby minimizing allergic reactions. Flavonoids prevent viruses from breaking into the nucleic acid of the cells by inhibiting the enzymes of the viruses. Flavonoids help out by scavenging free radicals that are produced during detoxification, and by inducing the enzymes that destroy epoxides.

534. Identification of 3'-methoxy-4'-nitroflavone as a pure aryl hydrocarbon (Ah) receptor antagonist and evidence for more than one form of the nuclear Ah receptor in MCF-7 human breast cancer cells

Y -F. Lu, et al., *Archives of Biochemistry and Biophysics*, Vol. 316, No. 1, January 10, 1995, pp. 470–477

Bioflavonoids can enhance some P450 enzyme activities and may provide some anticancer protection. Some bioflavonoids also work as plant estrogens.

535. Curcumin as an inhibitor of cancer

M. Nagabhushan and S. V. Bhide, *Journal of the American College of Nutrition*, Vol. 11, No. 2, 1992, pp. 192–198

Chili and its irritative compound capsaicin are cancer-promoting spices, while turmeric and its compounds, curcumins, have cancer-inhibiting properties. Curcumins change the activity of both Phase 1 and Phase 2 enzymes.

536. Curcuminoids as potent inhibitors of lipid peroxidation

Sreejayan and M. N. A. Rao, *J. Pharm. Pharmacol.*, 46, 1994, pp. 1013–1016

Curcumin, an antioxidant, has both antiinflammatory and anticancer properties, and its three variations are more active than α-tocopherol.

537. Nitric oxide scavenging by curcuminoids

S. Raq, *J. Pharm. Pharmacol.*, 49, 1997, pp. 95–97

Curcuminoids, from turmeric, have been shown to scavenge nitric oxide, which is produced by macrophages during inflammation.

538. Preliminary study on antirheumatic activity of curcumin (diferuloyl methane)

S. D. Deodhar, et al., *Indian J. Med. Res.*, 71, April 1980, pp. 632–634

The antirheumatic activity of 1200 mg of curcumin per day was comparable to that of 300 mg of phenylbutazone per day without any side effects.

539. Scavenging effect of extracts of green tea and natural antioxidants on active oxygen radicals

Baolu Zhao, et al., *Cell Biophysics*, Vol. 14, 1989, pp. 175–1'

Green tea has stronger free radical scavenging effects th?

C and E, while rosemary antioxidants and curcumin have weaker effects than vitamin C, but stronger than vitamin E.

540. Polyphenolic flavanols as scavengers of aqueous phase radicals and as chain-breaking antioxidants

Nida Salah, et al., *Archives of Biochemistry and Biophysics*, Vol. 322, No. 2, October 1, 1995, pp. 339–346

A number of phenols from plants were tested for their ability to protect vitamin E in LDL from free radical activity. The strongest was ECG, then EGCG, then EGC, then gallic acid, then epicatechin and catechin, all of which are found in green tea.

541. Effect of red wine ingestion on the antioxidant capacity of serum

Tom P. Whitehead, et al., *Clinical Chemistry*, Vol. 41, No. 1, 1995, pp. 32–35

Tea, onions, and apples are high in flavonoids with strong antioxidant properties and their consumption in large quantities reduces coronary artery disease. Red wine is high in phenols from the grape skin, which has flavonoid properties; the grape skin is not used in making white wine.

542. Cancer chemopreventive activity of resveratrol, a natural product derived from grapes

Meishang Jang, et al., *Science*, Vol. 275, January 10, 1997, pp. 218–220

Resveratrol is a phytoalexin found in grapes, mulberries, peanuts, and other plants. It is an antifungal in grape skins for the grapes, but in the body, it is an antioxidant. It stimulates Phase 2 detoxification enzymes, and inhibits the cyclooxygenase enzyme that converts arachidonic acid into prostaglandins, thus having an antiinflammatory effect greater than aspirin, as well as an anticancer effect.

543. Dietary linoleic acid-stimulated human breast cancer cell growth and metastasis in nude mice and their suppression by indomethacin, a cyclooxygenase inhibitor

Jeanne M. Connolly, et al., *Nutrition and Cancer*, Vol. 25, No. 3, 1996, pp. 231–240

Linoleic acid has been shown to stimulate breast cancer metastasis by conversion to arachidonic acid and then to PGE_2 by cyclooxygenase enzyme. This study showed that inhibiting cyclooxygenase inhibited metastasis. Products of arachidonic acid made by lipoxygenase enzyme have been shown to also play a role in tumour motility and invasion.

544. Increased green and yellow vegetable intake and lowered cancer deaths in an elderly population

Graham A. Colditz, et al., *The American Journal of Clinical Nutrition,* 41, January 1985, pp. 32–36

This study of Massachusetts residents 66 years of age or older showed that those who ate the most green and yellow vegetables had the lowest risk of cancer.

545. The flavonoids

Elliott Middleton, Jr., *TIPS,* August 1984, pp. 335–338

Certain flavonoids, such as quercetin, hesperitin, and catechin, have antiviral activity.

546. Myricetin and quercetin, the flavonoid constituents of Ginkgo biloba extract, greatly reduce oxidative metabolism in both resting and Ca^{2+}-loaded brain neurons

Yasuo Oyama, et al., *Brain Research,* 635, 1994, pp. 125–129

The antioxidant action of myricetin and quercetin, the flavonoid constituents of the extract of Ginkgo biloba, reduced the oxidation in resting brain neurons.

547. Antiviral substances in plants of the mint family (Labiatae). III. Peppermint (Mentha piperita), and other mint plants

Ernest C. Herrmann, Jr. and Louis S. Kucera, *PSEBM,* Vol. 124, 1967, pp. 874–878

"Extracts of various plants of the mint family (Labiatae) were studied for antiviral activity. Peppermint (Mentha piperita) extract had antiviral activity against Newcastle disease (NDV), herpes simplex, vaccinia, Semliki Forest, and West Nile viruses in egg and cell-culture systems. It contains a tannin with an affinity for NDV and mumps virus and a nontannin fraction with antiviral effects against herpes simplex virus. Aqueous extracts of sage (Salvia cyprea), marjoram (Origanum majorana), wild thyme (Thymus serpyllum), American pennyroyal (Hedeoma pulegiodes), Crea monda (Satureia sp.) and Spanish and French thymes (Thymus sp.) all exhibited some antiviral effects against NDV. The first 6 also exhibited some antiviral effects against herpes simplex. Hyssop (Hyssopus officinalis) extracts had activity against herpes simplex virus while rosemary (Rosmarinus officinalis), horehound (Marrubium vulgare), and catnip (Nepeta cataria) extracts were not detectably antiviral. None of these plant extracts produced an antiviral effect superior to that of melissa (Melissa officinalis) extracts."

548. Therapeutic effects of liver hydrolysate preparations on chronic hepatitis - a double blind controlled study

Kiyoshi Fujisawa, et al., *Asian Med. J.*, 26 (8), pp. 497–526

In Japan, approximately 600 patients with chronic liver damage from chronic hepatitis were treated with aqueous extract from liver, and showed improvement in liver function.

549. The benefits of aqueous liver extracts

Michael T. Murray, *American Journal of Natural Medicine*, Vol. 2, No. 10, December 1995, pp. 5–7

Liver extracts provide the best form of iron, heme iron, which is iron bound to hemoglobin and myoglobin. Heme iron is the most efficiently absorbed form of iron with an absorption rate as high as 35 percent. Nonheme iron supplements, such as ferrous sulfate and ferrous fumarate, have an absorption rate of about 2.9 percent. Liver extracts also contain vitamin B_{12} and folic acid, which play a role in increasing energy levels, among other things.

550. Loss of delta-6-desaturase activity as a key factor in aging

David F. Horrobin, *Medical Hypotheses*, 7, 1981, pp. 1211–1220

One of the characteristics of ageing is decreased activity of the enzyme delta-6 desaturase, which converts linoleic acid (LA) to gamma-linolenic acid (GLA). Other factors that inhibit this enzyme are diabetes, alcohol, and radiation. Decreased delta-6 desaturase activity can lead to immune and cardiovascular problems. Factors that improve its activity are moderate food restriction, vitamins C and B_6, zinc, and melatonin. This enzyme can be bypassed by using foods or herbs high in GLA.

551. The reversibility of cancer: evidence that malignancy in human hepatoma cells is gamma-linolenic acid deficiency-dependent.

Nola Dippenaar, et al., *SA Mediese Tydskrif*, Deel 62, October 30, 1982

Supplementation with GLA (gamma-linolenic acid) reduces the growth rate of human cancer cells in culture, which indicates that a deficiency of delta-6 desaturase may be an essential feature in the onset of malignancy.

552. The nutritional regulation of T lymphocyte function

D. F. Horrobin, et al., *Medical Hypotheses*, 5, 1979, pp. 969–985

Prostaglandin E_1 plays a major role in the regulation of thymus development and T cell function. By careful attention to diet, it should be possible to improve T cell function in a number of immune-related diseases.

553. The arachidonic acid cascade: an immunologically based review

Camila K. Janniger and S. P. Racis, *Journal of Medicine*, Vol. 18, No. 2, 1987, pp. 69–80

Lymphocytes, macrophages, and eosinophils are capable of producing eicosanoids (like prostaglandins) and also have receptors for prostaglandins. Leukotriene B_4 (LTB_4) stimulates movement and superoxide generation in neutrophils, eosinophils, and macrophages. LTB_4 has been found in the synovial fluids and tissues of patients with rheumatoid arthritis and also in the skin of psoriasis patients. Cystic acne and nodular prurigo are known to be high in leukotrienes, as well. Inhibition of prostaglandin production can increase leukotrienes. Products of arachidonic acid mediate a number of cellular functions and the immune system.

554. Ethanol and prostaglandin E_1: biochemical and behavioral interactions

John Rotrosen, et al., *Life Sciences*, Vol. 26, No. 22, 1980, pp. 1867–1876

Findings suggest a tentative role for PGE_1 (and possibly other prostaglandins) as a mediator of certain effects of ethanol, as well as the possibility that a functional PGE_1 deficiency may underlie the development of ethanol withdrawal symptoms.

555. NMDA receptors activate the arachidonic acid cascade system in striatal neurons

A. Dumuis, et al., *Nature*, Vol. 336, November 3, 1988, pp. 68–70

NMDA receptors activate phospholipase A_2 enzyme to begin the arachidonic acid cascade. They are stimulated by glutamate and inhibited by magnesium.

556. Salivary prostaglandin concentrations: possible state indicators for major depression

Seiji Nishino, et al., *J. Psychiatry*, 146:3, March 1989, pp. 365–368

Prostaglandins of the 2 series from arachidonic acid were higher in patients with major depressive disorder, and the more severe the depression, the higher the prostaglandin concentration. Patients on antidepressant medication still had high prostaglandin levels.

557. Elevated levels of prostaglandins E_2 and thromboxane B_2 in depression

Julian Lieb, et al., *Prostaglandins Leukotrienes and Medicine*, 10, 1983, pp. 361–367

A lack of prostaglandin E_1 (PGE_1) and elevation of prostaglandin E_2 and thromboxane B_2 in depressed patients indicate that prostaglandins play a role in the regulation of mood. A lack of PGE_1 might be associated with excessive arachidonic acid mobilization.

558. Prostaglandin production in chronic progressive multiple sclerosis

Judith A. Aberg, et al., *Journal of Clinical Laboratory Analysis*, 4, 1990, pp. 246–250

Chronic progressive MS showed higher production of prostaglandin E_2 but not of thromboxane B_2.

559. Possible role of prostaglandin E_1 in the affective disorders and in alcoholism

David F. Horrobin and Mehar S. Manku, *British Medical Journal*, June 7, 1980, pp. 1363–1366

Prostaglandin E_1 (PGE_1) may play an important part in the affective disorders, with an excess being present in mania and a deficiency in depression. Ethyl alcohol stimulates PGE_1 production whereas lithium inhibits it. Alcoholics will tend to have raised PGE_1 concentrations while drinking, but, because precursor supplies are limited, when alcohol concentrations fall, PGE_1 concentrations may fall sharply leading to depression. PGE_1 biosynthesis may be affected by nutritional factors including essential fatty acids, pyridoxine, vitamin C, and zinc. Nutritional approaches may be of value in both depression and alcoholism.

560. Does kinin released by pineapple stem bromelain stimulate production of prostaglandin E_1-like compounds?

George E. Felton, *Hawaii Medical Journal*, Vol. 36, No. 2, February 1977, pp. 39–47

Bromelain from pineapple stem activates a compound in the body that acts similar to prostaglandin E_1. This action does not seem to be caused by the main protein-digesting enzyme of bromelain.

561. Bromelain: a literature review and discussion of its therapeutic applications

Gregory S. Kelly, *Alternative Medicine Review*, Vol. 1, No. 4, 1996, pp. 243–257

Bromelain from pineapple stems has been shown to break up fibrin, reduce arachidonic acid eicosanoids, increase the amount of PGI_2 (prostacyclin) in relationship to thromboxanes, improve digestion of proteins, and inhibit metastases of cancer—with few side effects. Bromelain has many other benefits, as well.

562. Antimetastatic effect of bromelain with or without its proteolytic and anticoagulant activity

S. Batkin, et al., *Journal of Cancer Research and Clinical Oncology,* Vol. 114, 1988, pp. 507–508

Bromelain from pineapple has been found to retard tumour cell growth and inhibit the spread of cancer to other tissues. This study showed that the anticancer properties existed even when the enzyme activity of the bromelain was removed.

563. Thérapeutique anti-cancéreuse et bromelaïnes – Anti-cancer treatment and bromelaines

G. Gerard, *Agressologie,* 13, 4, 1972, pp. 261–274

Oral treatment with 600 mg of bromelain (from pineapple) per day caused remission of masses in a breast cancer patient and transformation of skin metastases in another breast cancer patient.

564. Redox modulation of p53 conformation and sequence-specific DNA binding in vitro

Pierre Hainaut and Jo Milner, *Cancer Research,* 53, October 1, 1993, pp. 4469–4473

The p53 protein controls cell proliferation and survival and suppresses tumours. Its shape is crucial for it to bind to DNA and carry out its function. Zinc appears to play an important role in keeping the necessary shape for p53 to bind to DNA. Oxidation, such as with peroxide, deformed p53, inhibiting its ability to bind to DNA.

565. Prostaglandins, glucose homeostasis, and diabetes mellitus

R. Paul Robertson, *Ann. Rev. Med.,* 34, 1983, pp. 1–12

Arachidonic acid is converted to prostaglandins and thromboxane of the 2 series by the cyclooxygenase enzyme pathway, and to leukotrienes by the lipoxygenase enzyme pathway. Glucocorticoids inhibit arachidonic acid metabolism and nonsteroidal antiinflammatory drugs (NSAID) inhibit cyclooxygenase enzyme. Experiments with aspirin with diabetics indicate that prostaglandins from arachidonic acid likely play a role in abnormal sugar metabolism in diabetes.

566. Prophylactic aspirin and risk of peptic ulcer bleeding

John Weil, et al., *British Medical Journal,* 310, 1995, pp. 827–830

Regular ingestion of aspirin may increase the risk of acquiring peptic ulcers.

567. Leukotrienes stimulate insulin release from the rat pancreas

Sumer Belbez Pek and Mary Frances Walsh, *Proc. Natl. Acad. Sci. USA,* Vol. 81, April 1984, pp. 2199–2202

Among the arachidonic acid metabolites, leukotrienes are involved in the modulation of secretion of pancreatic islet hormones and they preferentially promote insulin release.

568. The role of fatty acids and eicosanoid synthesis inhibitors in breast carcinoma

Masakuni Noguchi, et al., *Oncology*, 52, 1995, pp. 265–271

Western women get more breast cancer and have greater problems with it than Japanese or Eskimo women. This may be because Western diets are high in omega-6 polyunsaturated fatty acids whereas Japanese and Eskimo diets are higher in omega-3 polyunsaturated fatty acids from fish, primarily EPA and DHA fatty acids. EPA inhibits both cyclooxygenase (COX) and lipoxygenase (LOX) enzymes while DHA inhibits only prostaglandins. Omega-3 fatty acids from fish inhibit breast cancer growth while omega-6 fatty acids tend to promote it via increased synthesis of COX and LOX products.

569. Effects of dietary enrichment with eicosapentaenoic acid upon autoimmune nephritis in female NZBxNZW/F₁ mice

James D. Prickett, et al., *Arthritis and Rheumatism*, 26, 1983, pp. 133–139

Mice who genetically develop kidney disease similar to that of lupus were given fish oil, which greatly delayed the symptoms. It's proposed that the fish oil EPA was converted to prostaglandins and leukotrienes—by cyclooxygenase (COX) and lipoxygenase (LOX) enzymes—that are much less inflammatory than those made from arachidonic acid.

570. Chemoprevention of colon carcinogenesis by dietary curcumin, a naturally occurring plant phenolic compound

Chinthalapally V. Rao, et al., *Cancer Research*, 55, January 15, 1995, pp. 259–266

Prostaglandins of the 2 series, made by the COX (cyclooxygenase) enzyme system, modulate cell proliferation, tumour growth, and immune responses. LOX (lipoxygenase) enzyme products affect chemotoxic responses, hormone secretion, tumour cell adhesion, stimulation of tumour cell spreading, and tumour metastasis. Curcumin, by inhibiting COX and LOX enzymes, inhibited colon cancer with no side effects.

571. Lower ratio of n-3 to n-6 fatty acids in cultured than in wild fish

Trinette van Vliet and Martijn B. Katan, *American Journal of Clinical Nutrition*, 51, 1990, pp. 1–2

Wild fish contain more very-long-chain omega-3 fatty acids (EPA and DHA) than do pond-reared (cultured) fish.

572. Physical activity, all-cause mortality, and longevity of college alumni

Ralph S. Paffenbarger, Jr., et al., *The New England Journal of Medicine,* Vol. 314, No. 10, March 6, 1986, pp. 605–613

Harvard graduates' death rates were roughly half that for white males in the United States, except for cases of suicide. Graduates who exercised regularly showed decreased mortality rates compared to sedentary men.

573. Aging: prospects for further increases in the functional life span

Denham Harman, *Age,* Vol. 17, 1994, pp. 119–146

The "natural" maximum life span of 85 years may be reached by minimizing free radical activity. This can be accomplished by maintaining a healthy body weight, following a diet adequate in essential nutrients, supplementing the diet with antioxidants, and avoiding accumulation of metals in the body.

574. Caloric restriction and aging

Richard Weindruch, *Scientific American,* January 1996, pp. 46–52

In experiments with rats, restricting caloric intake—while still supplying nutrient needs—increases lifespan and youthful vitality. It also delays the onset of cancers of the breast, prostate, immune system, and gastrointestinal tract, as well as other diseases. Caloric restriction may slow the ageing process by lowering free radical production. Studies suggest that restricting calories can be beneficial even if it's not started until middle age.

575. The limit of human life, and how to live long

R. H. Dalton, *JAMA,* 20, 1893, pp. 599–600

"If the habit of taking nutriment in quantities adapted to early life is continued, the surplus left after the loss by waste is supplied must either be cast off with much greater difficulty as age advances, or deposited as fat among the tissues to impair their functions. This is inevitable, for as manhood wanes imperceptibly into old age, all the energies must participate in the decline, though failure may not be obvious at any particular time.

For some years past, reported deaths from "heart failure" have become frequent and fashionable among practicing physicians, and perhaps the reports may have been true, but not the whole truth, for it is probable that, in nine cases out of ten, the heart failure was secondary and brought on by an ineffectual effort of the stomach or alimentary tract to cast off indigestible matter clogging the way.

It would be well for physicians to recognize the significance of that wonderful aggregation of nerve cells constituting the solar and semilunar plexuses behind and contiguous to the stomach and bowels. They are the power houses sending forth energy to run the whole machinery of digestion; and when that power fails, the main link binding the whole fabric together is broken, and then of course the heart, as well as other organs, *must* fail. Hence the importance of regulating diet as age advances to serve nutrition according to the power of digestion remaining.

The morbid influence of habitual constipation on an organism, otherwise healthy, is an interesting study, but easily understood. The fecal mass having traveled down through the long digestive conduit, finally subsides into the colon and rectum in a complete state of decomposition—a mass of ptomaines to be seized by the active absorbents of these receptacles and thrown back into the general circulation, poisoning tissues wherever they go and defying the liver, kidneys, or any other emunctory to cast them out of the system. Congestions, inflammations, abscesses, and all the catalogue of pathological complications are liable to ensue. Most likely, a large majority of chronic diseases take their origin from this cause."

Index for Introduction Through Chapter 9

(Please note that the Research section has its own Index.)

Page numbers in **bold** indicate illustrations.

Index for Research

DOCQUE'S FOOD CHART

• WARMING

PROTEINS

Recommended

All or most of the time

salmon, sardines, mackerel, trout
cod
bass
sole
halibut
tuna
tempeh
soy yogurt
chicken breast
turkey breast
tofu
soy protein
soy milk

In Moderation

shellfish, herring, anchovies
eggs
lamb
low fat cottage cheese
low fat cheese
quark
veal
beef (low fat)
duck
pork
liver

PROTEIN/CARBOHYDRATE

goat's milk or yogurt
low fat milk or yogurt

• NEUTRAL (if salted with sea salt)

CARBOHYDRATES

Lightly cook: steam or stir-fry.

Recommended

Cruciferous Vegetables

broccoli
cauliflower
brussels sprouts
cabbage
collard greens
kale
kohlrabi
bok choy
turnips/rutabagas
mustard greens
radishes

Other Vegetables

tomatoes
swiss chard, spinach, romaine
nettle
watercress, endive
garlic, onions, leeks
artichoke
asparagus
green/wax beans
eggplant
okra
snow peas
zucchini, yellow squash
celery
fresh herbs
sprouts
cucumber
mushrooms

• COOLING

FRUITS (CARBOHYDRATES)

Fruit should be limited.
Select fruits that are in season for
your growing area.

Approx. glycemic index is shown in brackets

(n/a) = glycemic index not available

cherries (32)
plums (34)
grapefruit (36)
peaches (40)
apricots, dried (44)
pears (51)
strawberries (n/a)
raspberries (n/a)
blueberries (n/a)
blackberries (n/a)
huckleberries (n/a)
apples (52)
grapes (62)
orange (62)
kiwi (75)
bananas (76)
mangoes (80)
raisins (91)
pineapple (94)
watermelon (103)

FATS

avocado
guacamole

FATS

Recommended
almonds and almond butter
flax seeds
olives and olive oil
sesame oil
tahini
canola oil

In Moderation
mayonnaise (canola)
soybean oil
walnuts
brazil nuts (1 per day)
other legume & nut butters

Use Sparingly
butter
cream
cream cheese
sour cream
nonhydrogenated margarine

OTHER
ginger

• BEVERAGES
water
dandelion/herbal coffee
herbal tea
green tea
vegetable or chicken broth
ginger tea

STARCHES (CARBOHYDRATES)
Approx. glycemic index (in brackets)
soy beans (25)
peas, dried (32)
barley (36)
bean thread (37)
pasta (38 to 131) See ↑ ↑ ↑ ↑ ↑
lentils, dried (41)
kidney beans, dried (42)
black beans (43)
lima beans (46)
chickpeas, dried (47)
oatmeal (slow cooking) (49)
bread (50 to 100+) See ↑ ↑ ↑ ↑ ↑
navy beans (54)
tortillas (54)
chickpeas, canned (60)
pinto beans (55), canned (64)
barley chipati (61)
bulgur (68), frozen peas (68)
kidney beans, canned (74)
lentils, canned (74)
sweet potato (77)
buckwheat (78)
corn (78)
rice: brown or white, long-grain,
       & basmati (79-83)
new potato (81)
beets (91)
couscous (93)
millet (101)
carrots (101)
potato, baked (121)
parsnips (139)

Examples of PASTAS
protein-enriched spaghetti (38)
egg-enriched fettucine (46)
white spaghetti (52 to 59)
whole meal (53)
durum (78)
brown rice pasta (131)

Examples of BREADS
rye pumpernickel (58)
barley kernel (49 to 66)
oat bran (68)
rye kernel (71)
rye flour (92)
barley flour (95)
whole wheat (99)

Foods Over (100)
bread stuffing
kaiser rolls
melba toast

A balanced diet includes proteins, carbohydrates, and fats.
• **To Lose Weight:**
  Choose carbohydrates from the NEUTRAL column with a glycemic index of less than 60.
• **To Gain Weight:**
  Choose carbohydrates from the NEUTRAL column with a glycemic index higher than 60.

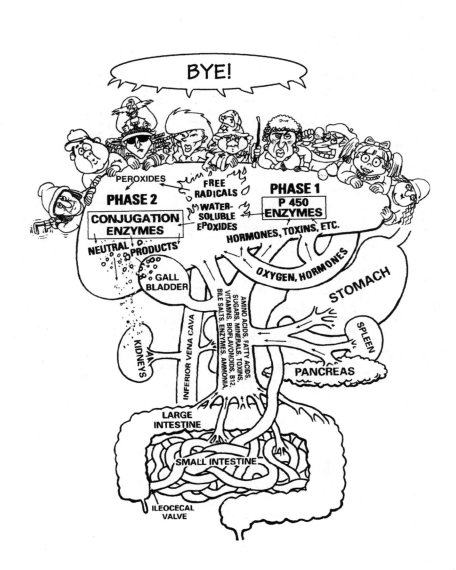

To find a Naturopathic Physician in your area,
please contact:

British Columbia Naturopathic Association
Suite 204–2786 West 16th Avenue
Vancouver, BC V6K 3C4
(604) 736-6646   Fax: (604) 732-3709

or

O.A.N.D.
(Ontario Association of Naturopathic Doctors)
304–4174 Dundas Street West
Toronto, Ontario M8X 1X3
(416) 233-2001

or

Canadian Naturopathic Association
303–4174 Dundas Street West
Toronto, Ontario M8X 1X3
(416) 233-1043

or

American Association
of Naturopathic Physicians
105–601 Valley Street
Seattle, WA 98109
(206) 298-0126

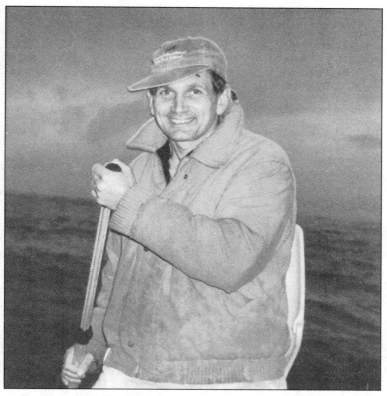

Dr. Matsen searching for EPA off the west coast of Vancouver Island
on his boat *Vagabond*.

Dr. Jonn Matsen earned his degree in Naturopathic Medicine at
Bastyr University in Seattle, Washington in 1983, where he later
sat on the Board of Trustees for five years. He has a thriving
practice at the Northshore Naturopathic Clinic, in North
Vancouver, British Columbia, which he has operated for the
past 15 years. His first book *Eating Alive: Prevention Thru Good
Digestion* has sold over 200,000 copies.